Embodying Culture

Studies in Medical Anthropology

Edited by Mac Marshall

Embodying Culture

Pregnancy in Japan and Israel

TSIPY IVRY

RUTGERS UNIVERSITY PRESS

NEW BRUNSWICK, NEW JERSEY, AND LONDON

LIBRARY OF CONGRESS CATALOGING-IN-PUBLICATION DATA

Ivry, Tsipy.
    Embodying culture : pregnancy in Japan and Israel / Tsipy Ivry.
        p. cm. — (Studies in medical anthropology)
    Includes bibliographical references and index.
    ISBN 978–0–8135–4635–3 (hardcover : alk. paper) — ISBN 978–0–8135–4636–0
(pbk. : alk. paper)
    1. Pregnancy—Japan.   2. Pregnancy—Israel.   3. Pregnant women—Medical care—
Japan.   4. Pregnant women—Medical care—Israel.   5. Medical anthropology—
Japan.   6. Medical anthropology—Israel.   7. Japan—Social life and customs.
8. Israel—Social life and customs.   I. Title.
    GN635.J2I914 2009
    612.6′930952—dc22   2009006025

A British Cataloging-in-Publication record for this book is
available from the British Library.

Visit our Web site: http://rutgerspress.rutgers.edu

Manufactured in the United States of America

To Avia, Sarahle, Shlomtsiyon, and Avigail

CONTENTS

ACKNOWLEDGMENTS

It is exhilarating to reach the point of writing to express my deep gratitude to all the people who supported and shared with me the pleasures and pains of a project with which I have been pregnant for over a decade.

I am deeply grateful to Meira Weiss for introducing me to the magic and wonders of anthropology. I owe an enormous debt of gratitude to Eyal Ben-Ari for his devoted mentoring, support, and invaluable advice throughout the many stages of this project. Very special thanks go to Elly Teman, without whose friendship, loving kindness, and intellectual companionship this book could not have been born.

I am grateful to the many anthropology students whose keen and honest questions challenged my thinking and impelled me to sharpen my arguments. Fruitful discussions with my colleagues Nurit Bird-Davis, Carol Kidron, Yoram Carmeli, Asaf Dar, and Yuval Yonai always bring forth fresh ideas. Special thanks are due to Amalia Saar, whose powerful feminist insights, continuous support, and inspiration have contributed immensely to the maturation of this project. Above all I am deeply indebted to the pregnant women and mothers who shared with me some of their most intimate experiences and kindly extended their hospitality. I am deeply grateful to the doctors who found time to discuss their ideas, practices, and concerns with me in the midst of their busy schedules. The women, their partners, doctors, birth educators, laboratory workers, and other care providers remain anonymous to preserve their privacy.

I thank my extended family, who supported me in various ways. My mother, Ruth Ivry, never ceased to bring me newspaper articles about pregnancy and women's health, and my sister-in-law, Ilanit Dado-Lensky, never ceased to pray for the successful completion of this book while lavishing upon me the miracle of her sisterhood. I am especially indebted to Miriam Lensky, my mother-in-law, who, together with Itamar Lensky, took upon herself the full care of our daughters during my field trips to Japan and who has always been ready to step into the breach and lend a hand. She and my mother have been meaningful and enthusiastic partners in raising the girls for the last twelve years.

I am grateful to the Truman Institute for the Advancement of Peace for its grants, which made the field trips to Japan possible. As a doctoral student at the

Hebrew University I was supported by the Department of Sociology and Anthropology. The rector's grant for excellent doctoral students was an immense help.

I acknowledge the following sources, where earlier and substantially different versions of some parts of chapters 1, 2, and 4 appeared as "At the Back Stage of Prenatal Care: Japanese Ob-Gyns Negotiating Prenatal Diagnosis," *Medical Anthropology Quarterly* 20 (4) (2006): 441–468; "Embodied Responsibilities: Pregnancy in the Eyes of Japanese Ob-Gyns," *Sociology of Health and Illness* 29 (2) (2007): 251–274; "'We are Pregnant': Israeli Men and the Paradoxes of Sharing," in *Reconceiving the Second Sex in Reproduction: Men, Sexuality, and Masculinity*, ed. M. Inhorn, T. Tjørnhøj-Thomsen, H. Goldberg, and M. La Cour Mosegaard, 281–304 (New York: Berghahn, 2009); and "The Ultrasonic Picture Show and the Politics of Threatened Life," *Medical Anthropology Quarterly* 23 (3) (2009): 189–211. I have benefited from the critique and suggestions of anonymous reviewers and from editors, including Helene Goldberg, Tine Tjørnhøj-Thomsen, Maruska La Cour Mosegaard, and Marcia Inhorn. I am indebted to Dick Bruggeman for his English editing of these early works and for his continuous support and encouragement.

The help of Kato Madoka, Kudo Masako, Yuriko Yamanouchi, Mitsue Uchida, Ukigaya Sachiko, Tsuchiya Mariko, Ishikawa Mizue, Michal Gerling, and Reuven Gerling in opening many doors for me with their introductions was truly invaluable.

I am indebted to the following individuals for reading previous drafts of this manuscript. Their comments and criticism helped to improve the book. These are Rotem Kowner, Edna Lumsky-Feder, Tomiyuki Uesugi, Limor Smamian-Darash, Dani Kaplan, Anat Rosenthal, and especially Noa Apeloig and Don Seeman. Special thanks go to Margaret Lock, Robbie Davis-Floyd, Delila Amir, Ofra Goldstein-Gideoni, Jennifer Robertson, and Amy Borovoy for their useful comments and suggestions as well as for their scholarship. I thank the anonymous reviewers of Rutgers University Press for their supportive treatment of my manuscript and their detailed suggestions; Alan Harwood, the Rutgers University Press series editor in medical anthropology for his close reading of the manuscript; and Adi Hovav, who patiently helped me over the hurdles of publishing a first book. I thank Junko Magid and Racheli Belifante-Afoota for the fine photographs that make up the cover art.

Rika Takaki Eini helped me prepare the 2007 field trip to Japan. Rika and Omi Morgenstern-Leissner aided me with the statistics and various references in the final revision. I owe an enormous debt of gratitude to Irith Friedman-Bernstein and Nirit Yardeni-Drori who were the most wonderful and devoted research assistants one could ask for. I can hardly imagine completing this book without their diligent, sensitive, and kind help. I am deeply grateful to Murray Rosovsky for his attentive English editing,

I thank my life partner, Itamar Lensky, for sharing with me the love for our daughters, and most of all I am grateful to Avia, Sarahle, Shlomtsion, and Avigail, who light up my life.

Embodying Culture

Introduction

Pregnancy, Cultural Comparison, Multisited Ethnographies

Conception

I conceived this study in the autumn of 1996, when, toward the end of a two-year study program as a research student at Tokyo University, I became pregnant for the first time. What I remember most vividly is an overwhelming and all-encompassing sense of becoming "different," which I felt constantly even though the pregnancy was not yet showing, and I continued my research and writing as before. I was twenty-nine by then, and although I used to think of myself as someone who had undergone at least a few powerful experiences (compulsory military service in the Israeli army, travel through East Asia, and studies in Israel and Japan), I could not recall any other experience that encompassed and over-whelmed me so intensely. Since 1996 I have experienced three more pregnancies and am now the mother of four daughters. The transformative experiences of birth and mothering, each with its own intensity and vigor, only strengthened my conviction that there is much more to pregnancy than merely the transitory stage to birth and motherhood.

Underlying this study was a sense of unease, curiosity, and fascination with pregnancy, and a wish to investigate and develop tools to better understand this way of being. Yet my initial positioning as an Israeli woman gestating in Japan turned this somewhat ontological bemusement with pregnancy in a specific direction: pregnancy as a cultural and social phenomenon captured my interest. The focus on "culturally constructed versions" of pregnancy came from my own everyday interactions with Japanese friends and colleagues, as well as my encounters with Japanese care providers. I particularly remember my conversations with Mr. Kobuta, a forty-five-year-old man with whom I practiced Japanese drumming for two years.[1] As soon as he learned that I was pregnant, he started talking to me about the importance of eating "good food." With sparkling eyes shining through his thick glasses, he explained on every available occasion how every bite I took went to the baby, and he frequently went on to tell me how the same is true of breastfeeding. Often he would remind me how wonderful (*subarashii*) it was to become a mother. Mr. Nonaka, the leader of our group, developed his own habit of reminding me when practicing the drums that "babies like the sounds of drums because it reminds them of mommy's heart beating." It struck me that Kobuta and Nonaka, who have never been pregnant themselves, "knew" so much about it. Moreover, the content of their knowledge and the system of categorization through which they conveyed their ideas about pregnancy stirred my curiosity.

Specifically, the notions of "mother" and "baby," which male and female Japanese friends used constantly, felt very strange to me. My encounters with Japanese care providers, particularly doctors' excitement about how "cute" my seven-week-old "baby" was, when referring to the shades of black and white on the ultrasound screen, raised very similar puzzles. Although at that time I had no experience of being pregnant in Israel, I could hardly imagine Israeli women and men, religious or nonreligious Jews, speaking of "babies" in the very early stages of pregnancy (I could hardly imagine Israelis speaking about their pregnancies at all at such early stages): "fetus" seemed to be a more appropriate word for what I was carrying. I started playing with the idea that the range of meanings that pregnancies carry might not be the same in Israel and Japan. At that initial stage I planned to investigate "Japanese versions of pregnancy." I set forth to "devour" my new field during the last four months of my stay in Japan. I took a maternity course at the hospital where I was receiving prenatal care, interviewed five women in the same course and two of the nurses who were giving it, bought myself ten different pregnancy guides and pregnancy magazines in Japanese, collected different types of medical records and government leaflets, and documented the responses of friends to my own pregnancy in a field diary.

In the course of interviews, Japanese informants would often ask me, in turn, questions about pregnancy in Israel, which I could answer only in a very vague and uncertain manner. When I told one of my informants that I did not know whether pregnant Israeli women underwent a specific prenatal test, she answered, "So you should find out and tell me when we get together again." Following this conversation, I realized that I had to learn more about pregnancy in Israel so as to be able to answer these questions. The very beginning of my comparative consciousness thus stemmed from fear of losing face in the eyes of my Japanese informants (who assumed that since I was a native Israeli I must know about these things).

Brief reflection on my thinking at that time may reveal that my fascination with "Japanese conceptions of pregnancy," and the process through which I singled out particular issues for problematization that guided my choice of materials to collect and observations to conduct, were all grounded in implicit comparisons. My fascination with the use of the concept "baby" in the early stages of pregnancy was because I was contrasting it with the "fetus." My fascination with the knowledge that Kobuta and Nonaka demonstrated was because I could not imagine Israeli men professing such ideas to an Israeli woman. I repeatedly compared "Japanese concepts of pregnancy" with the ways in which I imagined pregnancy being talked about, experienced, and medically treated in Israel. However, whereas my ontological fascination with pregnancy stemmed from my own experience, the feeling that "Japanese pregnancies" had something culturally particular about them was beyond experience. It stemmed from the implicit comparison between what I saw and heard in Japan and my "common sense" as a native Israeli-Jewish woman who by 1996 had had no experience whatsoever of gestating in Israel.

Toward the end of the second trimester of pregnancy, my partner and I returned to Israel. At that stage I imagined that returning to Israel would bring a feeling of familiarity about everything that had to do with the pregnancy. Shortly after arriving in Israel I went to see my ob-gyn, who was very friendly, just as I remembered him. He went over my translations of my Japanese medical records as an act of politeness, it seemed, and immediately administered an intensive raft of tests. One of them, he said, "is extremely urgent. You must go tomorrow first thing in the morning. I don't see why they didn't do such an important test." The important test turned out to be the triple marker—a screening test that uses a biochemical analysis of maternal blood to estimate the probabilities of chromosomal abnormalities in the fetus. I checked in the Japanese guides, but this "urgent" test was not listed as a prenatal routine. About a week after I underwent the triple marker I received a phone call from the laboratory urging me to make an immediate appointment with my ob-gyn, because, the secretary said, "The results are suspicious: they could predict all kinds of abnormalities in the fetus, and you must consult your doctor about what to do next." Although this had never happened to me before, the whole experience felt very familiar: I was scared, even terrified, but not surprised. What followed was four months of anxiety. My doctor urged me to have amniocentesis and voiced his disapproval when I chose instead to have an ultrasound scan by a specialist. After conducting a forty-minute scan, the specialist said that he could not give me a 100 percent guarantee that the fetus was healthy, but he thought that it was. I decided not to have amniocentesis, a decision for which I was heavily criticized by my ob-gyn. My anxieties subsided some weeks after I gave birth to a healthy baby girl.

Throughout these anxieties I could not stop thinking that this might not have happened if I had extended my stay in Japan. Nor could I stop thinking about what would have happened if my daughter had indeed been afflicted with a fatal disease. Had I stayed in Japan I might have discovered the problem only well after she had been born. And I had no idea how I would have reacted if the ultrasound expert had suspected that my fetus was abnormal. Would I then have had amniocentesis, or even considered an abortion?

In retrospect, I admit that these experiences molded my approach to the Japanese field. At least in the initial stages of the research, when observing Japanese arenas of pregnancy, I was actually looking for an arena of pregnancy that made possible an alternative, less frightening, more optimistic experience of pregnancy for women. However, as my fieldwork progressed I realized that any romanticization of Japanese ideas of pregnancy would be out of place. Pregnancy in Japan turned out to be at least as medicalized, supervised, and socially manipulated as in Israel. Yet whereas the Japanese medical regime is oriented to managing the woman to maximize fetal health, the Israeli medical regime is oriented to diagnosing the fetus directly. Whereas in Japan the experience of pregnancy is considered a part of motherhood, and women are given a sense of agency as mothers, in Israel, pregnancy is taken tentatively. Whereas in Japan the "socialization" of the child in utero is given weight equal to its genetic composition, in Israel the genetic makeup of the child is a primary concern of pregnant women, their partners, and their doctors. In fact, I discovered that the difference between the Japanese and the Israeli realms of pregnancy was that medicalization, supervision, monitoring, and disciplining developed in keeping with different theories about pregnant bodies and the women who are "in" them. These medical regimes, each embedded in its socio-cultural and political contexts, and the pregnancies that women experienced within them, were the matters I set out to explore. They proved far more complex than I had expected.

Pregnancy: Evoking a Meaningful Cultural Category

Significantly, this book is about pregnancy; and it is pregnancy as a meaningful cultural category that this book endeavors to illuminate. At the beginning of the third millennium it remains true that any living human being will have been gestated for some months inside a woman's body. This includes both premature babies and babies who have been conceived through surrogacy agreements. Not even "test tube babies" are actually gestated in test tubes. Yet how many of us acknowledge pregnancy as a significant part of our life histories? How many of us count the months of gestation when calculating our ages? Gestation hardly "counts" in Euro-American societies—people celebrate "birth" days. Discounting gestation might not be as obvious in societies with Buddhist traditions, in which gestation used to be counted as the first year of life. But even there, many people are enchanted by birthdays. From the perspective of the "gestator," however, such arithmetic might not pass as obvious: "birthdays" disguise and erase the long-term socio-cultural and personal project that predated them, namely, pregnancy.

The pregnancy that I mean is the rather "gray" and "undramatic" category into which most pregnancies still fit, even in postindustrial countries: typically a pregnancy conceived by women in their twenties or thirties via a heterosexual relationship and without medical intervention, and proceeding without any particular indications of health complications for the pregnant woman or the fetus, a pregnancy that many medical practitioners would categorize as "low-risk." This pregnancy is first and foremost a process of physical and social change and, as such, marked with fundamental uncertainties within any system of cultural categories. For this and other reasons, experiences of pregnancy might be very far removed from what the noneventual language that designates them as "expecting" suggests. Yet the social category of pregnancy seems gradually to be receding while issues of reproduction and its various fragmentations take center stage.

Human reproduction is capturing much attention in public discourse in many countries throughout the industrial world. Occasionally in these societies, reproductive scandals, paradoxes, and ethical dilemmas rear up: in Israel, ova stolen from women undergoing fertility treatments; British IVF clinics facing shortages of sperm cells; skyrocketing prices of ova "donated" by celebrities in North America; a Japanese municipality's refusal to register the genetic parents of twins that were delivered by a surrogate; petitions by an Israeli mother of a soldier who died in battle to use his sperm with a surrogate to bear her grandchildren. Such juicy scandals make reproductive cells, and the technologies that render them, visible, usable, transferable, commodifiable, and disposable, as the objects of an emergent public discourse on reproduction. Often one cannot help noticing that human beings are thus repositioned in relation to the cells (as their owners or kin, their donors, users, or commissioners). The human subjects that become the protagonists in such dramas are often those who experience reproductive disruptions. Very rarely, if ever, is public discourse preoccupied with the mundane experience of "normal" pregnancy.

The remarkably innovative body of scholarship in anthropological research on human reproduction has developed along similar lines, and has been hesitant to take up pregnancy as a meaningful unit of analysis, let alone its focus. Whereas a host of anthropological studies have problematized a wide range of reproductive issues during the female life cycle, anthropologists seem more fascinated with birth and other, often technologically oriented, reproductive dramas than with the process of gestation. With few exceptions, when gestation has appeared as the focus of recent studies, it has often been analyzed through the lens of women's encounters with the New Reproductive Technologies (NRTs). In fact, technologies of procreation, such as assisted conception and prenatal diagnosis, are becoming the ultimate perspectives from which to theorize the meaning of pregnancy.

Such a distribution of research perspectives appears somewhat incongruent with the realities of the field if we compare the incidence of "pregnancy" with that of "birth" and the utilization of NRTs. First, pregnancy is a much more common experience for women than birth. It is widely acknowledged that about one quarter of all pregnancies end in a spontaneous miscarriage (Layne 2003) and others are deliberately aborted. So most women become pregnant more often than they give birth, and at most the number of pregnancies can only equal the number of births for any one woman. Secondly, women spend much longer periods of time being pregnant than actually delivering babies. Thirdly, while biomedicine enables women to "skip" the experience of birth with the help of analgesics and anesthetics, the reality of pregnancy remains mostly "inescapable." Is it at all likely that this lengthy experience, which is both physical and social, is less influential or less intensive than the relatively short experience of birth?

The tremendous emphasis on encounters with high-tech biomedicine neglects the fact that all over the world many NRTs are still expensive options, virtually open only to the socio-economically privileged (Davis-Floyd and Dumit 1998, 7). Particularly when considering "assisted" conception, it should be borne in mind that most women conceive without any medical intervention. Moreover, whereas the advent of the NRTs suggests that human reproduction can be "assisted," "designed," and ultimately "replaced" by technology, in the absence of an "artificial womb" pregnancy remains the one stage of procreation where this is not possible: at present there is no substitute for pregnancy if one wants to give birth to a live baby.

While borrowing on conceptions and theoretical advances in scholarship on the anthropology of reproduction, and while sharing deep concerns about biomedicalization and technologization with this literature, I propose a project with a somewhat different focus, raising an alternative series of questions. This book places at the center of the analytical effort not biotechnology but *pregnancy*, as it is experienced and managed within its socio-cultural and political context at a particular historical moment. It does so while engaging in an explicit cultural comparison of two contemporary socio-cultural settings of gestation: Japan, my original field of study, and Israel, my own culture of origin. It asks how pregnancy is experienced and managed by women and their caretakers in these two societies; what kind of systems of knowledge are available in them with which to think about pregnancy; and what pregnancy means for women, their partners, their care providers, and policy makers in the two different settings, which are nevertheless both heavily medicalized.

Certainly, pregnancy does not mean one and the same thing for all members of any society, so inevitably this book attempts to piece together multiple perspectives on pregnancy—those of pregnant women, their partners and relatives, doctors and strangers—to obtain a broad socio-cultural understanding of it. Within this amalgam, biomedical practices and theories, hegemonic though they might be, are treated as part of the diverse landscapes of pregnant life. While working to integrate a multitude of perspectives on pregnancy, I attempt to extend the analysis of technologies beyond their "impact" on the experience and management of pregnancy to question the local sources of the authoritative position of biomedicine in two markedly different socio-cultural settings. Above all, however, this study is an attempt to contribute to the understanding of pregnancy as a biosocial phenomenon from the comparative perspective of two versions of medicalized pregnancy.

My exploration draws its analytical and conceptual tools from the growing body of feminist anthropological inquiries into human reproduction, and it is to the ongoing discussions in this field of scholarship that I would like to contribute. Below I account briefly for the theoretical trajectories of this literature that have informed my study, and present my own analytical and theoretical propositions. Clearly, the major concerns in social studies of reproduction have crystallized around concepts of power, knowledge, gender, medicalization, technology, and culture.

The Politics of Reproduction

Concern with the distribution of power in reproductive relations, and its effects on women's bodies and experiences, cuts across studies in the anthropology of reproduction. More specifically, studies of the new reproductive technologies have focused their concern on the power relations at work between biomedicine and women. In all these studies "biomedicine" is seen as a powerful body of technologies and knowledge yet scholars disagree about how power should be theorized. Two categorical ways of doing it in the social arena of reproduction can be identified. One is by the radical feminist approach that emerged during the 1980s, which sees biopower as a top-down, repressive structure that subjugates women.[2] The other is characteristic of ethnographically based studies of reproduction since the late 1990s that are influenced by the later works of Michel Foucault and tend to see power as interactively produced and in flux.

The radical feminist approach is powerfully encapsulated in the front cover illustration of the paperback *Test-Tube Women*, an anthology of cross-cultural contributions (Arditti, Klein, and Minden 1984). It depicts a dark-skinned, dark-haired, pregnant, naked woman, physically struggling to push away a blond man wearing a white gown, who is leaning forward, close to her, trying to connect a bundle of colorful electrical wires he is holding in his hand to her body. The overall impression given by this picture is of a rape scene, in which the doctor is raping the pregnant woman with his technology: it is a powerful expression of the concern inundating feminist anthologies and monographs of the 1980s and early 1990s engrossed with the implications of NRTs for women.

Feminist scholars and activists are often equivocal on the issue of NRTs, but many suspect that beneath the new set of "reproductive choices" lurk sophisticated techniques that can be used to subject women to further scrutiny and control via the technologization, commodification, and colonization of female reproductive powers. This feminist approach has fed anthropological accounts of reproduction in general, but I would suggest that studies of childbirth in America during the 1980s and early 1990s particularly echo this strong sense of technological rape. The overall picture from accounts of scholars such as Davis-Floyd (1992), Jordan (1978), and Martin (1987) is one of biomedicine as a repressive system of domination that alienates women from their bodies.

At the same time, consciousness of the repressive aspects of biopower draws attention to forms of woman's resistance to it. Anthropological accounts include a range of private and unorganized forms of resistance, such as those by women who delay going to the hospital as much as they can in order to be in labor while walking around in their home (see, for example, Martin 1987, 188–186), or who refuse amniocentesis offered to them by authoritative genetic counselors (Rapp 1999). Martin illuminates a range of women's responses to the biomedicalization of their bodies that range from lament, nonaction, sabotage, resistance, and rebellion, and Root and Browner locate women's behaviors in relation to prenatal norms of diet on a scale from compliance to resistance (Root and Browner 2001). Anthropologists also account for more organized and explicit forms of resistance, such as those of midwives in the home-birth movement (Davis-Floyd and Davis 1997).

Yet despite alternative birth movements, a range of private forms of resistance and the absence of proof that the Western obstetrical model has improved birth outcomes, evidence is sufficient to suggest that the hegemony of biomedicine remains in place. In the United States, according to the 2004 National Vital Statistics Report, 99 percent of all births were delivered in hospitals. In assisted conception, women seem to subject their bodies to painful and often costly treatments despite the relatively low rates of pregnancy achieved (Becker 2000; Franklin 1998). In prenatal care, the biochemical test of alfa-fetoprotein in maternal blood has become routine despite women's skepticism (Browner and Press 1995; Parens and Asch 2000; Press and Browner 1994). In fact, women seek "emotional reassurance" from their prenatal care (Browner and Press 1997, 116), expect care providers to interpret their sensations (Browner and Press 1997, 117), prefer these interpretations to their own intuitive knowledge of their bodies, and often seek more, rather than fewer, medical interventions (Davis-Floyd 1994; Lazarus 1997, 2; Sargent and Stark 1989).

The question of how biomedicine maintains its hegemonic position, not always formulated explicitly, thus remains an important locus of inquiry. This is precisely where alternatives to the top-down model of power relations come to mind. In 1991 Fay Ginsburg and Rayna Rapp proposed a "politics of

reproduction" as a basic theoretical point of departure for anthropological studies of the subject (Ginsburg and Rapp 1991, 312). By "politicizing" reproduction,
the authors suggest that power is not unidirectional, and they encourage
anthropologists to pay attention to the *multiple* loci of power in which reproductive relations are played out. On one level power is "structured and enacted
in everyday activities—notably in relations of kinship, marriage, and in inheri-
tance patterns, rituals and exchange systems" (Ginsburg and Rapp 1991, 312). On
another, local reproductive relations are simultaneously embedded in national
as well as international global politics, where the globalization of Western medicine is a typical example.

Thus, Ginsburg and Rapp's "politics of reproduction" goes beyond a mere
suggestion that "power" be emphasized in the study of reproductive relations by
having attention drawn to the multiple and intricate ways in which this "power"
is distributed and exerted. My study clearly follows their lead by attempting to
synthesize a broad picture of the multiple loci of power within which reproductive relations are played out in both Japan and Israel. I try and develop a model
of *the interactive production of authoritative knowledge*, a concept I review below.
This, of course, is not to deny the domination of biomedicine but to search for
its cultural and political basis as it figures in shared understandings of pregnancy. My approach is influenced by Michel Foucault's suggestion that, "If
power were never anything but repressive, if it never did anything but to say no,
do you really think one would be brought to obey it? What makes power hold
good, what makes it accepted . . . is that it traverses and produces things. . . . It
needs to be considered as a productive network which runs through the whole
social body, much more than as a negative instance whose function is repression" (Foucault 1980, 119). A model of multilayered and interactively produced
power relations frames the treatment of resistance quite differently because it
does not understand power in general or biopower in particular as necessarily
repressive. I find particularly useful Lock and Kaufert's suggestion that pragmatism rather than resistance or subjugation guides woman's relationships with
biotechnology (Lock and Kaufert 1998).

Following Lock and Kaufert's lead, my study attempts to locate local forms
of agency within their respective loci of power. My findings support the notion
of resistance as "shaped by the existing moral order, even while simultaneously
undertaking a reimaging and challenging of that order" (Lock and Kaufert 1998,
13). So while trying to show how forms of resistance are contingent on local
models of thinking and on local versions of authoritative knowledge, I also seek
to show how medical knowledge and standards of practice correspond to pregnant women's own assessment of its authority (Lazarus 1997; Root and Browner
2001). My purpose is to demonstrate the local dynamics by which pregnant
women and medical practice are mutually and actively constituted, being
informed by ethno-theoretical paradigms of thinking about pregnancy.

The Local Construction of Authoritative Knowledge:
"Environmentalism" and "Geneticism"

Concern with power is central to anthropological studies of reproduction, yet knowledge, that is, the nature of its truth claims, as well as its uneven distribution in society, are at least of equal concern. Women's quest for medical information and their felt need to become more "educated" have been identified as a particular characteristic of the experience of modern pregnancies (Davis-Floyd 1992; Sargent and Stark 1989). In prenatal arenas women and care providers understand medical information as a necessary tool in the project of taking decisions and sorting out new "reproductive choices." In this context, various scholars probed the differential accessibility of medical information to women across boundaries of class and race (Lazarus 1997; Rapp 1999) and its dependence on "scientific literacy" (Rapp 1999). However, Barbara Katz Rothman's problematization of the concept of "reproductive choices" itself raises questions about the means required to make choices, that is, about the whole practice of consuming medical information. Following Ruth Hubbard's suggestion that "As 'choices' become available, they all too rapidly become compulsions to 'choose' the socially endorsed alternative" (Hubbard in Rothman 1984, 27), Rothman recalls that "We thought that information would give us power. What we perhaps overlooked is that it is *power* which gives one control over both information and choice" (Rothman 1984, 26). Rothman's argument illuminates the problematic assumption that underlies the consumption of medical knowledge, namely, that this information is adequate, important, and absolutely necessary for pregnant women.

While this claim brings us back to Foucault's treatment of power and knowledge as mutually constituted through discourse and practice, anthropologists of reproduction have developed similar models of power/knowledge based on their ethnographies in specific reproductive arenas. Such is Jordan's concept of "authoritative knowledge," on which I draw here. By "authoritative knowledge" Jordan means "the knowledge that participants agree counts in a particular situation, that they see as consequential, on the basis of which they make decisions and provide justifications for courses of action. It is the knowledge that within a community is considered legitimate, consequential, official, worthy of discussion and appropriate for justifying particular actions by people engaged in accomplishing the task at hand" (Jordan 1997, 58). Rather than a substance that can be possessed, Jordan sees authoritative knowledge as a state that is "collaboratively achieved." Most importantly for my study, a body of knowledge has to "make sense" to become authoritative (Jordan 1997, 58). She stresses that there are "local versions of authoritative knowledge," which is always locally produced and displayed. Drawing on Jordan's analytical concepts, I explore two local versions of authoritative knowledge about pregnancy, in

Japan and Israel, whose orientations I call "environmentalism" and "geneticism," respectively.

In environmentalism I attempt to capture the huge range of somatic and emotional responsibilities that the Japanese regime of truth allocates to the pregnant mother while emphasizing that primary responsibility for fetal health lies in the bodies of pregnant mothers, and that their management of their bodies—which serve as the environment of the fetus—is crucial for the creation of a healthy fetus. In geneticism I attempt to capture a fatalistic theory that explains fetal health through genes and chromosomes that are independent of the pregnant woman's willpower. Responsibility to bear a healthy fetus, in the geneticist truth regime, rests with the mother, but she must rely on diagnostic technologies to be able to fulfill this responsibility to her family and to society. Yet it should be born in mind that while "environmentalism" and "geneticism" are crucial for understanding medical theories of pregnancy and their modes of care provision, they draw their power of reasoning from Japanese and Israeli paradigms of thinking about persons, and how they come into being, that go beyond biomedicine.

Indeed as Jordan shows, access to authoritative knowledge is uneven between doctors and women. Yet through comparative research I can go beyond analyses of differential accessibility between women and doctors, and beyond social class, to examine accessibility of different kinds of medical information *across cultures.* My findings suggest that large-scale flows of information are restricted by national political and cultural loci of power. In general, different kinds of medical information on prenatal care are accessible to these two groups of women. Israeli women, regardless of class differences, possess far greater access to information about prenatal diagnosis than Japanese women.

Such differences in accessibility have to do with the ranking of different kinds of knowledge in each locality (and with their adjacent moral economies, to which I return). Jordan claims, "for any particular domain several knowledge systems exist, some of which, by consensus, come to carry more weight than others" (Jordan 1997, 56). Here I examine not only the hierarchies between "folk" and medical theories about pregnancy, but also hierarchies that are constituted between different kinds of scientific truth claims within local versions of biomedicine: in the present case knowledge about the genetic and chromosomal factors of fetal health versus biomedical knowledge about environmental factors such as maternal nutrition. In this I have been influenced by Lock's analyses of Japanese medical theories of the menopause. As Lock shows, the majority of Japanese physicians and women associate menopausal syndromes with "disturbances in the autonomic nervous system" (Lock 1996, 98) rather than with hormonal changes, as, for example, Canadian doctors and women would claim. This, Lock claims, has to do with the affinity between the "holistically oriented physiological approach characteristic of Sino-Japanese medicine"

(Lock 1996, 98) and medical theories about the association between the endocrine system and the autonomic nervous system suggested in the 1930s by German doctors. Foucault's deconstruction of the concept of scientific "truth" is also helpful in this context. Foucault sees truth as an effect "produced within discourses which in themselves are neither true or false" (1980, 118) but which nevertheless produce a "truth regime." By integrating Jordan's concept of authoritative knowledge, drawing on Foucault's "regime of truth" and taking Lock's observations on Japanese medical theories as a cue, I try to identify the role played by socio-cultural perceptions of the body, the self, and social relations within their local political settings as they are forged in a specific moment in history, in the construction of hierarchies between different kinds of medical knowledge about pregnancy. Finally, I also opt to go beyond the delineation of cultural concepts at work to show *how* these truth regimes are produced within a range of social settings in each locality.

Themes in the Theorization of Pregnancy

Broadly speaking, at least two shifts seem to have occurred in the anthropology of reproduction. One, discussed above, is a shift from the study of biomedical power as a top-down repressive structure, which produces resistance in women, to a growing tendency to see biomedicine as an incoherent collection of practices and knowledge that women exploit while being influenced by pragmatic considerations. The other is a shift from the theoretization of how biomedicine "medicalizes" or "pathologizes" reproduction to the theoretization of NRTs as transforming and even revolutionizing reproduction. This line of argument is particularly dominant in relation to pregnancy.

First, scholars such as Rothman (1986; 1989), Sandelowski (1994), and Van der Ploeg (1995) claim that NRTs change the perception of women's bodies, transforming them into increasingly permeable and transparent entities. Secondly, NRTs are increasingly transforming the fetus into a person, producing in the process new categories of patients whose rights might conflict (Petchesky-Pollack 1987). Thirdly, scholars claim that NRTs transform the experience of pregnancy. Eugenia Georges states that the visual technology of ultrasound has replaced the realization of pregnancy through quickening (Georges 1996). Rapp (1999) argues that prenatal diagnosis forces women to cope with a new and complicated set of "reproductive choices" and moral dilemmas. Specifically, the technology of amniocentesis transforms women into what she calls "moral pioneers." When deciding whether to undergo a test that might endanger the life of a fetus or to have an abortion if it is diagnosed as abnormal, women are continuously in search of moral solutions (Rapp 1999). Similarly, Barbara Katz Rothman maintains that amniocentesis makes pregnancy tentative (Rothman 1986). Scholars like Strathern and Franklin go a step farther, saying not only that NRTs *redefine* reproduction but that their impact far exceeds reproduction itself, transforming our fundamental concepts of kinship and nature (see, for example, Franklin 2003; Strathern 1992).

The present study reexamines these assertions from a cultural comparative perspective. It asks questions such as: Are technologies transforming pregnancies in different localities in the same way? Are Japanese and Israeli pregnancies equally tentative? Put differently, under what kinds of socio-cultural and political conditions are NRTs being "allowed" to transform pregnancies? The explicit comparison allows me to ask further: Are the technologies transforming pregnancies, or are socio-cultural conditions transforming pregnancies through the technologies?

These are the sort of questions I shall be examining throughout this book in relation to contemporary Japanese and Israeli societies. In all, I shall ask: What is it in cultural theories of pregnancy, in the metaphors and concepts available in these societies to think about pregnancy, in the reproductive politics and emergent moral economy, that gives power to biomedical technologies, and how is this power given?

The comparative apparatus of this study, I believe, has been crucial for the formulation of these questions. I now move on to elaborate what is at stake in the comparisons it draws.

The Unavoidable Comparison

Above I noted that my initial plan was to study versions of pregnancy in Japan, and did not include any comparative aspects. But my positioning in the field set my mind shuttling back and forth between the Japanese and Israeli realms of pregnancy, and this shuttling, moreover, affected the way I singled out topics for research.

The role of implicit comparisons in stimulating interest toward a specific social phenomenon is not unique to anthropological pursuits. Nor is it unique in the analysis of social phenomena. As cognitive science informs us, comparisons are part and parcel of living in the everyday world: we compare, intentionally or not (Gingrich and Fox 2002, 6; Toren 2002, 188). However, as Fox and Gingrich (2002), Holy (1987), Nader (1994), Overing (1987), and Toren (2002) argue, comparisons are even more fundamental in anthropology. First, Nader reminds us, the discipline is rooted in a comparative consciousness, since historically, anthropology has explored "other" cultures. The concept of "otherness" at the basis of the anthropological endeavor has been constituted in relation to the (seemingly) unproblematic Western investigator (Nader 1994, 88). Secondly, as Peel argues, "comparison is implicit in any method of deriving understanding through explanation" (Peel 1987, 89). In the specific case of anthropology, to "understand" "other cultures," researchers rely on ethnographic descriptions literally made of translations. And since it is impossible to make "direct" or "exact" transcultural translations, anthropologists end up forming "arrays of judgments of sameness" (Barnes and Bloor 1982) that are again the products of intercultural comparisons. The position of anthropologists as interpreters of cultures to audiences from another culture practically compels some level of comparison. As Bird-David writes: "Any ethnographic work involves a kind of comparison; in a world of relativities we can only see something in relation to something else" (Bird-David 1996, 303).

One question, then, is not whether one compares or not, but whether the comparison is implicit or explicit: how conscious is the researcher of the preeminence of the comparisons s/he is making? Once I realized that I was comparing, I tried to use comparisons reflectively and to specify what it was that I was comparing, but the more reflective I became about making implicit comparisons, the more my "cultural logic" and "common sense" as a native Israeli were put into question.

The anxieties, into which I drifted during my first pregnancy, once I landed in Israel, were a key transformational experience in my understanding of research. First, I realized that although I could make sense of everything that had happened using my "native logic" and could even feel familiar with it, I was completely unaware of how far its consequences might reach in terms of experience. Secondly, it became clear that my being a native Israeli was not enough to supply me with a "license" to assume "what pregnancies are like" in Israel. Consequently, "the range of experiences of pregnancy of Israeli women" could no longer serve as an "Archimedean point." Thirdly, my curiosity about the "Israeli pregnancies" was increased. "Israeli conceptions of pregnancy," which I had taken for granted, turned out to be at least as intriguing as "Japanese conceptions." Moreover, the above events strengthened my feeling that the Israeli case is particular and cannot be generally conceived as grounded in "Western conceptions" (a point I shall return to later).

Finally, I realized that since it seemed impossible to stop my mind bouncing back and forth between "Israeli pregnancies" and "Japanese pregnancies," and since I lacked knowledge in both realms, there was no escape from investigating both, not only to save face in the eyes of my Japanese informants (who were eager to know how pregnancy was experienced in Israel), but first and foremost to cooperate reflexively with a mode of thinking that was already present in my research. In practice, this realization meant that I was now committed to creating two "distinct" ethnographies whose relationships were established only in my own mind.

In retrospect, my route to explicit comparison seems to illustrate the shift that has occurred in anthropology as a whole, from gazing at the "other" to "othering" one's own gaze. By making a commitment to explicit comparison, I attempted to go beyond "reflexivity" as such, and concomitantly to differentiate the Japanese and Israeli cultures in order to create a methodological apparatus where neither the Israeli nor the Japanese case can be taken for granted or serve as a point of departure: rather, points of departure shift back and forth. Ultimately, such apparatus rejects privileging the perspective of either culture under investigation.

I soon discovered that a comparative research apparatus also entails a particular mode of consciousness with far-reaching effects on every single aspect of research.

Comparative Consciousness as Analytical Inspiration

Two features characterize comparative thinking throughout this study: first, the shift of viewpoints back and forth between the cases; and secondly, the use of "differences" and "similarities" as "stimulants" for thinking and as "analytical resources." "Differences" are first identified at the level of empirical findings and trigger a series of sub-questions that propel the analysis up to the conceptual level in a zigzag movement between the fields. These sub-questions are used to illuminate the broad question that is the focus of this study: how is pregnancy experienced and socially managed in two different societies? However, as Howe argues, "Relations of similarity and difference are not given in the empirical phenomena themselves but are generated by people who act on them and decide, using criteria of their own choosing, to which class, category or concept they conform" (Howe 1987, 135). Therefore, it is necessary to specify what kind of "differences" and "similarities" were employed here.

Two types of "differences" generated the entire analytic process: differences in *how* similar practices are carried out, and differences in *how much and what kind of space* practices occupy.

These are "differences" between two sets of empirical findings that become particularly visible when set against "similarities." In the case of pregnancy, one of the most notable similarities between Japanese and Israeli practices is that pregnancy is medicalized in both. Many of the "activities" of pregnancy are framed within medical institutions and orchestrated by medical professionals trained in conventional (i.e., Western-style) medicine. As a part of this global trend, the majority of Israeli and Japanese women see ob-gyns while they are pregnant, in private clinics, maternity hospitals, or general hospitals. I focus on a visit to a clinic to exemplify the comparative work of differences.

Let us say that a visit to the doctor is launched as soon as the pregnant woman arrives at the clinic. From that moment, both Japanese and Israeli women participate in a number of procedures. The events listed below may take place in both cases, in whole or in part, and not necessarily in the order given here. The woman registers at a desk occupied by nurses or medical secretaries, sits for a while in a waiting room, then at some point is invited to enter the ob-gyn's office. Then the woman will typically talk to the ob-gyn, ask and be asked questions, have her blood pressure and weight measured, and have the doctor examine her physically. Finally the doctor or an ultrasound technician might perform an ultrasound scan for the woman. Following an array of some (or all) of these procedures, the woman will usually be invited to return to the clinic in a few weeks and/or be given forms to have additional examinations, such as blood or urine tests, carried out. "Thin" descriptions such as the above can be used to draw attention to the ways in which the pregnant body becomes bureaucratized, measurable, diagnosable, and objectified in both the Japanese and the Israeli context. However, a comparative consciousness would suspect that the meaning that is being conveyed through the practices, which construct the pregnant body as measurable (to take one example), might not necessarily be the same in the Japanese and Israeli cases.

This is exactly where the focus shifts to *how* similar practices are carried out. Take, for example, measurements of blood pressure. While in Israel the doctor or the nurse takes the woman's blood pressure, in many Japanese clinics (and usually in the larger hospitals), the woman is expected to check her blood pressure herself before entering the doctor's office, using a digital device situated in the waiting room, and bring the printed results to the doctor. In many cases there are digital scales for the woman to weigh herself, and again she herself hands the printout to the doctor. This comparison reminds us that different agents can carry out the same procedure of measuring blood pressure. Although the bodies of Japanese and Israeli women are "measured," the Israeli woman is acted on by others while the Japanese woman acts herself. The Israeli doctor's professionalism seems to cover acts that a Japanese doctor considers sufficiently non-professionalized for the patient to manage herself.

What can this distinction tell us about the agencies of Japanese and Israeli women? Of course, one cannot theorize on women's agencies on the basis of a single measurement. Illustrated here is the stimulus to the ethnographer's attention: noticing the difference sharpened my attention to other self-supervision practices. I noticed that many of my Japanese informants used to weigh themselves regularly at home and register minute weight gains. Some even kept diaries in which they registered weight gain, bowel movements, physical activity and food intake weekly and even daily. These women understood self-supervision as necessary for the health of their unborn babies. My attention to this self-supervision was heightened by the realization that Israeli women whom I observed and talked to were considerably less inclined to supervise their nutrition and weight, although they were at least as interested as Japanese women in giving birth to healthy babies. Instead, characteristic of their pregnancies was their wide use of prenatal diagnosis to detect inborn abnormalities. Could it be, I asked myself, that Japanese and Israeli women employ "different techniques" to ensure the birth of a healthy baby? And if so, could it be that these techniques are based on different theories of the development of healthy fetuses? What do "Japanese theories" say? What do "Israeli theories" say? What makes them different?

In the initial stages of the research, it was not clear to me whether the theories that I was looking for were "medical," "folk," or "private" theories of gestation, or maybe hybrids of medical and folk theories. I hypothesized that the medical theories of ob-gyns and of pregnant laywomen would differ. Medical theories would differ among doctors, as might "folk" and "private" theories among women. However, while carrying out more and more observations in both fields, my focus gradually shifted from tracing different kinds of theories to the ways in which these theories work together and facilitate the interactions that surround pregnancy. I came to view prenatal care as a cooperative enterprise between women and doctors. This idea first occurred to me when I noticed that some Japanese women would show their private records of weight to their doctors and consult them about their notes. The doctors expected their patients to supervise their own bodies, and many women cooperated with this expectation by keeping detailed diaries. Once my attention was drawn to "cooperation" I immediately tried to "think with," and even "search for" it in the Israeli situation.

In the initial stages of this study, I was beset by a feeling that the proliferation of prenatal tests in Israel is due to a "conspiracy" between the health ministry and the doctors against abnormal fetuses. From this perspective, women were merely the intermediaries in a eugenic enterprise. The cooperative dimension in the Japanese field led me to try and experiment with the concept of cooperation in the Israeli field. It made me realize that even if a conspiracy was indeed involved, there was no way of forcing women to undergo prenatal diagnosis (in the same way that there was no way to force Japanese women to supervise themselves). That many women with no prior indication of any fetal abnormality pursue additional testing, which is not reimbursed by health funds, suggests that there is more to prenatal testing in Israel than a conspiracy. The comparative framework directed my thinking to theories of pregnancy in terms of the shared cultural understandings between doctors and patients. Here again consciousness is situated *in between*. Both ethnographies discuss the practices of doctors and pregnant women, and both attempt to uncover the conceptions of pregnancy that define women's agency and doctors' authority, and to make sense of the interactions between them.

The comparative framework thus suggests going beyond criticizing the medicalization of pregnancy in both the Israeli and the Japanese case for subjecting the body to scrutiny, pathologizing pregnancy, and controlling and intruding into the body. Noticing differences in *how* the same medicalizing practices are carried out reminds one that different ways of using them can convey a diversity of meanings, construct different forms of agency, and make possible various systems of relationships, while retaining their medicalizing effect. Comparisons remind us that the meanings of biomedical technologies are not only *in* the technologies themselves: these meanings are assigned by those who practice and experience them.

Which brings us to the second kind of difference: in the "space" that practices occupy. "Space" relates to the centrality, conspicuousness, and elaboration that surround a practice. Observing Japanese and Israeli practices of pregnancy from a broader perspective reveals that although similar prenatal tests exist today in both arenas, they occupy different "spaces" in terms of frequency of use and the importance attached to each. A comparative perspective reveals that while the weight gain of pregnant Japanese women is checked and marked on a graph, and discussed in every prenatal visit, Israeli ob-gyns are much less consistent about checking their patients' weight gain. Some Israeli practitioners even said that they do not weigh pregnant women at all. By contrast, while Japanese ob-gyns are often reluctant to mention prenatal diagnosis even to older women, and discuss this issue hesitantly when it is raised, some of the Israeli ob-gyns I interviewed said that they offer prenatal diagnosis to each and every patient, regardless of her age.

Observing Japanese and Israeli women from the same perspective, it became clear that while the majority of the Japanese women who were interviewed were preoccupied with daily nutritional calculations, and took advantage of any opportunity to discuss the matter with medical and paramedical practitioners, my Israeli informants rarely had the chance to discuss these issues in medical arenas—not that nutrition is nonexistent as an issue in pregnancy in Israel. Rather, it belongs mostly in popular magazines and much less in medical contexts. By contrast, while Israeli informants from different socio-economic statuses were prepared to pay for expensive prenatal diagnoses in addition to the testing funded by health funds, my Japanese informants were relatively reluctant to use these technologies. So nutrition and weight occupy a large space in pregnancy in Japan, while in Israel the same is true of prenatal diagnosis. As stated, "space" here designates the relative degree of elaboration, centrality, and conspicuousness of a practice, and the concerns that sustain it. My awareness of the differences in the "spaces" that certain practices occupy encouraged me to pay attention to deemphasized arenas in each field and led to a broader mapping of both. The Japanese ethnography made me ask Israeli ob-gyns about their attitudes to weight and nutrition, and thanks to the Israeli ethnography, I started asking Japanese ob-gyns about prenatal testing.

Together, the differences in *how* similar practices are carried out and the differences in *how much space* these practices occupy bring out the particularities of each case and furnish empirical grounds to raise questions of a kind that would be more difficult to ask with one ethnography in mind. With just an Israeli ethnography, the popularity of prenatal testing would logically be addressed by questions such as: what is the dominant image of the body in Israeli society that makes Israeli women so preoccupied with identifying and disposing of abnormal fetuses? No substantial way would exist to add a question such as why Israeli women are so preoccupied with abnormal fetuses, and much less with the way they might be able to affect their fetuses themselves. Such a question automatically sharpens one's senses on issues pertaining to ethno-theories that explain how fetuses *become* abnormal in the first place.

In the same way, a Japanese ethnography alone would probably have oriented my focus to questions about the disciplining of women's bodies through the supervision of weight and nutrition. But the Israeli arena calls Japanese reluctance to use prenatal diagnosis into question. Keeping in mind the image of Japan as a competitive society that cherishes education (*gakureki shakai*), are not Japanese women concerned with the social and practical implications of raising an abnormal child?

Once this question had arisen, there was no other way but to go back to the field again, check figures and talk to people. A number of Japanese ob-gyns I talked to suggested that indeed few Japanese women subjected themselves to prenatal diagnosis. These practitioners claimed that if an abnormality was detected these women had abortions citing legal reasons for doing so. Such findings raised another, much broader question: can we assume that aversion to abnormal children is a universal trait, that most people are interested in disposing of them, and that the cultural variation is only in *how* to dispose of them and whether to talk about it openly or not. Or can we perhaps differentiate societies in terms of the "degree" of tolerance they show to abnormal children? Finally (returning to the focal point of this study), how can possible answers to the questions above illumine the position of pregnant women and the conceptions of pregnancy within these societies? It is in the stimulation of such questions (and not necessarily in their answers) that I see the value of the comparative apparatus.

As one may sense, the comparative thinking is maximally facilitated in areas where ethnographies *contrast* rather than "differ." Skocpol and Somers (1980) call such a comparative apparatus a "contrast-oriented comparative methodology." Contrast-oriented methodologists, they write, hold that "particular nations, empires, civilizations or religions constitute relatively irreducible wholes, each a complex and unique socio-cultural configuration in its own right" (Skocpol and Somers 1980, 17), though this attitude does not reject more general insights. Geertz (whose *Islam Observed* they mention as a contrast-oriented study) explains the purpose of his turning to comparative (anthropological) history as hoping to "stumble upon general truths while sorting through special cases" (Geertz 1968, 4). Skocpol and Somers argue that the "task of the contrast-oriented comparative historian is facilitated when maximally different cases within given bounds are chosen for comparison" (Skocpol and Somers

1980, 179). In this respect, Japan and Israel, as I elaborate below, proved a choice with a powerful theoretical thrust.

Why Japan and Israel

"Why compare Japan and Israel?" I am frequently asked. Underlying the question is not only skepticism about comparative methods, stemming, I think, from the connotations that comparative studies in anthropology bear on scientism, but also criticism of what "smells" of arbitrary choice; I suspect it would be less likely to arise were I to compare prenatal care in North America (or any other country designated "Western") and Japan. Anthropological literature is in fact replete with major works that compare Japan with the West (Benedict's *Chrysanthemum and the Sword* and Lock's work on menopause and brain death, to mention two very differently oriented but influential scholars). It is beyond the scope of this book to discuss the significance of some comparative choices being obvious while others need explanation; I would simply clarify that my positioning between the Japanese and Israeli cultures of pregnancy initiated experimentation with these field sites, but the emergent theoretical merits of this specific choice of sites for comparison sustained them as key components in the analytical design of this study.

To begin with, Japan and Israel share a number of important features. Both are non-Western, modern democracies, with highly industrialized and technologized societies and they share a militarized history—extending, in the case of Israel, to the present day. Medical care in both countries is regulated through national insurance, is readily available, affordable, and subsidized by the government, at a high technological level and commensurate with the most developed Western countries, and for the most part provided on a nonprofit basis. In both countries, health-care facilities are available in government medical centers, university hospitals, and private clinics, as well as in voluntary organizations, and medical professionals are trained to standards equal to those of other developed countries. Finally, of major importance to this study is that in both countries biological and cultural reproduction has clearly become the object of medical and social discourse and intervention. One can safely say that pregnancy and birth are highly medicalized in both countries: the overwhelming majority of pregnant women in Japan and Israel today enroll in prenatal care during pregnancy, and 99.4 percent of Israeli and 99.8 percent of Japanese women give birth in medical institutions.

Yet Japan and Israel also markedly differ in a number of important aspects. Though both are explicitly pro-natal, Japan's steadily decreasing fertility rate (a 1.24 rate was reported in 2007 by the Mother's and Children's Health and Welfare Association) is considerably lower than the Israeli rate of 2.9 (reported in 2009 by the Israel Central Bureau of Statistics), which is high compared with other industrial societies. Moreover while Japanese pro-natalism was constructed in the last few decades of the twentieth century, against the prospect of a "graying society," Israeli pro-natalism developed under the "demographic threat"—the discourse about Israel being a lone Jewish state surrounded by Arab nations with its explicit implications for the Israeli-Arab and Israeli-Palestinian conflicts, with which Israel's history was intertwined even before its own birth in 1948.

Governments' attitudes toward supporting fertility also differ: while the Israeli government subsidizes prenatal care (as well as assisted conception technologies) rather generously, the Japanese government leaves quite a large portion of prenatal care uncovered by national health insurance. Significantly, reproductive health-care providers in these countries are known for different kinds of achievements: whereas the Japanese medical system claims the lowest neonatal mortality rate in the world (1.4 per 1000 live births as reported in 2007) and is well known for its incubators, professional neonatologists, and smallest viable neonates, Israeli neonatologists have been fighting an increase in neonatal mortality and morbidity (infant mortality rates were 3.1 as reported in 2005). Instead, Israeli ob-gyns "have emerged as global leaders in the research and development" of fertility treatments (Kahn 2000, 2), and are also well known for their innovative contributions and expertise in the area of the prenatal diagnosis of inborn abnormalities.

The list of differences goes on and on: a government overburdened with security issues (Israel) and one that still has relatively minor security concerns (Japan); two differently oriented trajectories of militarism and colonialism, and two different historical positions vis-à-vis eugenic ideas and practice; a country that is relatively ethnically homogeneous (Japan) and an immigrant society (Israel); and two markedly different modes of gendered division of labor. Finally, Japanese people and Israeli Jews show a contrast between a culture in which polytheistic traditions are mixed with a strong Buddhist component in conceptions of life and death and one based on the monotheistic traditions of Judaism, as well as with their emergent moral economies.

In working with such complex sets of differences in the frame of "contrast-oriented" methodology, I do not mean to reduce the relations between them to "opposites" (cf. Robertson 2002a) I see Japan and Israel as two markedly different societies (in Skocpol's sense) within accepted ideas of modernity, constituting two complex, irreducible, socio-cultural and political wholes, each with its own trajectory of historical development. Note that the American culture of reproduction does not occupy any privileged position in this study as an "index case." Though major parts of the literature on reproduction do deal with American society, I aspire to contribute to the growing body of works focused on non-Western reproductive culture (Gameltoft 2007; Inhorn 2003; Roberts 2007) that identify North America as a special case.

To summarize, the comparative method applied here can be characterized as follows. First, it is *reflexive* in the individual and global sense, in the way it reflects (and stems from) the researcher's position with respect to the two field situations, and in the way it reflects the current tensions between globalization and local culture. Secondly, it is *qualitative*, bringing together two distinct ethnographies. Thirdly, comparison here is used as an *inspiring analytic resource* that sharpens distinctions, broadens the scope of ethnographies and generates conceptual questions, not as a means to "prove" grand universalist theories. In sum, the methodology used here is a reflexive, qualitative, contrast-oriented cultural comparison that uses systems of "differences" and "similarities" first and foremost as tools to think with in relation to two distinct social settings for pregnancy.

Multisited Ethnographies

As I discuss below, fieldwork in Japan and Israel bears a different character. Fieldwork in Japan was conducted during four intensive round-the-clock field stints: for the five consecutive months from December to April 1996, in January and February 2000, in February 2001 and in November 2007. These spells were supplemented with continuous e-mails and phone conversations, and dozens of exchanges of written letters with several of the people I interviewed and observed. Through these connections I was consistently updated about my informants' lives. Fieldwork in Israel was conducted between 1996 and 2003 and during the summer of 2006 as I went on periodic weekly excursions while living at home and working. Each of these different fieldwork trajectories—one characterizable as fieldwork at home and the other more similar to classic fieldwork (albeit in a globally connected world, which makes keeping in touch afterwards simpler)—shaped the data that emerge from each site. As I will make clear, my continuous presence at the Israeli field site did not necessarily make my entrance and access to it simpler than in my Japanese fieldwork.

All in all, this study it based on data collected through more than one hundred in-depth interviews and long hours of participant observations at multiple sites where pregnancy was being related to and socially negotiated (Marcus 1995). The "posited logic of association" (Marcus 1995, 105) among the string of specific sites is that of an imaginary "route" of pregnancy from a woman's perspective. I visualize pregnancy as a social path, a journey with "stations" on the way: it is precisely this route that I endeavor to "map," and its stations that were chosen as sites for data collection. Birth-education courses, medical check-ups and popular pregnancy guides are examples of such stations in both Japanese and Israeli society. When examining each site I was interested in discourse as well as practice, in narratives as well as visual and textual representations, in professional and nonprofessional perspectives, and in private and public negotiations of pregnancy. Such a research design understands pregnancy as a dynamic structure of interconnected practices and ideas in a constant process of production that occurs synchronically in multiple social arenas and by a variety of agents. By piecing together the perspectives of different agents acting in diverse social locations, I was hoping to paint a broad picture of the range of meanings of pregnancy as viewed from plural viewpoints and as articulated and practiced in two societies.

Medical Arenas

But soon after compiling a list of sites for my imagined pregnancy map I realized that their accessibility was differentially linked to my position with respect to each site. The obstetrical clinic—where ultimately I could witness how pregnant women are practically treated in a medical setting, and a station through which virtually all the Israeli and Japanese women I knew passed while pregnant— went onto the list early in the formative stages of the study. Gaining access to Israeli medical arenas was by far the most difficult task.

In the first stages of research the closest I got to observing doctor-patient interactions was when Professor Ravel, a senior ob-gyn who heads the ultrasound department in a hospital in the north of Israel, showed me into a special room housing his latest invention: equipment for demonstrating abdominal and vaginal ultrasound scans to medical students. There, in a little room, beside the screen of an ultrasound scanner, lay a life-size female model on the white sheets of a hospital bed, naked and ready to be scanned abdominally or vaginally. My host inserted the ultrasound transducer into the puppet's vagina and, while staring at the image of the "fetus" that was reflected on the screen, explained how, with the help of this device, students could learn to interpret ultrasound images correctly. I felt extremely grateful to him for showing me his invention, but at the same time a bit nauseous when looking at this ideally receptive, exposed, and penetrable model of the female body.

This was not the only invention that I encountered in the field. Israeli ob-gyns often mentioned Israeli inventions and were proud of the achievements of Israeli obstetrics and gynecology. Generally they were oriented to Western learning and often likened their achievements to those of their Euro-American counterparts. Many felt that Israeli obstetrics and gynecology was at the "cutting edge of prenatal diagnosis," as one ultrasound expert put it: "When we report our detection rates [of fetal abnormalities] at international conferences, Americans do not believe us." Clearly, Israeli professionals were fascinated with contemporary biomedicine.

Yet a number of senior ob-gyns commented on how clinical standards in Israel had shifted over the previous twenty years from a hands-on approach to an increasingly technologized and compartmentalized profession that turned the ob-gyn into a "mere technician of tests." Their statements, however, were accompanied by the display of much appreciation and fascination with the diagnostic abilities of the new technologies. One senior doctor admitted that he felt that the medicine that he and his colleagues had practiced thirty years before now seemed medieval.

However, to observe practitioners at work, enacting these cutting-edge procedures, seemed a forlorn hope at the time. Israeli doctors were reluctant to let me into their clinics as an observer, even after positive interviews. Quoting from the "Israeli patient's bill of rights," they argued that my presence would violate the patients' right to privacy and the confidentiality of the medical information communicated during visits. Such were the most common arguments against giving me an opportunity even to ask the patient herself if she agreed to let me be present. Another reaction to my requests was to refer me to the bureaucratic labyrinth of hospital authorities to ask for formal approval. I was not even allowed to sit in the waiting room of one of the labs where women undergo the triple marker. The head biochemist of the lab explained that many representatives of insurance companies, cosmetics companies, and other commercial dealers had tried to obtain his permission to speak to the pregnant women sitting in the waiting room. However, "I see my duty as blocking them. It is my very basic duty to secure the pregnant woman from anybody bothering her as long as she is in my territory. And you must admit, I don't need to supply anybody with reasons to sue me." Clearly, while using his patients as tokens, this practitioner echoed the defensive attitudes I encountered throughout the field.

Surprisingly, my route into the Japanese medical field was smoother, even (I often thought) too smooth. Judging from my experiences in Israel, I expected the Japanese medical arena to be similarly impenetrable. It began when an Israeli friend introduced me to her uncle, an Israeli man in his fifties, who was married to a Japanese woman and had been teaching English to medical students in a Tokyo teaching hospital for the previous twenty years. We met briefly one cold evening at a Jerusalem café. He listened to my request patiently and said that he would do his best to help. I gave him two papers that I had written, should anyone be interested in what I was doing, and we parted.

To my surprise, within weeks of his return to Japan he e-mailed me that I had been given permission to sit in the obstetrics and gynecology outpatient clinics and asked me to send my curriculum vitae and a short description of my research. I was more than grateful, but deeply puzzled: there were no forms to fill in, no certificates to provide, no bureaucratic procedures to go through. The head of the maternity ward who had granted the permission inquired about me only retrospectively, and the English-language teacher said that nobody read the papers I had given him. I was excited but did not really believe that I would be allowed to sit and watch doctors receiving patients. Maybe, I thought, I would be allowed into the waiting room, which seemed more than enough.

The day after I landed in Japan I went to the teaching hospital. The building was quite old, but the shiny corridors, white gowns, patients, and neon lights felt familiar. Dr. Hayai, an ob-gyn in his forties who worked in the obstetrics and gynecology outpatient clinics, was waiting for me as arranged in the staff relaxation room on the top floor of the building. Like so many Israeli ob-gyns that I had met, he looked very busy. He handed me a white gown to put on. We took the elevator down, and Dr. Hayai guided me through the maternity ward. He introduced me to ob-gyns we met on the way as "the Israeli professor of sociology" (although I had told him that I was an anthropology student). There was no opportunity for more than a short, polite exchange since all this happened in the course of a race through the corridors of the ward. I ran after him all the way, answering short questions, bowing and politely saying how pleased I was to meet the staff.

We reached the outpatient clinic. It was a corridor with brown leather sofas where the patients sat across from a row of white doors, each displaying a number. At the far left of the row was a curtained side entrance, apparently to the first room. Stepping through this curtain after Dr. Hayai, I was surprised to discover a long and open corridor running behind the row of doors. The space behind the doors was separated into cubicals where ob-gyns saw their patients and examination rooms, each equipped with a gynecological chair. Once behind the curtain I realized that these rooms had only three walls, the fourth side being open to the common corridor. Along the corridor, medical equipment and medical forms were arranged, and ob-gyns and nurses moved freely to and fro. A few more steps into the common corridor revealed two wide-apart naked legs and the person I later came to know as Dr. Yamada moving the ultrasound transducer between these legs while gazing intently at the ultrasound screen. I could see only the naked legs and the vagina between them; the rest of the woman was veiled behind a light brown curtain hanging from the ceiling and separating the woman's lower body parts from her upper body. Until that moment the closest I came to witnessing doctor–patient interactions was when I was shown the life-sized female dummy. Now the "penetrable female body" was made of flesh and blood, and I was standing there peering into the insides of a woman who had not given me her permission to do so. I was shocked, to say the least. Why had they let me in? Were Japanese doctors less concerned about their patients' privacy? Or was the connection between the patient's privacy and her body perhaps defined differently in Japanese culture, as Ohnuki-Tierney (1984) suggests? Better still, had they let me in because, as a foreign observer, I was supposed to be "harmless"?

Shocked though I was, I realized that I was indeed being permitted to observe. The doctors I observed saw about fifty patients a day, dedicating four to ten minutes to each. Japanese patients often came to see their ob-gyns alone. Even when their husbands accompanied them, they rarely followed their wives into the doctor's office and often waited for them outside in the waiting room. This was in sharp contrast to the Israeli arena, where husbands often accompanied their wives into the doctor's office, especially when their wives were being given ultrasound scans.

The interactions I witnessed in Japanese clinics were characterized by short "target-oriented" questions and answers. I saw patients going to see their ob-gyns with notes that they had prepared at home "not to waste the doctor's time," as one of my informants put it. Doctor–patient interactions were marked by gestures of respect. Often patients would refrain from continuous eye contact with doctors and bow when they left the room. Compared to the Israeli patient, the Japanese patient seemed much less threatening to her ob-gyn. In 2000 and 2001, I learned from the doctors that lawsuits against medical practitioners in Japan have increased slightly in the past decade, though they are still fewer compared with the United States and Israel. Lawsuits regarding wrongful births in particular are even rarer. While in Japan lawsuits against ob-gyns accounted for 15 percent of litigation against doctors in general from 1994 to 2001, in Israel ob-gyns are the most sued medical experts: 33 percent of lawsuits against medical practitioners between 1993 and 2002 were in the area of obstetrics and gynecology.

The absolute numbers might be even more revealing: in Israel, with a population of 7 million, 440 cases were litigated from 1993 to 2002; in Japan, with a population of 127 million, only 745 cases were litigated between 1994 and 2001. Toward the end of 2007 the Japanese media reported a sharp rise in lawsuits against ob-gyns. However, while in Israel a significant proportion of suits were and still are "wrongful life" cases—where parents sue doctors for failing to diagnose a fetal anomaly in utero—in Japan doctors are sued for delivery accidents and not for failures to diagnose inborn anomalies. The ease with which I entered the Japanese medical field is at least in part clearly due to the fact that Japanese ob-gyns still practice under fewer legal constraints than their counterparts in Israel or America.

My identity as a foreign woman, more specifically as a Jewish woman, also contributed to this smoothness: large stretches of the 2001 field trip were organized by a distinguished head of a maternity ward at a large medical center in Saitama prefecture, who, as I discovered later, felt great attachment to Jewish people.

Soon after I returned to Israel with my notes from the Japanese outpatient clinics, I discovered that they were much more than ethnographic data. They were also quite powerful keys to unlock medical arenas in Israel. Israeli doctors were more interested in speaking to me than ever before, because they were curious about Japanese prenatal care (although some rejected Japanese practices as outdated once they heard about them). I could now supplement my interviews with Israeli doctors with focused, comparative questions on specific medical procedures. I could now question Israeli ob-gyns about their reluctance to perform vaginal examinations by presenting them with the explanations I heard from Japanese doctors about their important diagnostic value, or tell them about the reluctance of Japanese doctors to offer prenatal diagnosis and wait for their reactions. I imagined a virtual discussion between Japanese and Israeli doctors about what prenatal care should include, what was considered important and worthwhile, and what was considered irrelevant. However, for me, the purpose of the discussion was not to discover the ultimate clinical "truth" but to sharpen my understanding of these practitioners' clinical attitudes by means of explicit comparison. This proved to constitute ethnographic capital in the process of co-producing ethnographic knowledge, especially in medical arenas.

Moreover, only after I returned from Japan did I manage to obtain permission to observe medical procedures in Israel. My entry was obtained through the exoticism that was associated with Japanese society, which turned out to be a source of attraction (pretty much like the role that my being Jewish played in Japanese arenas). Utilizing the capital of comparative studies, I received permission to observe obstetrical ultrasound screening and the procedures that surround amniocentesis for six months. Once allowed into the examination room, nobody bothered to robe me with a white gown, and patients were never asked to give their permission for me to be there.

All in all I interviewed fifty ob-gyns (twenty Israelis and thirty Japanese) whose ages ranged from thirty-one to seventy-two; nine of them were women. The ratio of male to female doctors reflects the statistical fact that although the portion of women ob-gyns is rising, in Israel and Japan obstetrics and gynecology is still a male-dominated profession (in both places 33 percent of ob-gyns were women in 2004).

Interviews were conducted in Japanese and Hebrew respectively, lasted from thirty minutes to four hours, were tape-recorded with permission and transcribed verbatim into Japanese and Hebrew respectively. Six Israeli ob-gyns did not wish to be recorded, so I took notes while interviewing them. All except three interviews were conducted at the practitioners' clinics and hospitals. The Japanese ob-gyns were from the Tokyo and Saitama area, the Israelis from the center and north of Israel.

Occasionally (especially when they were in a hurry) practitioners referred me to medical literature. Reading increasing numbers of journal articles and textbooks inspired me to initiate discussions with them on specific concepts and ideas that emerge in this literature. These conversations were ways to explore the meanings of what counts as authoritative knowledge, thus transforming the interviews into an interactive process involving the co-production of ethnographic knowledge, as indicated by Holstein and Gubrium (1997). I came to think of my goal in reading medical materials in terms of speaking a foreign language rather than becoming "knowledgeable" in obstetrics and gynecology. Like any language student, I focused on learning the "grammar" and "vocabulary" of this knowledge. As these materials proliferated, I began to consider them data in their own right.

One of my Japanese ob-gyn key informants, who was critical of my qualitative methods, insisted that questionnaires should be used to supplement my data and provide a wider perspective on the field. With his extensive help a ten-page questionnaire in Japanese was distributed to one hundred ob-gyns in the Saitama area; twenty-six were returned. The questionnaire basically included the initial set of questions about medical standards of practice that I had been using at the beginning of in-depth interviews.

Classes Taken during Pregnancy

Significantly, in both the Japanese and Israeli-Jewish settings, once pregnant, women and their partners become the target of educational activities of various types, of which the most popular are (what Americans call) birth-education classes. Such classes in both Japan and Israel form a somewhat less "strictly medical" site, where pregnancy is negotiated in a larger group of people (compared with the doctor–patient–patient's husband triad). In both the Japanese and Israeli cases, the instructors did their best to transmit medical knowledge in popular terms while using plenty of props—pictures, videos, and vivid illustrations, and tried to create a relaxed atmosphere in which the women and their partners were invited to ask questions and create friendly interactions. To facilitate this relaxed atmosphere, food and drink were offered to the participants during breaks.

In the Israeli case in particular, birth-education classes provided an opportunity to witness how male partners negotiate pregnancy in a public arena, as well as specific aspects of their relationships with their pregnant wives. In Israel I participated in five birth-education courses, each of seven to eight sessions, three held in hospitals and two in private homes. In Japan I participated in four "maternity courses" of four to five meetings each, three in hospitals and one at a municipal community center. I took notes of all the classes and interviewed two Japanese and two Israeli instructors.

Pregnancy Events

While the birth-education and maternity classes allowed a glimpse into negotiations of pregnancy in small groups of pregnant women and their partners, the site of Israeli "pregnancy events" opened a window onto how pregnancy is negotiated in a truly public sphere. The proliferation of "pregnancy events" throughout Israel during the 1990s can be seen as the reaction of medical institutions to growing public awareness of the plurality of ways to give birth, in particular to ideas of "natural birth." Medical centers are making active attempts to re-hospitalize birth on the patients' terms, utilizing "pregnancy events" as opportunities to explain and advertise their woman-friendly approaches to childbearing. In the course of these public negotiations of birth, the management of pregnancy itself has also entered the discussion, and it is on the negotiation of pregnancy that I focused while observing these events.

Pregnancy events are advertised in daily newspapers and child-rearing magazines under titles that associate them with pleasure and indulgence: "pregnancy and fun fair," "a Friday coffee," and "pregnancy fair" are examples of titles under which such events are advertised. The ads invite women to hear lectures from the best obstetrical experts and enjoy a nice breakfast free of charge. According to the organizers, hundreds of pregnant women participate in each event. My impression was that they came from a wide range of socio-economic strata and various levels of education, though I have no way of confirming these impressions statistically. The pregnancy events that I attended took place at various geographical locations throughout Israel. Some were held in hospitals, some in large community centers. "Pregnancy events" are always the joint enterprises of medical establishments and commercial companies, which market their pregnancy and child-rearing products at these events. To facilitate this commerce, the events are always held in large spaces. Cosmetic ointments to lubricate the stretched skin of a pregnant belly, pregnancy workout videos, maternity outfits, child-rearing magazines, baby carriers, water filters, and even amulets to protect pregnant women and future babies against the evil eye are only a few on a long list of commodities on sale at such events. While strolling among the stands, pregnant women and their companions are offered food and drink and given samples and presents of all kinds. However, the core of such "fun days" is a series of lectures by "master" medical practitioners who are well-known experts in their fields and/or hold senior positions as heads of maternity wards at distinguished medical centers. Lectures explore a range of reproductive topics from different medical perspectives. "The development story of the fetus," "obstetrical ultrasound," and "pain management in labor" are examples of frequent subjects. Lectures are accompanied by absorbing PowerPoint presentations, and the lecturers do their best to entertain their audiences with jokes and humorous pictures inserted into these serious presentations. In fact, more than once the boundaries between the "medical sphere" and the commercial and entertainment sphere become blurred.

I soon became "addicted" to pregnancy events, not only for their interesting combinations of the medical, the commercial, and the popular, but because they allowed my presence as an anthropologist to pass unnoticed. Since 1999 I have observed ten events throughout Israel, each lasting an average of three to five hours. One of the 1999 events was a two-day happening that lasted nine hours each day. I tape-recorded all the lectures presented on pregnancy days and also took notes of what was happening in the exhibition halls.

Five of the pregnant Japanese women I interviewed told me that they had participated in public lectures given by a famous ob-gyn. According to my interviewees, the focus of these lectures was the process through which maternal attachment developed toward the unborn child as part of the process of gestation. Unfortunately I was unable to attend such large-scale public events in Japan.

Interviews with Women

Finally, I tried to approach the terrain of personal experience of pregnancy by collecting women's narratives of their pregnancies. I conducted semi-structured, open-ended, in-depth interviews with twenty Israeli women and twenty-seven Japanese women who were pregnant or had had babies recently. Interviews were conducted in Japanese and Hebrew respectively, tape-recorded with permission and transcribed verbatim. In both Japan and Israel the women were introduced to me by friends or women I had met at birth-education classes or pregnancy events. Half were pregnant at the time of the interview and half had newborn babies. In Israel about one-third of the women I interviewed were pregnant for the first time, and the rest had one to three children. In the Japanese case most of the interviewees were pregnant for the first time or had just had their first child. In Japan and Israel, interviewees' ages ranged from the early twenties to the mid-forties, and they were diverse in terms of education and occupation. Generally, they can be characterized as urban lower- to upper-middle class. The Israeli interviewees lived in the areas of Jerusalem, Tel Aviv, and Kfar Saba. The Japanese interviewees lived in Tokyo and the Kamakura area, and in Saitama prefecture; half had grown up in different prefectures throughout the Japanese archipelago and still had families there. This is particularly significant, since eight of my interviewees returned to their natal homes toward the end of the third trimester to give birth there and be taken care of by their natal families. In the case of Israeli interviewees, I included in the analysis only those whose self-identification ranged from secular (non-religious) to traditional Jews. Except for one interviewee, they had all been born in Israel, though their parents or grandparents had migrated to Israel from different areas, including Middle Eastern countries, Eastern and Western Europe, as well as South and North America. Religious and ultra-religious Jewish women were not included in the data analyzed here, nor were recent new immigrants from Ethiopia and the former Soviet Union or women from the various groups of Israeli Arabs such as Muslim and Christian Arabs and Bedouins. Certainly, I encountered these women and their families in the course of my observations in various medical institutions, and doctors and nurses often told me about their interactions with them. Nevertheless, the relationship between these women and medical practitioners, as well as the concepts of pregnancy that they brought into these interactions, deserve attention in and of themselves.

I treat these issues in works based on further research (Ivry 2007a; Teman and Ivry n.d.). Similarly, since I did not interview Japanese women who live in agricultural areas, my findings are limited to women of the urban lower- to upper-middle classes.

Most interviews were conducted in the interviewees' homes and lasted from two to four hours. Often, in the course of the interviews, women presented me with various "pregnancy objects," such as ultrasound pictures and medical records, to illustrate and enhance their stories. Some also showed me the pregnancy guides that they read. I took these instances as opportunities to find out *what* kind of literature my informants were reading, but also *how* they were reading it. For example, I asked interviewees to tell me which parts of the pregnancy guides they read and which they skipped, and often a discussion of pregnancy guides would ensue. I used the woman's reflections on popular pregnancy guides in the same way that I used the comments of ob-gyns on textbooks and professional publications. Like obstetrics and gynecology textbooks, pregnancy guides also became a set of data in themselves. They provided an opportunity to examine popular images of pregnancy, as well as the process by which medical knowledge became popularized through the media. Reading through various kinds of pregnancy guides and discussing them with their readers, I could explore visual and textual representations of pregnancy and the ways women interpreted them. The interviewees who were pregnant at the time of the interview were interviewed again after they had given birth.

One of the Japanese birth-education teachers I contacted suggested that I should supplement my data with questionnaires, which she invited me to distribute to the pregnant women who were participating in her maternity classes. Consequently fifty questionnaires were distributed, of which thirty-five were returned. The questionnaires included the same initial questions that I had used in the in-depth interviews with the women.

Now that the major sites of fieldwork have been reviewed, I would like to remind readers about the initial commitments of this study: to investigate pregnancy while undertaking explicit cultural comparison. Although fieldwork was conducted at a variety of sites, the ethnographies that have resulted are not of obstetrical clinics, birth-education classes, pregnancy events or any other site mentioned above, but are two ethnographies of pregnancy drawing on scenes from a range of sites.

The multiplicity of sites gives rise to a system of cross references. Combined with the comparative apparatus, this helps identify in each locality the ideas that are negotiated *across* sites and are referred to by multiple and diverse agents. In this way I attempt to illuminate the trajectories along which ideas and practices of pregnancy develop *across* sites while reflecting and refracting a diversity of perspectives on pregnancy and pregnant women.

On Reading This Book

This book is divided in three parts: part one explores medical theories of pregnancy through the narratives and practices of Israeli and Japanese ob-gyns, and the second part explores the pregnancy experiences of Japanese and Israeli women while incorporating the viewpoints of their male partners, birth-education teachers, and media images into the picture. Part three pieces together the data presented in part one and two and uses cross-cultural comparison to reexamine the metaquestions of this study: What is pregnancy about in Japan and Israel? If it is about different things, what kind of social-cultural and political circumstances produce the differences? What are the implications of these differences to the ways in which pregnancy can be experienced and dealt with? And what can the Japanese and Israeli versions of pregnancy tell us about ethnographic ways to study human reproduction? The book has been written so as to preserve the comparative consciousness that is so central to its design. Thus the chapters are arranged to offer commentaries on each other: the first chapter, which explores the perspectives of Israeli ob-gyns on pregnancy, is followed by a chapter on the perspectives of Japanese ob-gyns; the third chapter, which explores Japanese women's experiences of pregnancy, is followed by a chapter on the experiences of Israeli women. Readers are invited also to read the chapters on women's experiences as commentaries on the chapters on doctors and vice versa.

Chapters one and two are based on data I gathered through participant observation in obstetrics and gynecology clinics and on a variety of narratives provided by ob-gyns during in-depth interviews. However, my focus of attention is less on the ob-gyns themselves as professionals and private persons as on pregnant women and pregnancy as reflected from their perspective. Thus, reading into narratives that account for their clinical practices, I initially seek to understand what kind of medical theories ob-gyns hold about pregnancy, and how they perceive the needs, interests, and state of mind of pregnant women. I explore how in each locality the archetypical images of pregnant patients that ob-gyns construct are directly related to their theories of gestation and fetal development. Moreover, I show how each medical theory of gestation is imbedded in a "metamedical" framework of thought, to use Worsley's terminology (Worsley 1982, 315), even though it is closely bound up with global developments in medical knowledge generally.

Set against the landscapes of local biomedicalization, chapters three and four are written so as to provide a sense of the local life-worlds of pregnancy and the way women experience their pregnancies in them.[3] These chapters juxtapose two ranges of pregnancy experience: Japanese women's experiences as they develop within an encompassing cultural paradigm of thinking about the pregnant body as "important," fragile, and in need of protection; and the experiences of Israeli women that develop within a general expectation that women will go about their roles as usual. Two significantly different types of imagined relationships between women and their fetuses arise in these different socio-cultural settings of gestation, complete with their emotional and practical implications on the lives of women. The final discussion draws on the contrast between the Japanese and Israeli arenas in order to reconsider the interplay of culture, biomedicine, and experience, and in particular, the implications of this interplay on women's agency and possibilities in each cultural setting when they navigate between their commitments to themselves, their families, and society.

PART ONE

The Doctoring of Pregnancy

1

A Risky Business

Pregnancy in the Eyes of Israeli Ob-Gyns

The National Politics of Reproduction and Israeli Prenatal Care

Israel, many scholars claim, is a pro-natal state, and Israeli pro-natalism is a powerful structure that draws on multiple cultural paradigms and political ideologies such as the Jewish religious imperative to "be fruitful and multiply," patriarchal familism, and Zionism (Portuguese 1998). Since its founding, and even before, the state has encouraged fertility among Jewish-Israeli citizens (Berkovitch 1997), intimating a link between the very existence of the nation-state and a high fertility rate. As a Jewish state surrounded by Arab countries and involved in almost continuous conflict, Israel has been preoccupied with the "demographic threat" (Sered 2000) and has tended to translate birthrates in Israel's chances of surviving a military conflict.[1] That the two population groups generally considered uncommitted to the Jewish nation-state—the ultra-orthodox and the Palestinian Arabs—have the highest fertility rates within the overall population has only worked to exacerbate the notion of the "demographic threat."

The financial support lavished on fertility-related issues by a state so overburdened with security is remarkable. A partial list of free reproductive health-care services for people covered by national health insurance includes heavily subsidized fertility treatments (until the patient has two children), free prenatal checkups, free hospitalized birth, and a "birth grant" [ma'anak leida]—a "bonus" that amounts to 20 percent of the average gross income paid by the state to mothers who have given birth in a hospital.

The social-science literature points to this state generosity as evidence of Israel's pro-natal regime (Birenbaum-Carmeli 2004; Gooldin 2008). It also indicates the enthusiastic embrace by medical experts and large segments of the public of NRTs (New Reproductive Technologies); Israel's having the highest rate in the world of IVF clinics per capita (Kahn 2000); Israeli couples' marked tendency to apply for fertility treatments less as a last resort than as a priority; and the institutionalization of surrogacy through the surrogacy law of 1996 (Teman 2001, 2003, 2010).

Adducing evidence from technologies of assisted conception, social scientists often associate the technologization of reproduction with an Israeli "cult of fertility" (an expression coined by Hazleton 1977). Yet the picture might change radically once the focus is shifted to a different set of reproductive technologies, which become conspicuous once conception has taken place, and these may not match ordinary notions of "pro-natalism" (Ivry 2010).

In 1978 the Israeli government enacted a (euphemistically entitled) Program for the Prevention of Inborn Abnormalities." The services offered under the plan were and still are free of charge. At first the plan dealt with lethal conditions such as Tay-Sachs disease. But soon the range of diseases screened widened (Weiss 2002, 80).

In a long interview, the former head of the program, a professor of genetics, described the introduction of new tests into the "national program" as intimately related to ongoing personal connections between leading scientists in the U.K. working on screening tests in the mid-1970s and Israeli geneticists. The latter, who directed the program, closely followed developments in technologies of genetic screening, importing them from all over the world. They quickly incorporated technologies for the detection of inborn genetic and chromosomal abnormality into routine prenatal care. A story I heard several times was that the alpha-fetoprotein (AFT) blood test, for neural-tube defects and the possible presence of Down's syndrome, was introduced by the Israeli Health Ministry shortly after its invention as a routine test when its credibility in diagnosing Down's syndrome was still only 30 percent. Since the initiation of the Program for the Prevention of Inborn Abnormalities, an increasing number of prenatal tests have been added to the "health basket" covered by national health insurance.

Adding to this picture the legislative system, together with the forces of the "free market," has taken prenatal testing a step further. In 1998, in a landmark judgment, for the first time a court convicted an ob-gyn who had acted in accordance with the guidelines laid down by the Ministry of Health. The plaintiff, a woman by the name of Yarkoni, who underwent all the prenatal tests in the "health basket" as recommended by her ob-gyn, none of which gave any indication of any fetal health problems, gave birth to a child with Dandy-Walker syndrome, an extremely rare genetic syndrome that causes mental retardation and paralysis. The plaintiff sued her doctor and her health fund for not informing her that she could undergo additional testing by privately paid experts that might have diagnosed the condition, in which case she would have had an abortion (Davies 1999). As stated above, the court declared the ob-gyn guilty. The precedent of the Yarkoni case placed medico-legal considerations right at the heart of gynecological practice. At present, a woman visiting an ob-gyn for an initial prenatal visit may be presented with an integrated list of about thirty or more prenatal tests, some of which are subsidized by her health fund (under specific conditions), others being expensive tests that she can pursue in government hospitals or private clinics. Some ob-gyns may ask her to sign a declaration that she has been made aware of the existence of all these tests.

Moreover, prenatal testing is "backed up" by the Israeli abortion law, which seems relatively liberal for a "pro-natal" state. The Israeli abortion law accommodates selective reproduction under an elaborate formulation of vague definitions. The law permits the abortion of defective fetuses, without specifying the kind of defect it refers to, and without setting a maximum time threshold beyond which abortion is forbidden (Amir 1995). Neither of these omissions has ever been a subject of public or parliamentary debate, even in the rare instances when abortion debates in the Knesset have momentarily managed to capture public attention.[2] In the mid-1980s several ultra-orthodox parties, which are a potent electoral force, tried to change the abortion law; but this was to erase the "economic clause" (permitting abortion in case of financial hardship of the mother), not to prevent "the murder of fetuses."

Adding to this picture is that virtually no criticism has been voiced by disability movements in Israel against the social meaning of prenatal diagnosis. The most vocal among these is an organization of army veterans wounded in combat, who do not affiliate themselves with other disabled people or evince any commitment to the rights of the nonmilitary disabled.[3] The "proliferation of publicly circulating representations of disability as a form of diversity," which Rapp and Ginsburg (2001, 534) point to in the context of postindustrial societies, is only starting to emerge in very limited segments of Israeli-Jewish society, namely, the ultra-orthodox and religious circles (who are formally opposed to abortion on rabbinical grounds), and is still quite unfamiliar among the nonreligious population.

Two of the diagnostic tests currently covered by national health insurance in a "low-risk" pregnancy are a second trimester scan against a "checklist" of the internal and external fetal organs for deformations and indications of abnormality, and a second trimester alpha-fetoprotein maternal blood test for probability of a child with a chromosomal or genetic anomaly; for the latter, state-funded amniocentesis is offered. In most cases doctors will also advise the woman to take more diagnostic tests, including a nuchal translucency scan and blood test at eleventh/twelfth week, a "checklist" scan at sixteenth week, and a second "checklist" scan at twenty-fourth week. Should suspicion arise about fetal health, women will face the decision of whether or not to undergo amniocentesis, with its 1/200 risk of miscarriage. This applies especially if they are over thirty-five, are terrified of having a disabled child, or have received "high-risk" results for the triple test.

Toward the end of 2007 the Israeli Ministry of Health and Welfare announced that it was withdrawing the general recommendation to women over thirty-five to undergo amniocentesis "since ultrasound screening has improved its diagnostic reliability." The stream of newspaper articles that followed were critical of the declaration: though they cited women and doctors with various attitudes to testing, the overall emphasis was on how amniocentesis "saved" the lives of women diagnosed as carrying a fetus with serious anomalies. Significantly, although the ministry withdrew its recommendation, the subsidy for women over thirty-five remained in place.

Generally, the average age of Israeli mothers at first birth has risen over the last decade; in 2007 it was 27.6 years for Israeli-Jewish women. The high percentage of births among Israeli-Jewish women aged thirty-five and over, accounting for 16–17 percent of births (Shohat et al. 1995, 967), and their high acceptance rate (67 percent) of prenatal testing (Davidov et al. 1994), is also a notable pattern. Sher et al. (2003, 420) report that 96 percent of secular Israeli women and 94 percent of traditional women take the triple test, and 94.4 percent of secular women and 62.5 percent of traditional women aged over thirty-five undergo amniocentesis. Many Israeli women under age thirty-five also have an amniocentesis, with or without indication of abnormality (Shohat et al. 1995) and often at their own expense, after they are made aware that amniocentesis is the only test, other than the less available CVS, that can give a diagnostic result of 95 percent accuracy.

Such women would pay privately for "in-depth" ultrasound screens and often for amniocentesis. During the last decade the prices have steadily risen: toward the end of 2007 a single ultrasound scan by an expert cost from NIS 600 to NIS 2200 ($150–$550) per scan per one fetus. Privately paid amniocentesis (for those not eligible according to the criteria of the Ministry of Health) was around NIS 4000 ($1000); note that average gross monthly income at that time was NIS 7700 ($1925).

Finally, according to Sagi et al. (2001) Israeli patients tend to terminate pregnancies upon diagnoses of relatively minor defects such as harelip, chronic sinusitis, or deformed feet, or upon unclear amniocentesis results, significantly more than patients in Europe and the United States (Sagi et al. 2001). During the last decade abortions were carried out in Israel legally until extremely late stages of pregnancy. Beginning in 1995, a woman who wished to undergo abortion after the twenty-third week of gestation had to appeal to a higher committee for late termination of pregnancy, in keeping with the regulations of the Israeli Ministry of Health. As of January 2008, such special committees discuss appeals from the twenty-fourth week of gestation.

However, statistical data published by the Israeli Ministry of Health attest that 95 percent of the 2007 applications were approved, and that approval rates have been steady since the late 1990s (Bureau of Information and Computing,

Israel Ministry of Health, November 2008, 20). Statistically, between 2000 and 2007 the abortion rate under the clause permitting abortions due to fetal abnormality ranged between 17.7 and 15.7 percent of all abortions, of which 1 percent were late abortions. In 2007, 89 percent of the latter were under the fetal anomaly clause (Bureau of Information and Computing, Israel Ministry of Health, November 2008, 22). The data reveal that in 2007, 51 percent of late abortions were performed at 24–26 weeks of gestation, 30 percent at 27–31 weeks, and 19 percent after 32 weeks. That the Israeli prenatal experts I spoke to claimed that their detection rates of fetal anomalies are higher than those reported by their Euro-American counterparts can be attributed at least in part to the fact that, as practitioners report, they continue to look for fetal anomalies till the end of term (unlike most Japanese ob-gyns, who told me that they stop searching after the twenty-first week of gestation). Thus, whereas in many places in the industrial world the law limits abortions to a certain gestational age, the Israeli context provides experts with a wider field of practice, since anomalies detected in the latest stages of gestation may still have a practical and legal solution, namely, abortion.

The above description, I think, provides some challenges to assumptions about Israeli society being "pro-natalist" or at least suggests that we should complicate our understanding of "pro-natalism" (I elaborate on this point later). From the point of view of the state, the above description highlights some inconsistencies and contradictions: why would a state so burdened with security expenses provide so many prenatal tests? Why would a state so preoccupied with birthrates and so threatened demographically be (relatively) liberal about abortions? It was with such questions in mind that I first approached the geneticists who had designed actions under the Program for the Prevention of Inborn Abnormalities.

The "Jewish Diseases"

When the directors of the Program for the Prevention of Inborn Abnormalities first agreed to speak to me, they asked me to explain the reasons for my research. When I told them that I was conducting a comparative study of Japan and Israel, they asked me what could possibly be different between these countries in respect of prenatal screening policies. I answered that the Japanese, for example, do not screen for genetic abnormalities as intensely as Israelis. Professor Shalem, sixty, a geneticist, smiled bitterly and said, "This is obvious; the Japanese do not have Ashkenazi Jews." He then handed me a list of diseases that Jews of different ethnic groups carry in relatively higher numbers. Indeed, I was struck by the sheer length of the list.[4] Professor Shalem went on to point out that every public-health policy has its own "program" suited to the problems of its own population; in Israel "We are simply tailored to deal with our own problems."

Various scholars who have written about genetic conditions that are common among Jews insist that "There are no 'Jewish' or 'Mediterranean' or 'Black' or 'Chinese' diseases, in a strict definitional sense. Gene frequencies differ among populations and therefore make for varying incidences of diseases in different populations" (Motulsky 1979, 425). For all that, the term "Jewish diseases" was in frequent use among the geneticists I spoke to. Far from being accidental, I believe this choice of words echoes the pivotal position that geneticists, particularly population geneticists, have come to acquire within the Zionist ideological apparatus: geneticists, I suggest, became trapped in Zionist attempts to define the Jews through a distinct biology, and an explicitly eugenic endeavor to heal the Jews of this biology.

Zionism, the political, cultural, and nationalist movement that aspired to restore the Jewish people to a homeland and "normalize" it as a nation among the nations, was concerned with the bodies of the Jews it wished to redeem in two significant ways. First, Zionism rendered Diaspora Jews as ill and aspired to create a breed of physically and mentally healthy "new Jews" (Falk 2006, 28; Weiss 2002). This illness, as the early European Zionists saw it, was acquired through long years of living under denigrating conditions: dark and airless ghettoes, the threat of persecution and occasional massacres, disconnection from land due to the prohibition against Jews' owning and cultivating land, and spending time bent over their rabbinical studies. Returning the Jews to the land and to agricultural work was perceived in the Zionist ideology as a collective healing mechanism.

Emerging almost simultaneously with the international eugenic movement, Zionism had an explicitly eugenic aspect (like the Japanese, European, and other nation-building projects of that time). Zionist leaders, educators, and doctors at the Jewish settlements in Palestine continuously borrowed ideas from the eugenic science of their time as early as the 1920s. Falk (2006) claims that eugenic arguments, including ideas such as the exclusion of Jewish potential immigrants who carried hereditary and other diseases, only gained strength during the 1930s, and eugenic consciousness did not diminish even when the Nazi government in Germany drew the scientific community after it.

Yet while Zionists were determined to cure the Jews, considering the huge diversity of cultural patterns, language, and physical constitutions that Jews of diverse ethnic origin exhibited, it was not at all clear how they could be defined. Religion could have served as a viable category, but Zionist ideology had a rather secular orientation. Zionism therefore became acutely preoccupied with supplying scientific evidence that the multiple communities of Jews to be regrouped in their homeland originated from the ancient Jewish nation that was exiled from its land and scattered throughout the world: proof was to be found in biological aspects that would characterize Jews as a distinct biological entity.

At the end of the nineteenth century, physical anthropologists attempted to identify biological aspects such as facial characteristics and the distribution of blood types as distinct, but toward the 1950s research on the biology of the Jews shifted from physical anthropology to population genetics, and concomitantly from facial characteristics and blood types to distributions of genetic diseases as markers of "Jewish" biology (Falk 2006).

Soon after the constitution of the state of Israel, waves of Jewish immigrants from Western, Eastern, Asiatic, and North African countries, as well as Holocaust survivors, streamed into the new state. The tensions in Zionist ideology grew worse: on the one hand, Jewish immigration was the realization of the dream of "ingathering of the exiles"; on the other hand, "hundreds and thousands of immigrants, many of them ill with diseases that required immediate hospitalization" (Davidovich and Shvarts 2004, 152) posed a health threat to the veteran Jewish population and placed a tremendous challenge on the local health system (Davidovich and Shvarts 2004, 152). The health-care system embarked on a series of preventive measures such as vaccination, along with an intensive project of educating the newcomers on a wide array of matters ranging from maternal–infant care, personal hygiene, posture, etc., while occasionally resorting to intrusive means culminating in sheer enforcement. These practices were of course not just health-oriented, they also aimed to "civilize" the newcomers and introduce them into the modern Zionist value system (c.f. Hirsch 2006). As Davidovitch and Shvarts argue, public-health policies clearly drew on "recommended" hygienic practices that were inherent to Zionist ideology during the early 1920s and the 1930s.

Although concern for prevention of venereal diseases, for vaccinations, and for public hygiene more generally somewhat subsided toward the 1960s (after the public-health policies largely succeeded in getting their message across), genetic diseases did not cease to capture the attention of politicians and health professionals, perhaps because they touched on the projects of both self-definition and self-purification, with which the state was (and still is) obsessed.

Faced with the real-life challenges of the "ingathering of the exiles," politicians and social experts became increasingly frustrated with the prospects of answering the question of "who is a Jew?" and it was hoped that the geneticists could point the way. The latter rose to the challenge, seeing it as an opportunity to contribute to the national effort of validating the "melting pot" ideology, but also as a unique professional opportunity to advance basic questions pertaining to population genetics and dynamics (Falk 2006, 173).

While identifying the unique research opportunities offered by the demographic conditions of Israel, Israeli geneticists rapidly became a leading professional community worldwide in the field of population genetics. Concurrent with their attempts to analyze the distribution of genetic markers in the population to illuminate theories about the distinctiveness of Jewish communities—a project that proved impossible, according to Falk (2006)—they discovered more and more (diverging) genetic markers and became more deeply committed to projects of eliminating genetic "Jewish diseases" in the Israeli population. The geneticists' frequent use of this phrase attests, I think, to their continued engagement in the eugenic and definitional endeavors of Zionism.

As Falk claims, genetics cannot "prove" that all the different Jewish communities stem from one distinct ancient population that was biologically distinct from the nations that surrounded it. Nevertheless, the ongoing efforts in genetic epidemiology have successfully formulated models to explain the clustering of specific diseases in particular communities; certain dynamics have been singled out. One of the ways recessive genetic diseases may spread among a particular population is intermarriage in a relatively small community. Many of these diseases, each of which is common among Jews of different ethnic origin, are currently thought to be connected to the way their observant ancestors lived in relatively segregated communities (in terms of marriage) for long periods (Bonne-Tamir and Adam 1992; Goodman 1979; Goodman and Motulsky 1979). In some communities consanguineous marriage was commonly practiced.

The case of the Jews can serve as an example of how culture interacts with biology. From the perspective of genetic epidemiology, the cultural condition of Jews (including environmental conditions) in the Diaspora seems to have led to the development of bodies with characteristic illnesses. This biocultural evolution of Jewish bodies reflects Lock's concept of "local biologies" (Lock, 1993; 1999), which returns the material body to anthropological consideration: "The biological and the social are co-produced and dialectically reproduced, and the primary site where this engagement takes place is the subjectively experienced, socialized body" (Lock 2001, 484).

Lock urges us to elaborate our analysis of the embodiment of culture by taking the material body into consideration. She reminds us that although the categories of local medical knowledge are indeed historically and culturally constructed, they also "correspond" with and are informed by the material body. Returning to the case of Jewish diseases, we might suggest that through biocultural interactions, Jews have developed specific biologies that exert profound influence on the lived experiences of pregnancy: they allocate pregnant women to the realm of what Rose calls "the asymptomatically or presymptomatically ill—those individuals carrying the markers or polymorphisms of susceptibility who are neither phenomenologically or experientially "sick" or "abnormal" (Rose 2001, 12). Note that in the case of pregnant women this presymptomatic illness is not necessarily even their own, yet as we shall see, it produces powerful anxieties. One should acknowledge that under the "truth regimes" of geneticism, Jewish couples have many more reasons to worry than Japanese couples.

Nevertheless, while "Jewish diseases" dominate the discourse of the geneticists that manage "the plan," my informants—ob-gyns and pregnant women—used this term to a much lesser degree. First, their concerns were with the less definite domain of "congenital abnormalities" (*mumim muladim*) rather than "Jewish diseases." Moreover, concern with fetal disability is broader than what is suggested by "Jewish diseases," as evident even in the health policies designed by "the plan": very soon after issuing the screening tests for Tay-Sachs, the well-known Jewish disease, the planners started promoting screening tests to diagnose various chromosomal conditions such as Down's syndrome, which are not particularly frequent in Jews.

The national biopolitics of reproductive bodies as expressed in policy makers' discourse described so far forms the "nexus of power" for reproductive relations; but the actual relations themselves must be explored for an understanding of the dynamics of Israeli prenatal care. We must look into the ideas that inform actual decision making about prenatal testing in the clinic, and locate the specific kind of dialectical relationship that exists between the material body and the social body.

The ob-gyns whom I describe in this chapter (like the pregnant women who are discussed in part two) do not merely practice according to the rules and regulations laid down by the state, the courts, and the medical community: they are purposeful agents who continuously negotiate and rethink their professional standards of practice among themselves and with their patients. Such negotiations are informed by assumptions about what gestation means physically and socially, and by a range of "affects and ethics" (Rose 2001, 9) or "moral economies" (Daston 1995) that constitute these assumptions and are constituted by them. So here I shift the focus from the national biopolitical nexus of power to the microphysics (cf. Foucault) of reproductive relations between ob-gyns and their patients inside and outside the clinic. Recall that persons with or without diseases are gestated in women's bodies, and that pregnancy is the somatic, experiential, and affective site in which the actual practice and narration of prenatal diagnosis takes place.[5] How is this pregnant body perceived by medical professionals? Who is the pregnant woman? What is she carrying? And how is she expected to feel about her pregnancy? And how is PND understood, communicated, and utilized within such understandings of pregnancy? Is there something "particularly Israeli" in the understanding of pregnancy that facilitates the enthusiastic embrace of PND?

Pregnancy and Its Discontents

I became friendly with Hannah, Dr. Ramon's secretary, during my repeated, month-long attempts to make an appointment with him. Hannah, a young law student who saw her role as blocking all possible intruders, would explain to me that Dr. Ramon was "bombarded" with patients and would not be able to see me that week. "The girls love him, you see"; he was so "cute and charming." Hannah insisted that this was not a joke and that some of the patients were clearly "in love" with him and kept coming back to see him whenever possible. Coincidentally, I ran into Ramon while I was strolling around a noisy and colorful exhibition hall during a pregnancy event the following week. I was standing in front of a sales counter selling workout videos for pregnant women, and a television set behind it was showing one of them. When a young doctor mentioned the importance of physical exercise during pregnancy, I heard one of the pregnant women clustering round the stand say to her friend, "There's Ramon, isn't he adorable?" The video opened with a shot of Ramon sitting in his leather armchair telling the audience, "It is well known to doctors that the births of Spartan women, who used to exercise wrestling and javelin-throwing during their pregnancies, were easier than those of Victorian women, who were only permitted to walk around their beds during pregnancy." Just as I was wondering about how he appeared to be so convinced about this piece of information, Ramon proceeded to invite Israeli women to follow the Spartan women and exercise right until birth. The next morning I told Hannah about my encounter, and asked whether Ramon emphasized physical activity during pregnancy. "Physical activity?" she replied, puzzled. "He does not have time to talk to patients about these things; anyway patients come here for something else. They are *hysterical* in this country, don't you know? They come here because they want to know that everything, everything is perfectly OK."

Ramon's expertise is in obstetrical ultrasound. Hannah had an array of metaphors to describe his superb diagnostic abilities: he was "eagle-eyed," operated like "radar" to spot defects, etc. In subsequent phone conversations Hannah insisted that some of his patients flew in from America and Europe just to be diagnosed by him. Once, she interpreted these special efforts: "Israelis live through wars; we cannot afford to be imperfect." "So that's why he talks about Sparta on the video," I joked, and she laughed. Two weeks later she arranged for me to see Ramon one evening after his office hours. I arrived just on time, only to be told by Hannah that he had had an unexpected emergency. I sat in the empty waiting room and stared at the big picture dominating the wall opposite. It was an advertisement by Aloka, a company that markets ultrasound devices worldwide. The picture featured a "transparent" pregnant belly gently embraced by a feminine arm through which the viewer could see a fetal profile as visualized by a three-dimensional ultrasound. The title said: "Aloka gives birth to perfection." If Aloka (not women) can give birth to the same perfection in any of the locations in which its products are used, why should any Israeli woman fly in to be diagnosed by Dr. Ramon?

Ramon, who became one of my key informants, explained his popularity among pregnant women in terms of his ability to understand their feelings and "what they really want." He often said, "It's hard to be pregnant; it's not an easy experience. An ob-gyn has to understand that." Ramon, like other ob-gyns I interviewed, claimed that Israeli women undergo much more prenatal testing than women anywhere else. Yet while the introduction to this chapter might leave the impression that the state intervenes to screen out inborn abnormalities, the medical practitioners I spoke to insisted that the overwhelming popularity of PND in Israel is due to public demand. More specifically, they often argue that Israeli women are "hysterical," an argument I repeatedly heard throughout the years I have been engaged in this research. The word "hysteria" is often used, by doctors, male partners, and relatives, and sometimes even by women themselves, to signify an anxiety about possible abnormalities in the fetus. Whenever hysteria came up, it was always in the context of undergoing numerous prenatal tests. Rarely was this word used to signify woman's anxieties about their own health.

I was especially surprised to encounter the conceptualization of pregnant women as hysterical one sunny Friday morning as I sat among an audience of five hundred pregnant women and their partners in the large hall of a community center in the course of a pregnancy event. After an hour meandering among stands selling maternity outfits, cosmetics, mineral water, and children's toys, the participants were invited to the first lecture, entitled "ultrasound in pregnancy," by Professor Bloch, the distinguished head of a maternity ward in one of the largest medical centers in Israel. Professor Bloch, aided by an impressive PowerPoint presentation of ultrasound videos, entertained his audience with a series of pictures of fetuses in "funny" positions. As he explained to me later, he wanted to "give the women a good time." Nevertheless he did not hesitate to tell the audience the following joke: "Question: Why do pregnant women have two eyes? Answer: One eye is to observe the ultrasound screen, and the other eye is to look at the doctor to see if everything [the fetus] is OK." I saw women in the audience smile faintly.

Deconstructing the above joke provides an opportunity to examine the image of the "hysterical" pregnant woman as seen through the eyes of an ob-gyn. First, it is implied (jokingly, of course) that women exist for the sole purpose of reproduction. Surprisingly, the evidence for this is not found in the anatomy of women's reproductive organs but in the parts of the body that are common to both sexes, namely, the eyes. (Even) the eyes, the joke tells us, have a different function in women, and are part of the reproductive project (otherwise, the joke implies, if women were not reproducers, one eye would suffice). Secondly, the woman is depicted as an external spectator of her own pregnancy and totally dependent on her authoritative ob-gyn. Most important, this grotesque image is not merely one of an anxious woman who depends on medical "assurance" but the embodiment of fear in a woman's body.

Significantly, the joke conveys "hysteria" in the context of the routine ultra-sound screening of a pregnant woman with no indication of any fetal problem. One more significant thing to bear in mind about "hysteria" is that it is a womanly state. Although pregnant women often visit their ob-gyns accompanied by their male partners, the ob-gyns I spoke to never described the latter as "hysterical."

Thus ob-gyns often understand "hysteria" as an underlying state of mind that might easily take over a pregnant woman or "erupt" at any moment. As Dr. Wolli, a forty-five-year-old prenatal expert at a large government hospital, told me: "Let's say that I am examining a woman and I tell her that maybe there is the tiniest problem [with the fetus]. Then they become completely blocked up [*nistamot*] and don't understand anything. This is an amazing phenomenon. Sometimes I explain [the nature of the fetal problem] for an hour, and without fail the next day I get phone calls: "Doctor, will he [the fetus] be able to live with it?" after I have already explained it for an hour. They simply shut down [*neetamot*] the moment you say there is a problem."

Wolli has an archetypical script that presupposes the existence of fear. His medical diagnosis merely brings out a latent anxiety. The way his account moves from describing how he examines "a woman" to how "they" become blocked up shows how much he sees the dynamics of "shutting up" as general. The Hebrew words he uses suggest a sudden inability to understand: "blocking up" of the head, shutting the eyes so much as to make the skull as a whole opaque (as his choice of the Hebrew root *atum* suggests). Like other ob-gyns I spoke to, Wolli can easily switch into speaking in his patient's own words. This ability to "switch" roles with the patients is evidence of how familiar he feels with the situation he describes.

However, compared with accounts of other ob-gyns, Wolli's account is quite mild. In Professor Bloch's account, patients who had an indication of a fetal problem not only "shut down," they can also "freak out." Bloch, cited above telling the joke, is a member of a special "high committee" dealing with patients' requests for late abortions. His accounts were more dramatic: "You should see how women insist [his voice rising] on late abortions, how they shout, 'bang on the table' and demand that you issue an abortion in the thirtieth week of gestation, and even later, and that you do it immediately, now! [voice rising higher still]. And because of what kind of defects . . . ? A cleft lip? Because some expert drove them crazy telling them that it might be an indication of other abnormalities as well. And they just would not take the chance."

Note the high frequency of verbs that indicate assertiveness to the degree of (barely controlled) rage and even violence. It seems as if "traditional" doctor–patient power relationships are being turned upside down, for in Bloch's account a patient can easily be driven crazy, thus turning into a physically threatening persona.

In the course of my observations I never encountered any of the extreme outbursts of tension that the ob-gyns described in their interviews, yet I could nevertheless feel this tension. In fact, twelve out of the twenty ob-gyns I interviewed were explicit about the strategies they had developed to alleviate this pressure. One very common strategy that I saw used in ultrasound screenings was to talk humorously about the fetus as human. Dr. Kishon, a fifty-year-old ob-gyn who practices privately, told me about an ultrasound screen he performed for a thirty-year-old pregnant patient. The patient, he said, was exceptionally nervous, and kept asking "Doctor, is everything OK? Are you sure everything is OK?" "And then," he told me, "a baby could be heard crying in the waiting room. There," said Kishon to his patient, "he [your fetus] is crying, can you hear?" He told me with a smile of satisfaction that the patient laughed, and explained that "humor is the only way I have discovered to deal with hysterics." There is no easy way to "quantify" the "hysteria" that the ob-gyns talked about. It is hard to tell how many "hysterical women" each ob-gyn has encountered in his or her overall career. Nevertheless, such cases predominated in the experiences of many doctors, and practical lessons were learned from them. The overall impression from doctors' accounts of pregnant women was that "hysteria" is omnipresent in the sphere of pregnancy; the question is only whether it is "latent" or overt.[6]

When I asked practitioners to explain why Israeli patients are "hysterical" they suggested that pregnancy "hysteria" had something to do with the "Jewish mother." One ob-gyn even went so far as to joke about Israeli women being afflicted with a "Jewish genetic disorder" producing hysteria. Such explanations locate the reason for "hysteria" in both women and their "Jewishness." Later I discuss the cultural paradigms of thinking at work in Israeli-Jewish anxieties; in the following sections I suggest that to understand why doctors expect women to become "hysterical" once they become pregnant, it is necessary to understand how they conceive pregnancy.

Pregnancy as a High-Risk Gamble

As medical anthropologists have shown time and again, in biomedicine any bodily process or condition can be understood as potentially pathological. Pregnancy is no exception to this rule. Rose argues that "the binary distinctions of normal and pathological, which were central to earlier biopolitical analyses, are now organized within . . . strategies for the government of risk" (Rose 2001, 7). These strategies, acting at a number of levels, differentiate risk according to groups of age, race, and descent, and culminate in the identification of specific individuals at risk. Rose observes that "demands for collective measures of biopolitical risk management, far from reducing, are proliferating and globalizing" (Rose 2001, 7). I would like to demonstrate a local tendency in the Israeli medical discourse on pregnancy to go beyond the differentiation of risk and instead to generalize the fatalistic notion of an omnipresent, undifferentiated risk. As Dr. Wolli told me: "Once I had a case [where] I discovered a [fetal] heart problem in a twenty-eight-year-old healthy woman. The ob-gyn in charge of the department called me and said, 'Well done [kol hacavod], I would never have discovered such a thing in a low-risk pregnancy.' So I told him, 'I don't know what a "low-risk pregnancy" is: every woman who walks into my clinic has a high-risk pregnancy.'"

The global medical system of categorization, Rose argues, differentiates two categories of pregnancy: "low-risk" and "high-risk." Specifically, the Israeli Association of Obstetrics and Gynecology defines a "low-risk" pregnancy as "a pregnancy with no prior indications (of health complications), in the course of which no findings indicate an increased risk of fetal and/or maternal morbidity or mortality" (Abramovich et al. 2000). Beneath these globalized categories lies the idea that pregnancy is a risky business: what differentiates one pregnancy from another is only the *degree* of risk. But in his above anecdote, Wolli dismisses the relatively positive category of "low-risk" pregnancy altogether: any pregnancy is risky by definition. Moreover, as noted earlier, although the "risk" is mainly to the fetus's health, not the woman's, Wolli talks about the disability found in the fetus as if it were the woman's disability [*matsati la mum balev*: I found *her* a heart problem], a typical way of talking among prenatal experts. Such phrasing reflects an understanding of fetuses with disabilities as afflictions of their mothers.

Understanding any pregnancy as risky, and defining risk to the fetus and regarding fetal disability as an infliction on the mother, I think, underlie doctors' expectation that pregnant women will become "hysterical." "Good" doctors, those whom patients speak of favorably, are those who, given the above definitions, are sympathetic to their patients. I heard Dr. Ramon, so popular among his patients, saying to them such things as, "Relax, I promise I'll tell you immediately if I find anything. You know me, don't you?" I never heard an Israeli ob-gyn giving a woman reassurance in phrases like, "The baby is healthy," which I so often heard Japanese ob-gyns saying. "It is obvious why not," said Ramon in one of our conversations. "You can never really know if the fetus is healthy or not. Honestly, it's not certain even after the baby is born."

I wish to emphasize that the notion of pregnancy as high-risk underlies the management of pregnancy, but it in no way dominates it every single moment. For example, it does not prevent doctors from celebrating pregnancies with their patients, especially when they have been long awaited. Dr. Zaken, sixty-four, a senior ob-gyn who was due to retire as department head when I spoke to him, told me how he celebrated pregnancy with a patient aged thirty-eight who finally conceived spontaneously after two years of undergoing fertility treatments. "I examined her internally, and while pushing the womb a bit higher with my fingers I made her feel her belly." He told me how surprised and happy the patient was to feel a "six-week-old little bulge." However, this did not prevent him from discussing amniocentesis with this patient later. He concluded: "I understood my own daughters, who both underwent amniocentesis at the ages of twenty-four, twenty-five. . . . After all, pregnancy is a gamble and you cannot blame them."

Dr. Zaken depicts a picture of pregnancy as a predetermined game of chance over which the gambler (the pregnant woman) has no influence whatsoever. She can only get rid of an unwanted outcome. Combining the notions of pregnancy and pregnant women as reflected in the above accounts, the image of the "hysterical" pregnant woman gradually becomes comprehensible. From the point of view of prenatal experts she may indeed be grotesquely hysterical, but rightly so. For although some practitioners may speak about her cynically, their narratives reveal their own conceptions of pregnancy as an almost unbearably dangerous gamble. If pregnancy is as dangerous as practitioners feel it is, perhaps pregnant women can never be "hysterical" enough.

Of major importance is that far from being confined strictly to clinical settings, notions of pregnancy as a high-risk gamble are in fact considered entirely legitimate ideas to express in public. The ethnography now moves to explore the medical discourse as heard in public: at pregnancy events. My aim in bringing this piece of ethnography is to illustrate how far notions of reproduction gone awry can go, first and foremost in order to convey a sense of the atmosphere that such ideas generate. Moreover, I wish to account for *how* these notions are actually produced. I chose to focus on pregnancy events precisely because, as public consumer-oriented events that market themselves as "fun" days designed to "indulge" pregnant women, they seem to be removed from notions of reproductive risk. Yet it was an opening lecture given by an ultrasound expert at one such pregnancy event that proved to be an ultrasonic horror picture show.

The Ultrasonic Picture Show

It was a sunny Friday morning in November 2002. After a short walk through the lanes of the medical center, following the signs "To the Pregnant Women's Day," I finally reached the neat plaza of a well-maintained building surrounded by greenery. Since I had come one hour ahead of schedule the plaza was still almost empty, but hospital workers were already setting up a buffet in the hall and the organizers were bustling about the assembly room. There I found Ms. Shein, an elegant woman in her mid-thirties, standing and looking at the huge placard hanging from the ceiling covering the wall behind the lectern. The placard featured the plump face of a blue-eyed baby about eight months old, with the words "To See the Unborn" (*lir'ot et hanolad*) written above the picture in thick black letters. The expression draws on a Mishnaic adage (unrelated to pregnancy): "Who is the wise man? He who sees what is about to be born" (*eizehu haham haroe et hanolad*); this expression idealizes those who engage in predictions of possible developments and plan their future steps accordingly. As I learned later, Ms. Shein worked in the public relations office at the medical center, and was therefore in charge of organizing the pregnancy events for the general public. She defined herself as a feminist: "I organize these pregnancy days for the benefit of pregnant women. I want them to feel good and have a nice morning. But I also think it is most important to see to it that they get correct and up-to-date medical information." Lectures on obstetrical ultrasound play a double role in this venture: Ms. Shein described them as both "fun" and "informative." As she and other organizers of pregnancy events often told me, a "pregnancy day" obviously should include a lecture by an ultrasound specialist.

An hour later the assembly room had filled up with about three hundred pregnant women and about twenty male partners. Ms. Shein warmly invited all the participants to be seated and welcomed them on behalf of the medical staff. Then she introduced the first lecturer: "Undoubtedly, one of the exciting moments in pregnancy is viewing the fetus in ultrasound. Ultrasound screening, which entered wider use during the late 1970s, has changed the face of gynecology and obstetrics and brought about a real revolution. Let me introduce Professor Cohen, who is the head of our ultrasound unit . . . and concurrently heads the disability clinic at our hospital." Observing the women in the audience moving uneasily in their seats, I felt that the idea of pregnancy as exciting quickly subsided when they realized that the "head of the ultrasound unit," who was to give the ultrasound lecture, was also the head of the "disability clinic."

Immediately on taking his place at the lectern, Professor Cohen responded to the introduction by "assuring" the audience that "I will do my best not to show you many disabilities today, only one or two examples; anyway it's unpleasant." "So don't show us any," a woman in the audience called out. Professor Cohen continued:

> We the experts, we the ultrasound people, began observing fetuses in the womb about twenty-five years ago, and with time we learned many things that even our embryology books still don't tell us. The things that we see in the womb are not in the books even today: all kinds of clinical indications and signs that have changed the face of medicine. Ask your ob-gyns what is the most significant thing that has happened generally in gynecology during the last two decades, and undoubtedly they will say, "The first thing that happened is that obstetrical ultrasound came into use." Anyone who worked in birthing rooms twenty years ago knows the huge difference in diagnosing now, in ways that I now wonder how we did it

then. For example, identifying twins during labor using X-ray. I remember an X-ray of twins in the birthing room, and they were identical twins, and not only identical, they were conjoined twins, and during the delivery, it was simply horrible what happened there, how they got out all completely torn apart.

Nowadays you [Professor Cohen used the Hebrew second-person masculine singular pronoun] do ultrasound, you identify it during the first trimester of pregnancy and I will show you the pictures. This is what makes all the difference. Nowadays we are wiser because we can see the unborn.

This proud metanarrative of biotechnological progress (achieved by an expert collective designated "we," so reminiscent of the ethos of progress narratives in Franklin's [1998] accounts of IVF) serves as the starting point for the narration of obstetrical ultrasound. However, I argue that neither progress itself nor its aim can be understood without the notion of reproductive catastrophe. Catastrophe is both the foil against which one is encouraged to measure progress, and the reason why such progress is necessary in the first place. The horrifying example described above of "what can happen in a world without obstetrical ultrasound" (evidence of progress) is only one example of a pattern repeating itself throughout this and other lectures. Another of the professor's examples was how, in the course of an amniocentesis fifteen years before, he had witnessed how "the needle went through the head of the fetus and they evacuated amniotic fluid." To "calm" his audience (while completely disregarding the fact that the latter catastrophe was caused solely by technology itself), he assured them that "Today things like that would never happen since every procedure is conducted "under vision."

I heard Professor Cohen giving this same lecture three times at three different pregnancy events. Particularly striking was his apparent assumption that it is legitimate to tell such horror stories to pregnant women, even though he was fully aware of the terrifying effect they were bound to have. However, that such representations "go public" also suggests that they are based, at least to some degree, on shared understandings by doctors and patients. In fact, it tells us much about how far terrorization can reach undisturbed. Otherwise it is hard to explain why Ms. Shein made sure that Professor Cohen's lecture always came first on the schedule, and why the woman mentioned earlier voiced the only protest I heard against this lecture. At one of the events, technical problems with his laptop prevented Professor Cohen initially from making his PowerPoint presentation work. After a twenty-minute delay, involving continuous attempts to solve the problem and Cohen's rejection of an offer by Professor Navon, the next lecturer, to change places with him until the problem was resolved, Professor Cohen told the audience: "I wanted to speak to you about the most important thing in gynecology and obstetrics. Ultrasound is the nerve center of any maternity department, with twenty-one thousand screenings a year. I don't know how to give a lecture about obstetrical ultrasound without pictures, but I will try. This is a pity though, because I wanted to show you pictures of fetuses masturbating in the womb."

I shall return to the "masturbating fetus" later. At that point one of the people in the audience, the husband of a pregnant woman, offered to help, saying he was a computer technician. Within a few minutes the presentation was up and running and the ultrasonic picture show started. Nobody, neither the audience nor the organizers, was willing to forgo the lecture on obstetrical ultrasound.

Cohen's lectures were also saturated with ultrasound pictures of deformed fetuses that he had integrated into the thematic flow of the lecture. These alternated between pictures of humanlike fetuses doing humanlike things (which were supposed to make the audience laugh) and images of anomalous fetuses. An example is Cohen showing the audience ultrasound pictures of fetal male and female sexual organs, leading to a brief, humorous account of a fetus he had screened masturbating for fifteen seconds. The audience duly laughs; but he then immediately follows this by telling them that this particular fetus died in the twenty-eighth week of gestation because of a heart problem. "Maybe he died from this [masturbation]," adds Professor Cohen, laughing as he proceeds to show a series of pictures of fetuses with deformed sexual organs, discussing each deformation at length. Another example is Cohen pointing out to the audience "how nicely you can see small details like the fingers and the toes," after which he shows pictures of fetuses with six fingers.

Since for each and every "normal" organ he discusses Cohen shows pictures of the same organ deformed (with no indication of how rare they are), the overall impression of the lecture is that a myriad of deformations and abnormalities occur all the time and that each and every organ may be subjected to deformity and abnormality. A partial list of disabilities and fetal deformations discussed in detail and shown on the large screen includes cleft lip, hernia, distorted sexual organs, extra fingers, fetuses with two heads (a form of conjoined twins) and more. It is noteworthy that the visibility of deformed fetuses in Cohen's PowerPoint presentation stands in sharp contrast to the relative absence of people with deformities in the Israeli public sphere (either because the public sphere is largely still physically inaccessible to people with disabilities, in spite of recent attempts to improve access, because their status and rights are still the subject of debate within the legal system, or because a multitude of implicit and explicit symbolic mechanisms enforce their distance from the collective of "the fit").[7]

Returning to Cohen's lecture: along with the numerous deformations and abnormalities the audience also learns about new tests that can be performed to detect them (with the clear implication that abortion of these fetuses is an acceptable solution to the problem). Although some of these tests are irrelevant for many of the women in the audience, who are approaching full term, the expert spares no effort to recommend them "for the next pregnancy." Still, he is sure to warn the audience that undergoing multiple screening throughout gestation can never give the woman and her supporters absolute "assurance." He explains that although for the detection of some abnormalities a first-trimester vaginal ultrasound screening is recommended, the patient must bear in mind that vital organs, like the heart and the brain, have not completely developed, so to detect problems in them, an additional screening in the twentieth week, during the second trimester, is advised. Yet even this cannot provide assurance: "The subject of dwarfism—well, this is something you can miss in earlier screening . . . and even in later scans, because sometimes shortened limbs become apparent only in later weeks, and sometimes they are discovered only when fetal weight estimation is done in the thirtieth week, so take it into consideration."

The audience is made aware of numerous tests offered for their consumption; at the same time, people are told that the apparent limitations of these tests "should be taken into consideration." But the following statement, I think, delivers the knock-out blow to the idea of obstetrical ultrasonography as "assurance." Cohen shows the audience a clear fetal profile and says: "Look how beautifully you can see, you can really see the tongue, those of you who have especially good sight can recognize the lens of the eye. Look how nice. If we can see a lens it says that the fetus has an eye but it does not say that he can see because we can't see the optic nerve."

First, Professor Cohen's fascination is clearly not with fetuses but with the ability of ultrasonic devices to display detailed images of them. Secondly, whereas the narrative of abnormality detection relies on the "panoptic" illusion (cf. Foucault 1977) of ultrasound's enhanced vision, it transpires that not all disabilities are visually observable. The collapse of "assurance" also adulterates the pleasure that might come from seeing even the most "beautiful pictures" that ultrasonography can provide, not to speak of the idea of "psychological benefits" of maternal–fetal bonding discussed by Taylor (1998).

Finally, speaking of "beautiful pictures" such as those shown on three-dimensional ultrasound scans, Cohen says: "Look at these faces; here is a fetus that has laid down his head and has gone to sleep "on" the womb; look at the lips and the nostrils, really very nice pictures. But you should bear in mind that three-dimensional ultrasound is a gimmick, and see it the way it is: it does not always have any additional diagnostic value."

To conclude this example, I suggest that Cohen's lecture illustrates how far the idea of reproductive catastrophe can go in public discourse. His lecture powerfully illustrates a metamessage saying that no assurance can ever be given about a fetus's health and prospects of living; this can be done only well after birth. Women are understood—and are told to understand themselves—as being in the process of carrying a potential fetal catastrophe. In this sense the lecture echoes Professor Bloch's witticism about pregnant women having two eyes. Ultrasound is presented as a diagnostic tool that can help prevent fetal anomalies as one type of catastrophe. Presented under such an overarching metamessage, all alternative interpretations of the images of deformed fetuses are repressed. Deformed fetuses are presented as one category in bulk, with little consideration of categories such as "minor anomalies" and "serious anomalies." Anomalous fetuses are warned against, rather than "nurtured," "cared for," "healed" or "saved." In its potential to generate terror and anxiety, Cohen's lecture parallels *The Silent Scream*. But that video attempts to generate terror to scare women away from abortion; Professor Cohen's ultrasonic picture show is likely to have the opposite effect, namely, to frighten women away from pregnancy.

Significantly, Professor Navon's lecture, focusing on issues of nutrition during pregnancy, was always scheduled after Professor Cohen's. In the three events that I attended at this medical center, Navon opened his lecture thus: "There is a division of roles between me and Professor Cohen: he frightens you a little and then I calm you down. Usually it works well. We are graduates of the Shabak [Israel's General Security Service or secret police]. He "shakes" [a euphemism for the physical violence the Shabak uses when interrogating detainees] and then I come and put things in order. Because he is the one who finds the disabilities and I am the one who maybe is trying to prevent them, he gets his share of problems, but I will try to give you the more optimistic approach."

Using the Shabak euphemism was Navon's way of breaking the tension his predecessor had generated by trying to make the audience laugh, in which he succeeded. His borrowing of metaphors from conflict-saturated life-worlds of physical violence in Israel is one more pattern that I found throughout pregnancy events, particularly when lecturers tried to alleviate tensions, or simply to entertain the audience.[8]

Moreover, Navon was proposing an alternative approach to pregnancy: one less about genetic and chromosomal fatalism (presented by Cohen, his predecessor) and more about women's agency in forging fetal health. Professor Navon focused on the description of a new nutritional supplement, a "cocktail pill" for pregnant women, which he is helping to develop. However, relatively little information was given to the women about how to "take charge" of their health while pregnant by consuming the ideal calorific intake or through balancing different nutrients in a meal.

The order of the lectures by these two medical experts (Cohen's always coming first), together with Navon's cautious way of presenting his professional endeavor as "maybe preventing" fetal disabilities, suggests an implicit hierarchy between the knowledge systems that focus on "nutrition/prevention" and "detection/diagnosis," respectively. This hierarchy is also reflected in the audience's different reactions to the two lectures. The women and their partners sit quietly throughout Cohen's lecture, but once the topic shifts to more preventive issues people tend to pay less attention, whisper, joke, and even leave the room to indulge in the buffet outside. The kinds of foods and drinks offered at such buffets include sweets, fried food, and coffee—precisely the sort of foods that preventive discourses emphasizing nutrition as a factor in fetal health tend to warn against (Markens, Browner, and Press 1997; Root and Browner 2001). While Navon enthusiastically urges the women to "contribute to the future health of the fetus by taking care of your diets now," coffee is being served to the women in the hallway and consumed by them uninterruptedly.

Of course, the disabled fetus is not the only fetal image present in the public sphere. The image of what I call the quasipersonified fetus—one that at first might seem quite similar to the one reported by scholars working in America—is found in the public discourse about ultrasound. Except that the meaning of this image takes different directions. This brings us back to the notion of the "gimmick" that Cohen and other ob-gyns I interviewed used during ultrasound scans when they referred to doctors' strategies of small talk about the fetus in terms of a human subject. For example, at a lecture given on 14 July 2003 on a pregnancy day at a medical center in the south of Israel, Dr. Gil showed his audience a series of ultrasound pictures of fetuses in different positions and gave them "humanizing" titles. One fetus holding her fist against her face he called "the boxer," another, who was sucking his thumb, was presented as the "sucker," and another, captured moving his hands and legs as if driving a car, was called "the driver"; Dr. Gil also showed a picture of a fetus making the gesture of "the finger," as well as twin fetuses kicking each other's heads while "playing soccer." Toward the end of his presentation, however, he told the audience about a pair of twins whose ultrasound picture showed how their umbilical cords had become tightly wound around each other in the womb. He said that these twins had been saved due to this prognosis, and the recommendation to deliver them by cesarean section; then he showed the wound umbilical cords just after birth. This presentation is an example of a more lighthearted sort of discourse on obstetrical ultrasound. Yet even this relatively optimistic presentation included at least some examples of possible reproductive catastrophe preempted by technology. When Dr. Gil finished his presentation and the next lecturer was being announced, I overheard the couple sitting next to me saying to each other, "What bullshit!" Having seen them earlier out of the corner of my eye intimately hugging, and the husband massaging his wife and stroking her belly throughout the talk, I had expected them to enjoy it: this couple looked as if they were "connected" or "bonded" to each other and to the unborn baby in a way that reminded me of the idealized American discourse of maternal–fetal bonding described in Taylor's work. However, as they told me later, both husband and wife thought that this "baby talk" before birth is totally out of place. Is he trying to make idiots of us?" asked the husband.

This couple's response to Dr. Gil's attempt to "humanize the fetus" echoed the insistence of my ob-gyn informants that, as a forty-six-year-old ultrasound expert I call Dr. Shalev said, "There is a mutual understanding between the patients and the doctors that this blah blah of 'Hey look, the baby's waving good-bye to you' is a joke. Both parties know what ultrasound is for." As Alan Dundes reminds us "people joke about only what is most serious" (Dundes 1987, viii).

Playing with Subjectivity

Ultrasound picture shows illustrate how far notions of reproduction gone awry can go uninterruptedly in the Israeli public sphere or in other words: how far the terrorization of pregnant women can reach. They also clearly show, that ultrasonography in Israel has not become engaged in anything similar to the "social project" through which "fetal subjects" are "discursively created and politically deployed" (Kaufman and Morgan 2005, 329). Fetal images have become entangled in what I have come to recognize as a "politics of threatened life": where "life" stands typically for the pregnant woman and "threat" for the fetus. Thus, ultrasound picture shows can be read as instances of the politics of threatened life at work (Ivry 2009b). To fully understand the power and impli-cations of this politics, first it is necessary to analyze *how* it works: and ultra-sonic shows provide a particularly condensed case to examine. To begin with, the messages of ultrasound picture shows are grounded in a general conviction about the importance of ultrasonography and a deep fascination with its prod-ucts. Ultrasonography embodies progress (cf. Sarah Franklin 1998), the offer of which can hardly be refused. As the large placard implied, wise people cannot turn down the offer of technology; they cannot afford *not* to see the unborn (through ultrasonography, which was introduced to the audience as "the most important thing that has happened in obstetrics and gynecology").

This message is reinforced, I think, by the ultrasonic shows generating a notion of nature as bound to make serious mistakes. True, doctors are often careful to warn patients about the limitations of ultrasonographic diagnosis, but their warnings are formulated in terms of the limits set by nature on tech-nology (the heart has not developed fully), and much less in terms of the limits of the technology itself, or of the professionals who practice it. Doctors were seldom reflective about their own role in the interpretation of fetal images, so that the possibility of a diagnostic mistake was more or less dismissed. If only women submitted to the panoptic gaze throughout their pregnancy often enough and long enough, any fetal anomaly (should one exist, and on condition that it was observable: "We can't see the optic nerve") would be discovered sooner or later.

The general assumption that major anomalies can be diagnosed through ultrasound holds fast: when on 27 September 2005 a pair of conjoined twins connected at the chest and heart were born to an ultra-orthodox couple, the hospital spokesman declared that as far as they knew, the mother had not had prenatal checkups, and the birth of conjoined twins was a total surprise to the medical team. The first wave of responses in the public media blamed the parents for their misfortune, assuming that they refused diagnostic tests on religious grounds. These assumptions were soon refuted when the parents responded that they had undergone three ultrasound scans, none of which revealed the problem. This story reflects how the possibility that a severe condition could escape the panoptic gaze of ultrasound was inconceivable for medical professionals and media interpreters. Thus, women's testimony about their ordeal as they decide to keep a pregnancy that medical professionals diagnosed as anomalous, only to find out postpartum that the baby is healthy, receives negligible coverage in the Israeli media (which otherwise highlight the horror scenarios) and remains confined to anti-abortion materials, whose public visibility is limited in Israel.

Ultrasonic shows are fully explicit about the diagnostic purposes of fetal ultrasonography, in sharp contrast to Janelle S. Taylor's accounts of the rhetoric that situates ultrasonography as a technology to "reassure" fetal health, prevalent in American clinical settings (Taylor 1998). Here, the deformed fetus, as well as other scenarios of reproduction gone awry, are made very explicit.

Significantly fetuses are represented as separate from their mothers and carry the authority of visual knowledge in the same way that Taylor (1992) and Petchesky-Pollack (1987) pointed out for their American counterparts. However, this authority is used to convey different meanings: rather than a personified fetus entitled to fetal rights, Israeli professionals tend to *play* with subjectivity, sometimes even cynically. The signification of fetal images becomes unstable: even if in a fleeting instant they appear human, they might collapse into deformation or a joke. The image of the deformed fetus is often narrated as if it were the embodiment of reproductive catastrophe—just the thing technology promises to prevent happening. Rather than "endangered childhood in need of protection" the fetus comes to represent danger itself, the one that women and ultimately society should defend themselves against.

In the Israeli medical discourse, worst-case scenarios loom notably large. But the catastrophic impression of these scenarios depends on a strategy that leaves little, if any, space to alternative interpretations of how the fetal images could be read. The absorbing PowerPoint presentations flashing images in rapid succession leaves little space for contemplating either the meaning of the deformed fetal images or the very choice of the images themselves: the rarest of all images that professionals encounter in their daily practice receive a degree of visibility disproportionate to their rate of occurrence. Ultrasonogaphy, in our case, uses the authority of visual knowledge to give shape and magnitude to a vague category of "disability" in a way that mutes its diversity and social circumstances.

Thus while the representation of the American fetus as separate helps anti-abortionists in their attempt to adorn it with individual rights, the Israeli version of fetal imaging reminds us that in a different socio-cultural setting separateness can also open up the distance required to keep it a potential candidate for abortion.

As a concise conceptualization of how ultrasonic shows work, I suggest that they *illustrate* a meaningful social script of reproductive misfortune. The ultrasonic shows described here distance fetal images either through humor or through overrepresenting deformed fetuses; they mute considerations of the diversity of disability and contemplation of its meaning; they explain the need for prenatal diagnosis; and most importantly, they frighten, and perpetuate anxiety—an effect powerfully reflected in the accounts of my women informants analyzed in chapter four. Israeli uses of fetal images remind one that they can lend themselves equally to a wide range of social projects, widely deviating from the deployment of "fetal subjects." Later I suggest that they draw their power from ideas, practices, and experiences that go beyond biotechnology. At this stage of analysis, however, let me go back to the clinic to account for how, with such powerful ideas in mind, doctors negotiate with their patients and colleagues the actual practicable standards of prenatal diagnosis.

Negotiating the Guidelines

Soon after the Yarkonis sued their ob-gyn for not discussing with them the possibility of privately paid screening in the course of a pregnancy that met the definition of "low-risk," the Israeli Association of Obstetrics and Gynecology (IAOG) conferred in order to lay down a "unified basis for relating to medical issues in obstetrics and gynecology," as the committee wrote in an introductory paper (Abramovich et al. 2000). After much debate the IAOG published a series of papers that specify regulations and standards of practice for a range of medically managed situations such as birth, monitoring low-risk pregnancy, monitoring high-risk pregnancy, etc. Nevertheless, fifteen of the doctors who spoke to me were dissatisfied with the standards and seemed to be continuously rethinking and revising their personal practical standards. I shall use the question of amniocentesis in a "low-risk" pregnancy as one example of this process of rethinking.

Amniocentesis is not on the IAOG list of tests administered routinely in a "low-risk" pregnancy. However, according to these guidelines, all women under thirty-five with "low-risk" pregnancies should be referred for the triple marker, "whose results will be the grounds to decide whether to perform a kariotype"

(Abramovich et al. 2000). The woman will be recommended to undergo amniocentesis only if the triple marker results are below 1:380 (meaning that one in 380 women who had the same result will be diagnosed as carrying a fetus with a disability), in which case the test is subsidized by the health fund. In fact, amniocentesis is recommended and performed on women under thirty-five with no prior indications from the triple marker test.

All twenty ob-gyns I interviewed said that with women over thirty-five there is no question about urging them to undergo amniocentesis: as Dr. Salomon, forty-five, an ob-gyn, told me, "In such cases I merely follow the regulations." This stands in sharp contrast to the Japanese ob-gyns, for whom it was hard to decide whether to discuss amniocentesis with women *over* thirty-five, even though they, too, were required to do it by the regulations laid down by the Japanese Society of Obstetrics and Gynecology. For Israeli practitioners the unresolved question seemed to be whether to offer amniocentesis to women *under* thirty-five with no prior indications from triple marker results.

Dr. Shalev, fifty-five, an ob-gyn who practices in a government hospital, as well as in his own private clinic, said that he felt obliged to raise the subject of amniocentesis "delicately and in a strictly informative way. I never tell a patient: 'You have to undergo amniocentesis' or 'You have to terminate the pregnancy.' I explain to her the risks and the chances, I tell her that there is such and such rate of miscarriage following amniocentesis; she should go home and decide with her partner."

I present his statement here because I heard it so many times from a large number of younger and older ob-gyns working in different medical institutions. Here Shalev is trying to convey a sense of the "pure," "value-free," and "emotion-free" style he has of raising the issue of amniocentesis with patients.

However, four out of the twenty doctors I interviewed (two of whom work in central Israel and two in the north) felt strongly that amniocentesis should be recommended to all pregnant women. Three of them emphasized that although the triple marker gives quite good indications, it has a rate of false negative results that cannot be ignored. This means that some of the women whose triple marker results indicate a low probability of their carrying a fetus with a disability will nevertheless be carrying one. Generally the ob-gyns I spoke to tended to refuse to deal head-on with ethical considerations that surround the test itself and the postdiagnostic abortion it implies. Dr. Melamed maintained: "A woman has the right to consider, at a relatively early stage of the pregnancy, if she is willing to get herself involved in such situation (of raising a child with a disability). This is a philosophical question, an ethical question, but we will not get into it now. She is the one who will live with it; she has to decide."

As Rapp (1999) and Rothman (1986) both indicate, here is an instance of pushing women to the frontiers of difficult reproductive decisions while using the language of reproductive rights. The underlying assumption in Melamed's narrative is that it is mainly women who are responsible for raising their children; although they cannot "prevent" chromosomal and genetic abnormalities in their children, they are the ones who are obliged to decide whether they wish such children to be born, with the implication that if they do decide to bear a child with a disability it is "their" problem. Dr. Lahover, fifty-six, an ob-gyn, did not mention the triple test, nor did he mention any ethical problem, while fervently maintaining the idea that amniocentesis is an issue of money versus peace of mind.

> For example, on the issue of amniocentesis, I offer it to every woman of any age. I explain to her, of course, that there is a risk of miscarriage, etc. But I offer it at any age. This is obviously a matter of the financial situation. It's obvious. Until twelve years ago they would perform amniocentesis on women over thirty-seven, and then the Health Ministry lowered the age to thirty-five. In the U.S. in most states it is thirty-two. It is a financial matter. I explain to people that it is an economic issue. If a woman is prepared to have the test performed by a doctor who is paid privately, that, in my opinion, would give her the greatest assurance that the fetus is healthy. For some thousand shekels she can have peace of mind, she can sleep peacefully. And of course, you see we discovered problems in low-risk groups, problems [because of which] we had to terminate pregnancies.

Lahover rejects the categorization of pregnancies by age groups (pretty much in the same spirit that Dr. Wolli rejects the categorization of pregnancies as "high-risk–low-risk"). Whereas offering amniocentesis to women over thirty-five seems to be a universal trait in most postindustrial Western countries, what I call into question here is the extension of this offer to all pregnant women and the reduction of the decision on whether to have amniocentesis to pure economics.

Such narratives silence a long list of issues that surface once amniocentesis is mentioned to patients: first, that a medical procedure is being performed on a woman's body, and that patients express their fears of painful invasive medical intervention. Similarly, the possibility that the fetus might be hurt by the needle that is inserted into the pregnant woman's belly—an anxiety that patients voice—is again absent from consideration. Moreover, for women under thirty-five the chances of losing a healthy child due to amniocentesis are statistically higher than the chances of detecting any abnormality in the fetus. Precisely here, as I shall suggest later, cultural perceptions of pregnancy take over, while doctors ignore the "universal and objective" system of medical knowledge in which clinical considerations present themselves as being grounded. The silence about "rates and risks" in relation to younger women reflects an order of priority in Israel in which life with a disability is more frightening than death. Finally, ob-gyns never mentioned to patients that two women have died in the past five years from infections caused by amniocentesis. Instead, Lahover mentions the rare cases of fetuses with abnormalities that were detected in women under thirty-five. This line of narration calls for a further problematization of the medical understanding and use of statistical data (a point I return to in the final discussion).

In contrast to how practitioners often dismiss the "economics issue," journalists in daily newspapers tend to emphasize the sizable financial profit that prenatal experts make from enacting an "industry of anxieties" (Kotets-Bar 2002). Without doubt, PND is good business in Israel, as attested by the sums noted above in the introduction to this chapter.

Nevertheless, my impression is that the ob-gyns I spoke to were seriously engaged in an attempt to provide their patients with "the best medical care possible." In other words, I argue that the silences in Dr. Lahover's narratives are not professional conspiracies against women but the medical implications of wider public awareness. Actually, like many of his colleagues, he takes health ministry recommendations and professional guidelines as minimal standards. Dr. Wolli, who was quoted above dismissing the category of "low-risk pregnancy," said explicitly that his position on amniocentesis for women under thirty-five simply stems from his positioning himself on his patients' side, which he understands to be almost opposed to the interests of the state of Israel (which has fixed thirty-five as the formal threshold): "I do not calculate the financial implications for the state of Israel. I am trying to give you the best care. The fact that you came to my private clinic means that you are telling me that you want the best. So who looks for such problems in a low-risk pregnancy? I don't know any low-risk pregnancy.... My attitude is not cost effective." Note how "best treatment" translates into maximization of the notion of risk.

In the same spirit, Dr. Reuven, forty-nine, an ob-gyn, said: "The health funds and the health ministry provide all the things that are written in the IAOG papers only because the public has twisted their arms. As it is we do more [testing] than they do in other places in the world, but it is still not enough."

So Reuven sees the structure of prenatal care in Israel, far from being enforced by governmental interests, as forcibly imposed on care providers by the Israeli public. His perspective inverts the traditional notion of power relations among state, medical-care providers and patients, rendering the last the most potent agents that forge pregnancy care. The range of negotiations accounted for here suggests that the diagnostic technologies did not "create" a new tension around gestation (cf. Laqueur 2000), but rehearse and exacerbate a preexisting fatalism surrounding it. This might explain why the existence of formal standards of practice did not satisfy the ob-gyns I spoke to. As

Dr. Lahover concluded, "Age thirty-five is not sacrosanct, and the health ministry regulations are not the word of God."

Envisioning the Worst

Whereas the accounts thus far have described the negotiations of PND in cases where no medical indication of any fetal problem exists, now we may consider briefly how practitioners deal with cases where a specific fetal health problem is indeed suspected or detected. I am particularly interested in the emotions that arise in ob-gyns when practicing, and in the emotions that they try to elicit from their patients.

A common concern of most of the ob-gyns I spoke to was how to make sure that the patients *deeply* understand *all* aspects of the suspected fetal health problem and their implications for their lives as parents of an anomalous child. Common to the explanation techniques is their attempt to make the disability and its consequences as "tangible" and as "realistic" as possible.

One practitioner told me how he sends women to visit institutions for handicapped children to see older children with the disability with which their fetus was diagnosed. Another said that when she senses a difficulty in decision making, namely, to have an abortion or not, she invites a pediatrician and together they explain to the couple the consequences of bringing up a child with the specific disability diagnosed in their fetus. In 2002 one of the general hospitals in central Israel, headed by Professor Cohen cited above, initiated a "disability clinic" where soon after a "suspect" diagnosis is made a couple are invited to consult a battery of professionals. These include a genetic counselor, a pediatrician, a neurologist, and others, depending on the disability. The attempt to illustrate the emotional "cost" of bearing an abnormal child peaks in a technique developed by Professor Gilad, fifty-four, an ob-gyn, which is supposed to help women "quantify" the consequences of doing so.

I heard Professor Gilad deliver a lecture before the ob-gyns of a maternity ward at a departmental colloquium at a large teaching hospital in the south of Israel in January 2000. The somewhat provocative title of his talk was "Is liberal amniocentesis justified?" The question Gilad raised was whether amniocentesis should be offered to all women free of charge without the precondition of the screening test. Gilad gave his colleagues a broad introduction, enumerating and explaining medical, statistical, and economic considerations, and comparing Israeli standards with medical practice in countries such as Britain and the United States. Toward the end of his lecture he told the audience that up to this point he had set forth the problem from the financial perspective of the state and the makers of health policy; now he would approach the problem from the "patient's viewpoint." He then expounded a "linear-analog scale of grief" which he had constructed. He told the audience how he presented the scale to his patients and asked them to estimate the potential grief of raising a child with a disability as against the grief of abortion. Gilad asserted that his initial data showed that women expected the grief caused by pregnancy termination following the diagnosis of fetal abnormality to be greater than the grief experienced during a lifetime of raising a defective child (regardless of the anomaly diagnosed). Again, Gilad's scale does not include the possibility of losing a healthy child in the process of diagnosis. He concluded from his data that for the state and the Ministry of Health, subsidizing amniocentesis for all pregnant women would indeed be inefficient and economically counterproductive, but for the patient a "mandatory" amniocentesis was absolutely justified.

As soon as Professor Gilad finished speaking, Dr. Schwartz enthusiastically stepped in to "validate" his analysis and conclusions: "A few years ago I treated a twenty-seven-year-old patient in her first pregnancy. She wanted to undergo amniocentesis. She was a young woman, everything was OK. [I asked her,] 'Why do you want to undergo this test?' She said: 'Listen, doctor, if I have a miscarriage [due to amniocentesis] I'll be angry with you, maybe I'll sue you and think that you were no good, but after a year this will pass. I'm young, I'll conceive again and I'll bear a healthy child. But if, say, even one in a million, that a Down's [baby] were born, my life would be over . . . ' She had a Down's baby."

A rare case like this thereby becomes an iconic story to explain a particular style of medical practice. This is because the story fits neatly into the scheme of catastrophe: the least expected worst-case scenario coming true. And it has a happy ending: the patient was cautious enough to expect the worst and prevented it from happening. So there is a moral: always be cautious, even when the chances involved are no more than scares. Two assumptions at the heart of this story "smooth" the liberal use of amniocentesis that is implied here: first, parenting a child with Down's syndrome means the end of the parents' own lives; second, women, being natural reproducers, may easily abort and conceive again. I suggest that this apparent facility with conceptions and abortions echoes a particular kind of pro-natalism: one that is torn between concerns about the number and "quality" of children born, and almost complete disregard of the consequences of these tensions for women. In any case, the ease with which conceptions and abortions seem to be accepted may make invasive testing even more appealing to younger women.

After Schwartz had told his story, the ob-gyns around the table began to whisper and debate among themselves the issue of liberal amniocentesis. My neighbor, a young intern, murmured that Schwartz was the doctor who had "killed a patient with his amniocentesis, so he is telling these stories to justify himself." His neighbor answered that even so, one could easily imagine this story happening in reality. The department head dismissed his colleagues and thanked Dr. Gilad for an "interesting and brave lecture." With such iconic stories in mind, how do ob-gyns understand patients who refuse to undergo PND?

Challenges to the Tyranny of PND

The way many ob-gyns reacted when asked about patients who refuse PND partly (or wholly) often impressed me with its intensity. Dr. Levi's response is one example of such emotional intensity. Since at present his daily encounters are mainly with secular women, who (like himself) regard PND as almost mandatory, he went back to his experience as an intern in Toronto for examples: "When I was working in a hospital in Toronto, I used to see women there, every second or third woman in the waiting room, with some kind of defect[ive child]. Things you do not see here. I was shocked. You perform an ultrasonic screening, and you tell her that the head of the fetus is filled with water. So she tells you, 'But there is a 20 percent chance that he will not be retarded.' 'But there is an 80 percent chance that he *will* be retarded [voice rising].' No! I get mad with that. Maybe I am fucked up but I don't see what is so happy about having a child with cerebral palsy. I personally could never mentally cope with such a child."

The emotions reflected in Levi's expressions are powerful. He would expect a woman in this case to become (legitimately) "hysterical," seek a second opinion, and eventually terminate the pregnancy. Women who "take chances," he told me, create an immense fury in him. Even when the patient tries to speak "his language," he cannot tolerate her alternative interpretations of the statistics he confronts her with. Later, Levi told me about his service in public hospitals in Israel, where the patients who refused PND were mainly ultra-orthodox Jews (a pattern clearly evident in the studies of Sher et al. [2003] and Remennick [2006], as well as findings from further research by Elly Teman and myself).

Although Levi claimed to have understood their refusal as rooted in religious belief, he would still hassle them.[9] He told me how, over the years, he had acquired "self-control" and learned how to "accept patients who act in a way I would not have acted." However, the concept of "self-control" emphasizes the degree to which he experiences his feelings as initially difficult to control. This intensity is directly connected to his inability to understand such patients. If women who make excessive use of PND are designated "hysterical," into which category may women who refuse it fall?

Dr. Zaken, who has worked as an ob-gyn for the last thirty-five years, told me: "If I explain to a woman over thirty-five about amniocentesis and she does not take it seriously, and then from nonsense, from sheer neglect, all kinds of *things* are born that could really be prevented, that is frustrating" (emphasis added).

Zaken sees the reasons for refusal as stemming from a lack of seriousness and neglect. Interestingly he refers to disabled fetuses as "things" rather than "children with disabilities." Rather than ultra-orthodox patients, he told me, he concentrates on women from "low socio-economic backgrounds who lack the tools to make such judgments."[10] As a senior doctor, he remembers the days before PND gained its present popularity, when more children with chromosomal and genetic abnormalities were born, and when parents often refused to take children with abnormalities home.[11] His recent experience shows that "nonserious" patients tend to return at later stages of gestation and ask for late abortions. He concluded that it is better to prevent such scenes "before the fetus is separate and has acquired the status of a person: then you cannot touch it." When I asked when the fetus becomes separate, Zaken replied that this only happens after s/he is born.

Dr. Kahn added more categories in which patients who refuse PND can be placed. When I asked him how he felt when a woman comes to give birth with an incomplete pregnancy-monitoring file (a situation I chanced to witness twice), he said: "I count to ten . . . what can I tell her? That she's dumb? Sometimes I say that it is irresponsible not to use what the twenty-first century has to offer."

Like Dr. Levi, discussed above, Dr. Kahn exercises "self-control," which reflects the depth of his resentment at patients who refuse PND. He recognizes two categories; the second of these (one where he can afford to be explicit to the woman) is "irresponsibility." In his narrative, responsibility is not defined in respect to the unborn child but to the degree of "compliance" with the new, progressive "offer." Actually, in Kahn's narrative there is no realistic choice but to accept the "offer."[12] The first category of "dumb" is simply a reference to the implicit idea that a woman must lack intelligence if she refuses testing. In this context, I understand the need to "count to ten" as reflecting a deeply felt urge to express anger at the patient's stupidity. When Kahn resorted to specific examples, he only mentioned ultra-orthodox patients (which testifies to how rare refusals are from secular patients). The fact that their refusal stems from religious beliefs did not "exempt" them from his contempt. He explained to me that ultra-orthodox parents who raise abnormal children face even greater difficulties than their (rare) secular counterparts, as the mere existence of such a child in a family limits the choice of marital partners for any of its children who are healthy.[13]

Dr. Ravel, a religious person himself, told me that even with the ultra-orthodox, he does not give up easily if he thinks that amniocentesis is absolutely necessary. He keeps a list of rabbis to whom he refers religious couples according to their religious affiliation. That practitioners expected ultra-orthodox patients to refuse PND, but seemed not to feel any less angry over their refusal, might have something to do with the implied message that they read into such refusals. As Dr. Harel told me: "Their [ultra-orthodox patients'] doctor is the rabbi, not me, and sometimes that brings me to my wit's end. . . . You see, the doctor is the executing arm of the rabbi. She will do as I say, not because I said it but because the rabbi happened to think like me. This is infuriating."

The above narrative is less concerned with the consequences of PND refusal for the lives of mothers and abnormal infants and more with the preservation of power relations that are based on the superiority of medical knowledge to other forms of knowledge. Infuriating for Harel here is the threat to the hegemony of medical expertise.

Who Is "Entitled" to Refuse?

Under very specific circumstances ob-gyns become tolerant of unconventional decisions. As Dr. Nave stated of his patient: "She is entitled to make a decision but this should be a wise, intelligent [*nevona*] decision. . . . I mean on the basis of deep reflection [*shikul da'at*]. If a woman, let's say, went through IVF and she is thirty-six, and she tells me—and she thinks that one out of two hundred amniocenteses results in a miscarriage, and there have been two cases of death following the tests . . . You know, so she has reached the conclusion; her decision is such that she is prepared to take the risk. This is legitimate, this is OK."

Nave considered the case of "a precious pregnancy," one achieved through assisted conception technologies and/or after a long period of failing to conceive. A woman who carries a precious pregnancy is entitled to resist amniocentesis, provided that she proves her intelligence. But this merely emphasizes the "disposable" nature of naturally conceived pregnancies. Only in the context of a "legitimate" unconventional decision does the threat to the life of the woman herself arise as a fact to be considered. As another practitioner commented, "Of course nobody tells you that [women have died following amniocentesis], because people will not undergo amniocentesis. No one can afford to spare the life of the woman." Note also that for the decision to be considered legitimate the woman (not the couple) who makes it has to take the risk *upon herself*, which implies exempting society from the consequences that such a decision might bear: it is her own business.

Dr. Levi, whose intense emotional resentment at anomalous children was quoted above, gave me another example of the "legitimate" refusal of a patient of his, who practiced in Holland as a doctor and was forty-four at her first pregnancy: "She did her pregnancy monitoring at my clinic and she did not want to undergo amniocentesis. She would say to me, 'So what if a mongoloid is born?' I told her, 'What do you mean, "So what?"' So she says, 'I come from a culture where they treat mongoloids very nicely. Mongoloids are nice people, aren't they? They give love and affection, they are not delinquents, and I don't have to worry about what will happen to them after I die. So what? Do I need a perfect blond child who will leave home at the age of seventeen to get into drugs, delinquency and crime?' This is the reality that she knows, you see. I can understand that."

Here is an obviously intelligent person, a doctor, behaving unconventionally and able to give a self-confident explanation for it. Under these circumstances Levi, who was shocked to see women with disabled children in his Toronto waiting room, is able to understand. Interestingly, while the patient quoted earlier, who was "merely" intelligent, had to "back up" her decision by citing rates of miscarriage versus her scant chances of conceiving again, a pregnant medical doctor is "free" to challenge the widespread perception about people with Down's syndrome (in this particular case) by reminding Levi of such people's merits; she challenges the very notion of "risk." Moreover, she points out the vital significance of the cultural context of disabilities. However, Levi fends off the argument by "othering" the cultural context, thus exempting himself from the challenge it poses to his own perceptions of children with Down's syndrome.

The archetypical images of pregnant patients presented thus far contextualize each other. At one pole stands the "hysterical" woman who is "overinformed." At the opposite pole stands the image of the lightweight, irresponsible, negligent, even stupid patient, who is not equipped to make proper judgments. Whereas both images are conceptualized in negative terms—juxtaposing the "hysterical woman" with her opposite image suggests that since she *is* responsible, serious, can visualize worst-case scenarios, and is equipped to make judgments—she is the preferred patient after all. Although she might become obsessively preoccupied with PND, the reality of her obsessions reaffirms the hegemony of medical knowledge. The notion of pregnancy as a high-risk gamble correlates with a specific microphysical surveillance focusing on the fetus, but it also correlates with a specific "emotional posture" in the pregnant woman, namely, "hysteria." Yet while ob-gyns often perceive "hysteria" as preceding their style of care provision, a state of mind to which they merely respond, the analysis above suggests that they play a substantial role in reproducing and exacerbating women's anxieties, first and foremost through their powerful illustrations of scripts of reproduction gone awry, embossed with their stamp of authority. Bear in mind, however, that such ideas and practices follow "logically" from the fatalistic model of gestation.

Liberalizing Weight Gain

So far, the embodied aspects of pregnancy that have been discussed and visualized are only those of the fetus: the pregnant body itself is missing. As I mentioned above, my observations show that the issues of nutrition and physical activity are relatively deemphasized in prenatal medical routines in Israel, although routine weighing is included in the IAOG's regulations for the management of high-risk pregnancy. This might not always have been the case. Two senior ob-gyns said that when they graduated from medical school about thirty years before, routine weighing was a required part of prenatal care. According to these practitioners, weighing was emphasized especially at community health centers [*tipot halav*], where nurses, not doctors, were the main health-care providers. These nurses, they claimed, conducted more systematic weight-gain monitoring and advised on nutrition. However, according to

Schenker and Elchalal the number of women undergoing prenatal care in such community health-care centers is rapidly decreasing, and there is a tendency among pregnant women of all socio-economic strata to undergo prenatal care at ob-gyns' private clinics or at the clinics of health funds (Schenker and Elchalal 1998, 94). What has happened to the supervision of weight gain and nutrition?

The last seven editions of *Williams Obstetrics*, a well-known textbook taught worldwide, discuss at some length the contribution of a list of nutrients to the formation and development of the fetus in a chapter entitled "Antepartum: Management of Normal Pregnancy" (see, for example, Cunningham and Whitridge 1997, 233–240). It goes into great detail about which nutrients a pregnant woman should consume while pregnant and how much in each case. It then proceeds to cover a range of issues under the title General Hygiene: exercise, travel, bathing, clothing, and care of teeth are a few examples (Cunningham and Whitridge 1997, 240–244). It also treats the issue of weight gain during pregnancy, citing a wealth of medical literature that connects excessive weight gain with birth complications that culminate in an increased rate of cesarean sections and various pregnancy complications (Cunningham and Whitridge 1997, 233–235). The American prenatal education classes described by Markens et al. (1997) seem consistently to follow the approach suggested in the textbook and in the National Health recommendations. The American best-selling pregnancy guide, *What to Expect When You Are Expecting*, is accompanied by a pregnancy cookbook, written and edited by medical practitioners. As we shall see later, Japanese practitioners are even more concerned than their American counterparts with the dimensions of the pregnant body and have at hand ideal weight thresholds and calculations of ideal nutritional intake.

By contrast, in a Hebrew textbook edited by Schenker and Elchalal (1998) nutrition and weight gain are treated briefly, and I found no reference to issues such as "clothing" or "care of teeth" (Schenker and Elchalal 1998, 89–90). Similarly, unlike their Japanese and American counterparts, Israeli ob-gyns I interviewed and observed paid relatively little attention to weight-gain monitoring or guiding pregnant women with "low-risk" pregnancies to healthier diets. Nor did they ensure that paramedical health-care providers took up this role. When I raised the issue of weight gain, many practitioners often said that they did not deal with it. Even when the nurse weighed the woman regularly and recorded her weight on each visit, they rarely spoke to the woman about her weight. What characterizes Israeli ob-gyns' accounts of monitoring weight gain and nutrition is their criticism of the practice and reluctance to carry it out. For example, Dr. Heller, thirty-nine, an ob-gyn, said, "I don't weigh women; it gives me no additional information whatsoever." When I tried to understand specifically what kind of "additional information" he had in mind, he said: "It will not tell me the relationship between the size of the fetus and the volume of amniotic fluid, whether the fetus is developing and growing. And this is really what I would like to know."

Dr. Heller is focused on the well-being of the fetus. The implications of weight-gain patterns for the woman's quality of life, as well as for problems that may arise in the process of giving birth, were not an immediate concern for him in a "low-risk" pregnancy. Later I shall suggest that this focus cannot fully explain the irrelevance of the pregnant woman's body. Rather, a cultural theory of fetal development that excludes the mother's "somatic responsibility" may account for such irrelevance.

Whereas Heller dismisses the need to weigh women, other ob-gyns criticize the imprecise nature of weight measurements. Dr. Levi's statement is an example: "Some of my colleagues, and myself, never weigh the patient. I observe how the pregnancy is progressing, if a woman comes to me and she is skinny and all of a sudden she looks twice as big, this might be a problem. But the thing is, if you come to me in the morning and I weigh you, and the next time you come to me, in the evening, the difference between evening and morning weight can easily be two kilos, but you haven't gained two kilos during that day. So the whole issue of weighing . . . I think it is not my responsibility. In my view you should weigh yourself by yourself at home routinely at a fixed hour and in fixed conditions."

Levi is not arguing here that information obtained from weight-gain monitoring is unnecessary; he does not weigh women because of the inaccuracy of the measurement. But note that he pushes weight-gain monitoring to the extreme of imprecision by being content to estimate it merely by looking at the woman once a month. It is interesting to juxtapose his attitude to women's weight gain to the seriousness with which I saw him estimate the fetus's weight using ultrasound measurements during the final weeks of gestation. The latter are well known in the medical community for their imprecision, with the possibility of more than 10–20 percent standard measurement error. His final argument, however, concerns whose responsibility is it to monitor weight gain. Inspired by accounts of Japanese practitioners who emphasized weight-gain monitoring as highly important, I asked him directly if any medical indications existed of the correlation between excessive weight gain, large fetuses, and birth complications. He answered: "Mothers are bigger today. Look at my children—relative to me they are bigger; I am bigger than my father. The generation is changing because people are becoming bigger and fetuses are becoming bigger because the economy has changed, the conditions of life have changed, so fetuses are bigger. A while ago, when we discovered a four-kilo fetus, we got hysterical—we sent her immediately for a cesarean section. But today? If I find a fetus of 4.2-kilo during an ultrasound screening, I ring the birthing room and ask them, would you like to induce labor? They say, "No, let it progress a little bit. So the fetus will be 4.3—if she gets stuck during delivery we'll help her, we'll operate."

Levi is aware of the connection of excessive weight gain, larger fetuses, and complicated deliveries, yet unlike the case of suspected fetal abnormality, here he is prepared to "take chances." His "relaxed" attitude is directly connected with the way he understands his professional responsibility, which is firmly based on particular worst-case scenarios. Then "we" can "help." The physical and mental costs that women may have to pay for such invasive medical procedures called "help" hardly arise. The above definition of responsibility also marginalizes the role that women can play in preventing such situations from evolving. Dr Valah, thirty-five, a female intern, admitted that she had not been socialized into taking special care of the nutrition and weight of women with "low-risk" pregnancies. When I asked her about the lengthy passages in which *Williams Obstetrics* takes up the issue of nutrition, she reflected, "Maybe we should pay more attention to that issue; I really never thought about it enough. I guess that we assume that in the present state of nutrition in Israel there are no cases of undernourished women, that there is nothing to worry about concerning nutrition, but maybe we should learn more about this."

Especially interesting in this context were four ob-gyns who perceived a correlation between excessive weight gain and later complications, and even said explicitly that the monitoring of weight gain was indeed necessary. One of these, the head of a maternity ward, told me, "I keep a record of the patients' weight gain. The nurse weighs them, much to their dismay. I keep a record but I only speak to them about it when I have to." This practitioner took the view that he was sparing his patients the inconvenience of discussing an unpleasant matter. Dr. Ramon, the popular ob-gyn for whose services women fly to Israel from abroad, was one of the practitioners who explicitly thought weight-gain monitoring important during pregnancy. He said that he explains to the patient the importance of maintaining a moderate amount of weight gain once, at the first visit, but, he said, "I cannot educate her, I cannot tell her what to do; she will do whatever she wants." Ramon's statement below might reveal how he imagines the physical experience of pregnancy, which guides his "liberal" approach:

> I only weigh patients who ask me to weigh them. I just recognized that for many women this weighing thing is a traumatic experience. Most women gain way beyond any proportion: twenty kilos, thirty kilos. If I start weighing them, they will stop coming to me. My cousin told us how much she hated to go to my father (who was also an ob-gyn) because he used to weigh them routinely. It is a very complicated matter from a psychological perspective. What is fashionable, as you know, is to be skinny, and most women have to make a lot of effort to achieve their ideal weight. So while

they are pregnant, women do not feel sexy—the body is deformed [*mit'avet*] anyway, and there are all these pregnancy cravings, so why watch your weight? And also the husband becomes very tolerant toward this food festival because at last she is giving him a child. . . . So they lose control and eat and eat. So I cannot tell her what to do. I cannot educate her.

In the above statement we at last encounter an embodied model of pregnancy. For the first time, too, sexuality surfaces and the male partner is brought into the picture. However, "returning" pregnancy into the body does not seem to help pregnant women acquire a more positive image. Once again the pregnant woman is represented as grotesque, except that here her huge "deformed" body, not her anxieties, makes her so. Significantly, Dr. Ramon expects pregnant women to feel less attractive when pregnant. Once again pregnancy is represented as a chaotic process of losing control, though this time it is because of the inability to control the dimensions of one's own body and one's own eating habits, not the child's "quality." With such an image in mind, Ramon assumes that women prefer not to discuss weight and that there is no point in suggesting any kind of effort on a woman's part to watch her weight. Recall that Ramon is very successful in generating a feeling of empathy toward his patients. His success might prove that giving up weight monitoring is a good strategy in attracting patients, albeit sometimes at the price of women's well-being.

None of the doctors who raised the issue of weight gain and nutrition with patients said that they discussed their implications for the fetus's health or for possible complications in the process of birth. This suggests that they consider worst-case scenarios correlated with excessive weight gain less dangerous than worst-case scenarios correlated with fetal genetic and chromosomal abnormalities. This differentiation reflects the general devaluation of the role of gestation in fetal development. American sociological literature conceptualizes weight-gain regimes in pregnancy as forms of social control, drawing on data suggesting that a wide range of weight gain (for women who begin pregnancy at a normal weight) is acceptable and unrelated to "pregnancy outcome"; from this perspective the attitudes of Israeli practitioners to weight gain might be mistakenly interpreted as "liberating." My own interpretation does not rule out a strong dimension of social control in weight-gain regimes. However, while bearing in mind that social control can take on myriad forms, I wish to illuminate the problematic nature of addressing weight gain only in terms of "pregnancy outcomes." This, in my view, is an extremely "feto-centric" perspective on pregnancy, almost "product oriented." One of my main points is that pregnancy is not only about fetuses or babies; there is a woman in the pregnant body, and her physical and mental well-being are often undercut once she sets off on the adventure of pregnancy. While statistics that correlate "pregnancy outcomes" and weight gain "allow" a wide range of weight gains, the statistics that correlate weight gain and cesarean sections indicate quite a clear correlation. No statistics, to my knowledge, have attempted to quantify women's quality of life and sense of well-being as related to weight gain. Well-being becomes an especially bothersome question in the Israeli case, where women, as described in chapter four, are expected to go about their duties as usual. In the Israeli case, women often speak bitterly about their experience of "dragging" rather than "carrying" a heavy pregnancy. Japanese doctors, whose accounts are set out in the next chapter, suggest that gaining less weight reduces the likelihood of having a cesarean section and makes pregnancy easier to carry. This, of course, does not make Japanese weight-gain supervision a "power-innocent" practice, as I show in that chapter. Rather it shows that Japanese ob-gyns are concerned about the pregnant women's well-being as part of their attempt to secure the fetus. My main point is that the expression of medical authority here has much to do with cultural paradigms of thinking about pregnancy, women, and fetuses, and not necessarily with hard numbers (whose meanings and the methods through which they are manufactured should be always carefully considered).

Gestation and the Key Scenario of Catastrophe

What has emerged from the analysis carried out so far is a fairly distinct version of a medical theory of pregnancy, complete with its moral economy. According to this theory, pregnancy is basically a chaotic process in which nature is liable to make mistakes, and it is this dangerous process that biomedicine must handle. In fact, what was described above is a local medical scheme of pregnancy, an interconnected set of ideas, categories, medical standards of practice with specific emphases, and characteristic emotional postures that patients and doctors may legitimately assume under specific circumstances. One can visualize this scheme as an open-ended flow chart in which certain medical practices and diagnoses bring forth certain "responses" from the patient and yet another set of medical practices. Anxiety caused by the likeliness of reproductive catastrophes and notions of "risk" play a central role in this scheme.

However, "risk" has assumed a particular local meaning here. Indeed, as Lock writes, "Increasingly, people everywhere adopt the concept of risk and become familiar with the disease nosologies of biomedicine" (Lock 2001, 483). Moreover, in the specific case of pregnancy, the works of Rothman, Rapp, and Browner and Press illuminate the role of "risk" in making pregnancy seem increasingly problematic to American women. These writers point out that the emergence of PND has made pregnancies increasingly problematized. A similar process has taken place in Israel more or less simultaneously. However, that Israeli standards of practice might go well beyond the global differentiation of risk, that patients' refusals to undergo testing are so rarely tolerated, that PND has raised no meaningful public criticism, and that it is considered justified to show "horror picture shows" (complete with their lack of political correctness and insensitivity toward the emotions of pregnant women) at public events illuminate the cultural particularity of prenatal diagnosis in Israel and take us beyond biomedical technologies to factors that shape the problematized nature of pregnancy in Israeli culture. I suggest that to understand the worst-case-scenario-oriented thinking so prevalent in the ethnography, one must explore broader Israeli-Jewish key scenarios of catastrophe so prevalent in Israeli-Jewish social life. These ideas go beyond reproduction to the core of the collective national identity of Israeli Jews and generate the self, both as an individual and part of a collective, as threatened by catastrophe.

The idea that terrible catastrophes—either physical, spiritual, or both—are around the corner predominates in parts of the collective Jewish memory and reestablishes itself through the commemoration of key events in Jewish history. In Jewish canonical narratives that predate the constitution of the state of Israel, the threat of extinction is usually countered by a miraculous redemption/salvation brought about by God and thus the relief from the threat is commemorated. Examples include the enslavement of the Israelites by Pharaoh followed by the Exodus from Egypt celebrated at Passover; a temporary relief in the bitter struggles for national and spiritual independence from Hellenistic rule that is celebrated in Hanukah; and the inversion of the magisterial verdict to exterminate all Jews in the Persian Empire that is celebrated in Purim.

It is beyond the scope of this study to provide a full historical and cultural account of the evolution and diversity of Jewish narratives of existential threats. However, it is clear that when Zionism absorbed this scheme of thinking into Israeli state narratives, it transformed it in significant ways. In fact, toward the beginning of the twentieth century, the Zionist movement put forward the constitution of a Jewish state as the most recent form of redemption from the age-old threat of Jewish extinction. The role of the state as redeemer appeared to be vindicated soon after the Holocaust, as refugees sought sanctuary in the Jewish state. Since the constitution of the state of Israel, the notion of redemption took on alternative trajectories, one of which has been the military as a symbolic substitute for the redemptive power of God.

However, with the rise in the late 1970s of public and scholarly criticism of the military and the militarization of Israeli society—only to intensify during the first and second Intifada—the "threat/redemption" formula appears to have jettisoned the latter part of the scenario, where catastrophe now looms large as a lone key scenario, powerfully transforming the worldview of those who have difficulty believing in divine redemption into one of pessimism. As Gerald Cromer (2006) points out, the *threat* of terror transcends terror events themselves and becomes a key notion to think with, an index case against which claimants, regardless of their political positions, weigh other unrelated issues.

Within such fatalistic conceptions of threat in mind, genetic fatalism makes much sense. The medical attitudes that have been analyzed here reflect an understanding of pregnancy that tends to "leave" fetal health to the mercy of random, unpredicted genetic and chromosomal breakages, to underestimate the role of women in fetal development, and to focus less on the health of the pregnant woman herself than on the fetus she is carrying. The deemphasis on supervising weight gain and nutrition is one example of the practical implications of this understanding of pregnancy.

From the vantage point of the threat/redemption scheme, it seems that the ultrasound experts quoted in the ethnography (to take one example) were trying to situate themselves and their technologies at the redemption side of the scheme. At the same time, in a narrative process that parallels the weakening of the notion of redemption, they again and again remind their audience that no assurance can be given. Thus, the hovering presence of reproductive misfortune throughout the ethnography has to do with the readiness of Israeli Jews—medical practitioners and lay persons, as I discuss later—to think with the key scenario of "threat": to imagine that the worst is about to happen and to devise strategies to defend oneself against it (i.e., to undergo invasive testing and abort fetuses with minor anomalies).

It is important to bear in mind that the doctors whose thinking and practices I have discussed in this chapter, although acutely aware of medico-legal constraints, were trying to provide their patients with the best medical care, according to their own understanding of what is best and according to what they expected most patients to pursue. The standards of practice that are described here constitute best practice under the regime of reproductive catastrophe. It is medically illustrated phobias of fetal catastrophe that give Israeli practitioners their preoccupation with discovering imperfections in the fetus in the best interests of their patients, while also making them less tolerant of patients' unconventional decisions and less interested in ethical debates about PND.

2

The Twofold Structure of
Japanese Prenatal Care

The National Politics of Reproduction and Japanese Prenatal Care

A History of Twentieth-Century Obstetrics and Gynecology (1999) [*Sanfujinka
nijûseiki no ayumi*], a book by a long list of Japanese ob-gyns addressed to the
medical community, introduces prenatal diagnosis, among other advances in
obstetrics and gynecology. However, when amniocentesis is introduced as a
technology to diagnose Down's syndrome (among other anomalies), the writers
warn that "Mongolism is a pejorative term that demeans the Mongol race as a
whole; therefore we use the term 'Down's syndrome'" (Sato 1999, 199). One
should bear in mind here that the Japanese consider themselves Mongoloids.
Then the authors proceed to remind readers of the "moral problems" (Sato
1999, 200) surrounding the test, and to assert that "nowadays prenatal diagnosis and genetic screening are limited to patients for whom there is a high
probability of carrying lethal diseases such as Duchan's muscular dystrophy or
hemophilia" (Sato 1999, 200). This cautious medical discourse echoes the criticism against the social implications of PND that emerged as soon as it became
available in private clinics in Japan, and persisted throughout the 1990s. Social
scientists (Matsubara 1997, 1998, 2000; Nakajima 1992; Saitô 1992; Tsuge 1992),
medical practitioners and ethicists (Hiroi and Saitô 1996; Nakatani 1996a,
1996b), as well as print journalists (*Asahi Shinbun* 1997a, 1997b), were all concerned with the eugenic implications of PND. As I suggest later, PND currently is
located backstage of prenatal care. Nevertheless, eugenics has not always been
a shameful word in Japan. Eugenic ideologies and policies were part and parcel
of Japanese nation-building strategies in the first decades of the twentieth
century (Frühstük 2003; Robertson 2002b).

However, as Robertson notes: "Eugenics, in the sense of instrumental
and selective procreation, was hardly a new concept in *fin-de-siècle* Japan"
(Robertson 2002b, 195). Strategically arranged marriages and adoptions were

key strategies in securing the continuity and genealogical integrity of households long before the institution of counseling agencies to encourage "eugenic marriages" in the first decades of the twentieth century. On a different level, abortions and infanticide were widely practiced in the Tokugawa period (1600–1868) when pregnancies occurred in extramarital relations or in response to economic inability to raise more children. Especially in the case of poor villagers, infanticide decisions were often enforced on parents by the village head, and executed by the midwife. Expressions such as "thinning out the plants" (*mabiki*) and "child-returning" (in the sense of sending back to the gods the present one was given) (*kogaeshi*) are euphemisms for an array of rather gruesome techniques of abortion and infanticide (Jolivet 1997, 117–123). Modern eugenics, oriented to building a modern Japanese nation, was different in the scope of its ambitions and in its social implications.

Looking back to the Meiji era (1868–1912), one observes the emergence of a sense of demographic threat intertwined with national pro-natalism as a prominent orientation of Japanese population policies. By 1853, when Commodore Perry forced Japan to open itself up to the world, extensive parts of Asia had already been colonized by the West.[1] National leaders feared that Japan would be next and were already thinking about birth rates in terms of "military preparedness" (LaFleur 1992, 119). Acting from this sense of threat, the Meiji government did not hesitate to intervene in its citizens' reproductive decisions (not unlike other European states of that time). In 1907 it outlawed the formerly widespread practices of abortion and infanticide (Hardacre 1997; Jolivet 1997; LaFleur 1992). Between 1920 and 1940 the population grew from nearly fifty-seven million to seventy-three million (LaFleur 1992). Increasing the size of the Japanese population was indeed a major goal but the government was also explicit about improving the quality (*soshitsu*) of the people's constitution, in the language of the eugenics protection law discussed below. As in European societies of that time, the urge to "improve" the physical constitution of the population was firmly connected to an upsurge of nationalism, imperialism, and militarism; in prewar Japan it also had to do with a national sense of racial inferiority to Westerners, inflated by an acute foreboding of military attack. How exactly the Japanese population might be improved to meet national challenges became an important question, to which Japanese eugenicists offered multiple answers.

"Eugenics" (*yûsei*)—literally superior birth—came to stand for a broad range of ideas and strategies. One set of ideas was oriented to maximizing the procreation of eugenically good stock (such as counseling agencies to "encourage" "eugenically" sound choices of marital partners) (Otsubo and Bartholomew 1998, 547; Robertson 2002b). Another group focused on minimizing the proliferation of a broad category of "unfit."[2] This, in turn, consisted of "environmental" public health-oriented approaches that attempted to improve the conditions of procreation through educational endeavors to implement advances in sanitation, nutrition, and physical activity, thus to eliminate infectious and venereal diseases (the latter was broadly referred to as *minzoku eisei*, or public hygiene); and "genetically fatalistic" approaches centered on the elimination of "hereditary" diseases (*idenbyô*) through sterilization and induced abortions.

However, viewing Japanese population policies broadly yields one particular eugenic orientation as predominant: a gynocentric–maternalist (but non-feminist) eugenics that endeavors to improve "the conditions surrounding *female* reproductivity instead of advocating sterilization as a way to reduce the reproduction of the unfit" (Robertson 2002b, 199). It should be clarified that by characterizing Japanese eugenics as gynocentric, neither Robertson nor I, who use her terminology, mean to imply that such eugenic orientation is more benign, but rather to delineate a specific logic of action. For later discussion, it should be borne in mind that women's health and education became the focus of attention in the specific context of eugenic endeavors to cultivate reproduction.

So while the "National Eugenic Protection Law" (*Nihon kokumin yûsei hogo-hô*) enacted in 1940 (modeled on the Nazi German sterilization law of 1933) explicitly stated its purpose as being to "ensure the improvement of the national character," and legalized induced abortions for persons with a predisposition to malignant familial hereditary diseases (*Kôshû Eisei Hôsoku* IV, 141–142), the number of people who were sterilized was fairly small (Otsubo and Bartholomew 1998, 558). Except for the specified cases, abortion remained a criminal act, which reflects the actual goal of the law to tighten control of fertility among the healthy population. Along with the subjugation of fertility to criminal justice, the government devised powerful discursive strategies, seeking to sanctify motherhood as an important patriotic obligation of women (though at the same time expecting women to contribute to industrialization and economic growth, as well as to the war effort in various ways; I return to this point later). Attempts to bind women's reproductive capacities to national goals were to persist until the end of World War II (LaFleur 1992, 120) and well beyond—to the beginning of twenty-first century, as I show below.

The end of the war marked a turning point in population policies. The government was as interested as before in directing fertility according to national goals, except that now Japan's leaders were alarmed about population expansion. Since Japan had been totally defeated and economically devastated, the national goal now was economic recovery, which was threatened by the baby boom that followed the repatriation of Japanese soldiers immediately after the war. This pushed policy makers to decide that the legalization of abortion was the only way to lower population growth (Norgren 2001, 50). In 1948 abortions were legalized, and in 1949 a clause permitting abortion for reasons of economic hardship was added. Consequently the early postwar years were marked by a steep upsurge in abortion rates. Again the government achieved its goals: according to the statistics of the Japanese Ministry of Health and Welfare, in the 1920s the average Japanese mother had 5.24 children. This figure shrank to 3.65 during the 1950s, immediately after the war, and steadily declined further to 2 during the 1960s (Sonoda 1990, 23–24).

However, as early as the late 1950s declining birthrate and rapid economic growth became confirmed trends and Japanese officials, concerned about labor shortages, began to back away from family planning (Norgren 2001). Moreover since the postwar years, life expectancy in Japan has lengthened considerably and is at present the highest in the world for women. During the 1980s this "health miracle" (Steslicke 1987, 24) increasingly came to be seen in Japan as a mixed blessing. Current statistical forecasts predicting that citizens aged over sixty-five will constitute a quarter of the population in the coming decade are often cited in the media to foreshadow a grave national crisis. Japanese welfare policy makers expect the family to take primary responsibility for the care of the elderly at home (Lock 1996, 1993, 1999). So unless more Japanese children are born to help out, care for an increasing number of elderly people will fall on the shoulders of a disproportionately small number of middle-aged women (mostly), making such care an increasingly heavy burden on the family. Accordingly, since the closing decades of the twentieth-century public concern with the shrinking size of the Japanese family has had less to do with the threat of military conflict and more with the very different matter of the "graying of society" (kôreika shakai). This has not notably eased the pressures exerted on women to reproduce.

On January 27, 2007, Yanagisawa Hakuo, minister of health and welfare, made a statement that created a scandal in the media. His statement gives an idea of how acutely policy makers feel demographic concerns and the alarming ways that such anxieties formulate women's citizenship. Expressing his deep concern over the growing numbers of pensioners, Yanagisawa went on to say that since the number of "birthing machines" (umu kikai) (referring to women aged fifteen to fifty) is fixed, "The only solution [to the demographic crisis] is that women will [favor us by] bearing one more child." Once again "mother machines" (cf. Gena Corea) are being called upon "to help out" in a national crisis.

Compared with the success of prewar governments in manipulating fertility rates according to national "needs," during the second half of the twentieth century such attempts failed badly, especially in light of the apparent success of Japan's postwar governments in managing society in other areas. As Garon argues, they obtained "not simply passive compliance from the people but the enthusiastic participation of many private groups in its ambitious programs to manage society" (Garon 1997, xv). The persistent drop in birthrates is an exception to this rule. Why has the Japanese government failed to "encourage" birth among Japanese women?

To begin with, government subsidies for prenatal care are surprisingly low for a state that wishes to improve fertility rates. Each prenatal examination (out of the fourteen recommended to women in a noncomplicated pregnancy) may cost between 5000 and 10,000 yen ($42–$85) for women who are covered by national insurance, depending on the examinations carried out and the type of medical institution. Prefectural governments offer on average 2.8 free checkups to a woman per pregnancy. In addition to the sums that women will have to pay for each checkup, they will also pay between 121,000–170,000 yen ($1026–$1442) for the delivery and between 35,000 and 50,000 yen ($297–$424) for a five-day hospitalization after a normal birth. Part of these sums will be reimbursed after the baby is born. The logic of this system is that pregnancy is not an illness. This contrasts strikingly with the case of Israeli women, who do not pay for at least five routine prenatal checkups, for any blood and urine test, for amniocentesis, if they are eligible, or for birth (whether vaginal or cesarean), and are granted a "birth grant" if they give birth in a hospital.

The Maternal Body Protection Law (*Botai Hogo Hô*), which replaced the Eugenic Protection Law in 1996, does not really facilitate population growth. From the 1950s the Eugenic Protection Law became the locus of a confrontation among family planners, feminist and nonfeminist women, the religious, right-wing parties, the disabled, and doctors (Norgren 2001, 53). The last-named emerged as a powerful interest group throughout the socio-political negotiations on the revision of the law and played a major role in designing Japanese sexual culture. The regulation, added to the law in 1949, permitting abortion in case of the mother's financial hardship (the "economic clause"), was pushed forward by Taniguchi Yasaburo, an ob-gyn and conservative representative in the Upper House. Norgren describes how the Eugenic Protection Law practically gave ob-gyns a monopoly on abortion services and created "an institutionalized incentive for ob-gyns to work to maintain and expand access to abortion" (Norgren 2001, 44). Since the 1970s ob-gyn interest groups have played a major role in blocking attempts by pharmaceutical firms to legalize the pill for contraceptive use. While maintaining abortions as one source of their livelihood, ob-gyns helped to make them an acceptable and widely used "contraceptive." So although the "economic clause" has come under attack throughout the last four decades, when the Eugenic Protection Law was finally revised in 1996 this clause remained in place.

The Maternal Body Protection Law prohibits abortions for eugenic reasons; this is the only aspect of the law for which revision was consensual. In fact, eugenic sterilizations had already become rare from even a few years after the war, and very few abortions were registered under the eugenic clause.[3] The new law institutionalized a public state of mind that generally took abortions to be a means of choosing when to have children rather than what *kind* of children were born. To this day abortions are available practically on demand in Japan, under the Maternal Body Protection Law, as under its predecessor. This should be borne in mind when considering the medical management of pregnancy in Japan: the assumption underlying prenatal care in Japanese medical institutions seems to be that a woman who goes to them for prenatal care wants her pregnancy. Otherwise she would have found a way to dispose of it earlier.

Once one enters the realm of prenatal care, medical initiatives appear to be upside down. Japanese officials have failed to "encourage" birthrates, but Japanese ob-gyns and neonatologists strive to "make the most" of their patients' pregnancies. The medical system works to minimize two of the main causes of neonatal mortality: premature birth and postnatal complications in newborn babies. Currently, with neonatal mortality at 1.4 per 1000 live births, Japan reports the lowest rate in the world, a statistic that many ob-gyns cite proudly (Kaneda 2007, 61). The strategies for defining and calculating these figures might be questionable, but it is manifestly clear that they are highly valued by their producers and that much effort is exerted to improve them. Comparing the Japanese achievement with the unsuccessful attempts to attain lower neonatal and infant mortality rates in Europe and America, one wonders what it is about Japanese prenatal and neonatal care that has brought about such improvements.

Before presenting my perspective on the questions raised so far, let me note that the above survey reveals a set of inner tensions, inconsistencies, and contradictions in which all reproductive relationships are played out. Specifically, the dual role of Japanese ob-gyns reflects a confusing pattern of reproduction: an affluent society with a pro-natal government is threatened by shrinking birthrates compounded by a "graying process"; its medical institutions are dedicated to lowering infant and neonatal mortality, while at the same time practically providing abortion on demand. How may such a confusing reproductive cultural politics be understood?

A host of studies have contributed to understanding this politics—from the broad perspective of government reproductive policies (Takeda 2005), the vantage point of religious and social politics of contraception (Coleman 1983; Hardacre 1997; LaFleur 1992; Norgren 2001), and the "postnatal" perspective on the "conditions of mothering," in Jolivet's (1997) terminology. This last tends to focus on the social organization of childcare and on the disadvantaged position of working mothers (Jolivet 1997). The stage of pregnancy is a missing link in the continuum of reproduction, ethnographically and theoretically.

Pregnancy shifts the focus to reproductive relationships on the "microphysical" level. If fertility is a national "resource," pregnancy reminds one that fetuses are gestated in women's bodies, whether they will be aborted or turned into the neonates whose mortality and morbidity doctors are seeking to lower, and that the state and the doctors have to deal with these women. Moreover, as the review above suggests, the role of ob-gyns can hardly be underestimated, as either interest groups or individual practitioners, in the day-to-day management of pregnancy; in this medicalized society women are expected to visit the clinic periodically during their pregnancy, and medical information is popularized through the public media. Yet few empirical ethnographies exist to date that illuminate how these powerful agents of reproduction think and act. I contend that, as the representatives of authoritative knowledge and the agents who manage the genesis stages of parenthood directly, ob-gyns can reveal a lot, not only about social conceptions of pregnancy: they can also illuminate assumptions concerning the *embodiment of motherhood* that underlie the broader organizational framework of parenthood in Japan.

The Frontstage of Japanese Prenatal Care

Framing Japanese Prenatal Care

The basic division of pregnancy into low-risk and high-risk is well known to Japanese ob-gyns. However, the phrase *hai risuku* is written in *katakana* (a Japanese phonetic system of writing that is preserved for foreign words). What seems to be more common is the division of pregnancy into "normal" (*seijô*) and "abnormal" (*ijô*). Yet, some medical discussions of the concepts reveal a perception of this set of categories as a dynamic continuum rather than a binary set. In the opening paragraphs of the volume about normal pregnancy (*seijôhen*) in a recent edition of a famous Japanese obstetrics and gynecology textbook, the authors warn against hasty categorization of pregnancy as "abnormal," even when there has been a move away from what they consider the norm.

> There are circumstances in which such a division [into normal and abnormal] *cannot be made clearly.* Sometimes a pregnancy proceeds completely normally and then . . . temporarily in one week 500 grams are gained. We should not declare that the pregnancy has entered the category of pregnancy toxemia; rather we must think about a median sphere [*kyôkai ryôiki*: literally a borderline sphere between normal and abnormal]. But even if we divide pregnancy into three categories: normal, border sphere, and abnormal, pregnancy can shift between these three categories, and it is the role of the physician to judge by the medical examinations [to which category a pregnancy belongs]. (Magara and Araki 2000)

The above discussion attempts to portray pregnancy as a process in motion rather than an either/or situation. The reluctance to rush to categorizing pregnancy as "abnormal" is most significant here; if pregnancy is basically "normal" it requires care rather than scrutiny.

Indeed, the idea of care (rather than "diagnosis") dominates the medical management of pregnancy from the outset. Whereas Israeli pregnancy monitoring is structured more as a schedule (in which fetal anomalies can be detected at each stage of the pregnancy), Japanese prenatal care is basically designed as routine activity "alongside" the development of "normal" pregnancy. Pregnancy guides commonly include a table of prenatal testing divided into categories such as "tests carried out on each visit" and "special tests." The "special tests" are further categorized between those available at most hospitals and those only available at major medical centers or teaching hospitals. However, routine tests remain the core of all the variations in these tables, and this "core" is the initial focal point of my exploration.

A prenatal routine consists of measuring the patient's weight gain, abdominal circumference, and fundal height (measured with a tape measure from top of the pubic bone to the top of the uterus). Her blood pressure and urine are checked an average of every three weeks when she goes to see the ob-gyn. In addition, ultrasound screening and internal vaginal examinations are performed at different frequencies, depending on the clinic. These tests form the main focus of the style of prenatal care that I observed.

The "Noisy" Ob-Gyn: Weight Gain and Authoritative Speech

I sat in the waiting room of the obstetrics and gynecology outpatient clinic, where I had arranged to meet Dr. Oikawa for an interview, browsing through gaudy maternity magazines. On the wall opposite was a colorful placard of the food pyramid, with a digital scale just below it. Stepping onto the scale was the first thing that women did before sitting down to wait until their names were called. At last Dr. Oikawa, a tall man in his fifties, came out of his office. We were already on our way to the cafeteria downstairs when Ueda-san, the nurse who was working in the room next to Oikawa, ran after us and called him back. She was uncertain about what calorific and nutritional intake she should advise for the patient he had just seen, since the weight recorded has been written unclearly. Dr. Oikawa returned to his office. The patient, a woman in her twenties and five months pregnant, was sitting there and nodded politely when he came in. She handed him her maternal monitoring card and he went over previous weight registrations, muttering to himself. As he told me later, he had gone over the figures a few minutes earlier, when he had seen the patient, and was doing so again "just in case" he had failed to recognize a problem. Then he said that the weight gain was "exactly right" (*pittari*) and praised the woman for having "improved" from the previous visit. "Ueda-san felt insecure in taking the responsibility on herself," he explained to me later. Oikawa and Ueda-san seem to regard weight gain and nutrition in pregnancy as highly serious matters, sites at which "deviations" from the required norm can be "exactly" measured and repaired, while heavy responsibilities are played out.

Dr. Oikawa, like the majority of the ob-gyns I interviewed, described himself as extremely exacting and fussy (*urusai*, literally "noisy") and strict (*kibishii*) when speaking to patients about the need to control their weight. Many ob-gyns I interviewed explained that they were simply following standard practice as laid down in the Handbook of Mother-Child Health (*boshikenkôtechô*), a medical record of prenatal care that I shall discuss later. All the ob-gyns I interviewed (thirty) and those who filled in a questionnaire (twenty-six) wrote that they had never skipped registering their patients' weight gain.

Unlike the Israeli ob-gyns, who were reluctant to discuss weight gain and tended to marginalize its importance, Japanese ob-gyns had a lot to say about the importance and strategies of "weight supervision" (*taijûkanri*) or "weight control" (*taijû kontorôru*). They frequently offered their own theories based on personal experience and systematic measurements and observations about how and why weight gain *must* be controlled (not only watched). Although I addressed my questions about weight gain in a general way—"Do you talk to your patients about weight gain?"—occasionally interviewees understood that I was after the ideal weight gain *threshold* they recommended. As Dr. Shimazaki, a female ob-gyn in her mid-forties, told me, "I think that the ideal weight gain is seven kilos. The baby is three kilos, one kilo placenta, one more kilo the amniotic fluid, breasts, blood volume . . . so altogether about seven kilos. But never more than ten."

The ideal weight gain is not an arbitrary figure but rather a carefully calculated quantity. With similar precision, other practitioners calculated thresholds of six or eight kilos, which they enthusiastically advocated. Notable in thinking in terms of thresholds is the way it standardizes physiological aspects of gestation. I usually felt the self-evidence of the "threshold logic" when I was asked by ob-gyns, as a matter of course, what the weight-gain limit in Israel was, and how much weight I was *allowed* to gain when pregnant. Practitioners found it hard to believe that I had undergone four pregnancies hardly ever being weighed, and that my ob-gyn never discussed weight gain or nutrition with me.

Some practitioners presented a more complex attitude to standardization, explaining that they calculated ideal weight gain individually for each patient. Such calculations were made according to guidelines published by the Gynecological Society. These set out ranges of weight gain for patients with different BMI (Body Mass Index). The Japanese gynecological community, which is highly ambiguous on issues of prenatal diagnosis, goes into minute detail to explicate ideal ranges of gestational weight gain.

Other practitioners even theorized the *rate* at which weight should be gained. Whereas Dr. Kuromaki, thirty-nine, an ob-gyn and head of the maternity ward in a government hospital, explained that "In principle I think she should not gain more than one kilo per month," Dr. Yamaguchi, forty-five, an ob-gyn who runs a private clinic, prescribed a rate of "half a kilo per month in the first trimester, seven hundred grams per month in the second trimester, and one kilo per month in the last trimester."

Dr. Yoshiaki, who practices at a large government hospital, suggested a combination, an elaborate notion of weight gain, integrating a nonstandardized concept with regard to rate:

> I follow the standards set by the Japanese gynecological society. They specified a table of values calculated according to BMI. Using the table one can specify how much the ideal weight gain should be for a particular patient from her initial weight and height. So after I calculate her BMI, I tell her the ideal weight gain to aspire to: you should gain, say, two kilos until the twentieth week, and during the remaining twenty weeks you may gain another four kilos. I tell her, "Let's aim at this [pattern of weight gain]." I say that from the very beginning, and I tell her to hold herself [*osaeru*]. I say, "Make an effort; try hard from now on" [*gambatte*].

The fact that Yoshiaki "tailors" an individual weight-gain pattern for each patient does not leave much space for individual diversity. He told me how, at the first prenatal visit, he plots the ideal weight-gain pattern that he has calculated with a red pen on a graph contained in the patient's handbook. Then he explains to the patient that after each future prenatal visit she should add the point that represents her actual weight on the graph with a black pen and try to stay as "close to" the ideal graph as possible. Yoshiaki's graph illustrates the threshold to the woman in a very visible and measurable way. Who is the pregnant Japanese woman that the whole enterprise of weight-gain control envisages?

In many urban hospitals women routinely weigh themselves on digital scales before entering the doctor's office on a prenatal visit. On entering, the woman hands the printout to the doctor, who records her new weight on the table in her medical-monitoring record. The woman is expected to plot the new dot on the graph (contained in the same handbook). She is also expected to modify her everyday behavior in accordance with the thresholds and graphs: to "hold back" and "tame" her appetite. A key Japanese concept used by Dr. Yoshiaki summarizes this expectation: the pregnant Japanese woman is encouraged and expected to *gambaru*, "make an effort."

The notion of *gambaru* can be traced throughout the Japanese life cycle; it emphasizes effort as the key to personal and communal achievement. Hendry explains *gambaru* as "the general ability to try as hard as possible in whatever one does" (Hendry 1986, 83–84). A number of scholars have pointed out the dominance of *gambaru* as a cultural model of "character building," and as the explicit and implicit trajectory along which educational projects endeavor to organize their activities (Amanuma 1987; Ben-Ari 1997; Singleton 1989; White 1987). *Gambaru* may stand for various kinds of effort, ranging from the mental to the physical, but it is often linked to withstanding and controlling physical needs (Ben-Ari 1997, 83–92) and is thus especially applicable to instructions such as those discussed above. In directing pregnant behavior along *gambaru* lines, doctors evoke a rich array of cultural scenarios calling for making an effort, together with the sense of achievement and the emotional rewards that can be expected to follow. *Gambaru* used in the medical rhetoric of prenatal care also suggests that the proper "education" of new mothers is one of its implicit goals. In the course of such endeavor, medical personnel are positioned as coaches to the women, who are supposed (ideally) to develop the spirit and character of a mother through a personal prenatal ordeal.

When doctors wish to provide extra care they will ensure that women are given detailed and practical instructions on how to nurture themselves during gestation. Dr. Ootsuma, fifty-six, a female ob-gyn who teaches at a medical school and practices at a maternity hospital that she established herself, told me:

> As an ideal, six to seven kilos is very good. I tell them that when I lecture at the maternity class; I speak to mothers about the importance of controlling weight. Then I have the nutritionist come along and give them *exact* directions about how to construct a meal, with all the necessary calorie calculations and nutrient distributions. Then, they are asked to bring to the next class an exact daily report of every single thing they ate, inserted in a timetable. The nutritionist goes over the table and checks it, showing women with problematic eating habits where their problems are, and having them bring another report the next time.

The narrative above recalls the descriptions of prenatal classes given by the Health Maintenance Organization in California as reported in Markens, Browner, and Press (1997), but with one major difference. While American women were "required to fill out charts . . . and were asked many questions about their own daily food intake" (Markens, Browner, and Press 1997, 357), Japanese women were often required to mend their ways and bring recorded "evidence" that an improvement had indeed taken place. The above narrative is also special in the scientific precision whereby it aims to manage the complex compound of balanced nutrition and weight gain. Specifically this strict nutritional supervision has made Ootsuma's hospital a highly reputable institution. Later I learned that she was particularly popular among Japanese women who were married to Pakistani men. These women, who convert to Islam, adopt various food taboos, and Ootsuma told me that they become very anxious once they have conceived. As she told me, "This [food] is forbidden, that [food] is forbidden, so how are they going to support this life? So they come here and we help them: this is our specialty, we manage to combine the foods that they are allowed to eat to get the best nutritional value, and indeed the babies born in this hospital are usually very healthy." In contrast to Israeli ob-gyns, whose reputation depends on their ability to check whether the fetus is healthy (or not), Ootsuma's reputation depends on her help in "growing" or "making" healthy babies. That her patients warmly recommend her hospital suggests that the Japanese emphasis on nutrition and weight is grounded in a shared understanding between doctors and their patients, or what we might call "public demand." In all the maternity classes in which I participated, whether given by hospitals or by municipal centers, a few nutrition classes were included as part of the curriculum. The pregnant participants, who are generally attentive but very quiet in other sessions, become excited when it comes to these lessons. They ask specific questions, take notes, and reflect on potential problems. In short, the cult of weight-gain control seems based on a shared understanding.

Since ob-gyns regard the mission of controlling weight gain as both important and feasible they openly describe how, when the patient does not seem to be doing her best (she is not *gambaru* enough), they demand her cooperation. Dr. Kojima, forty-eight, head of the maternity ward in a general city hospital, told me: "I attribute much importance to weight checks to the extent that often pregnant women weep in the waiting room of the clinic. But there is nothing to be done about it [*shô ganai*]. If I realize that she has gained too much since the previous visit, I ask 'Why?' It is not because I get angry; rather I ask her objectively. 'Maybe you're hungry? Maybe you've been eating a lot at night? Maybe you've been eating sweets?' I want her to become self-conscious, to understand what has gone wrong, and to make an effort to mend it."

Here the narrative is concerned with gaining weight in terms of right and wrong behavior within a context of correcting improper behavior. Kojima's statement implies that he is familiar with colleagues for whom the importance of controlling weight justifies expressing anger with patients in similar situations. Moreover, it seems that patients are easily driven to tears, even without being scolded. Professor Tadanori, the head of a maternity ward in a large hospital in Tokyo, said that although he records weight gain in his patients' maternity records, he tries his best not to scold them, because his heart breaks to see patients crying in the waiting room. The tendency of patients to cry suggests that they share the doctor's understanding of the importance of weight-gain control, and dread the consequences of failing to control it. Anxieties surface here, just as in the narratives of Israeli ob-gyns; but whereas the Israeli-Jewish anxieties are arrayed around notions of the inevitability of genetic and chromosomal "accidents," the Japanese anxieties reflected here focus on different notions and ranges of worst-case scenarios.

From the description above, Japanese ob-gyns, unlike their Israeli counterparts, seem preoccupied with the patient's body, particularly its dimensions. Japanese prenatal care is obviously not unique in its desire to control weight or in its production of thresholds and prenatal education classes; yet the particular strictness and conviction with which the need to control weight is communicated to patients call for interpretation. What kind of worst-case scenario underlies Japanese ob-gyns' strict supervision of weight gain? In what kinds of theory on the physiology of gestation and fetal development is the cult of weight supervision grounded?

The Causal Theory of Gestation

The range of reasons given by Japanese ob-gyns to explain their emphasis on controlling weight gain contains many that are similar to those listed in Western medical textbooks.[4] Yet the most typically feared consequence of excessive weight gain in Japan is having a big baby, which is widely known in medical literature as macrosomia. Still, a big baby as understood by Japanese ob-gyns might not accord with definitions of macrosomia in international literature, as the following conversation illustrates.

After an elaborate monolog in which the aforementioned Dr. Kojima described how he strictly enforces supervision of weight gain on his patients, he asked me:

KOJIMA: How is it in Israel with weight supervision?

TSIPY: Some of the doctors I spoke to do not weigh their patients at all.

KOJIMA: Is that because most women are skinny?

TSIPY: No. Doctors complain that some women gain twenty kilos and even more.

KOJIMA: But you [Israelis] are also taller, aren't you, over 160 centimeters? In the case of the Japanese it is different. Clearly the dimensions of the pubic bone and the birth canal are absolutely parallel to the height. . . . People who are 160 centimeters tall can deliver even a four thousand-gram baby. Certainly there are cases when the baby is over forty-five hundred grams and it can end up in a shoulder distochia and a difficult delivery [nanzan], but for Japanese if they are 150 centimeters tall, it becomes difficult to deliver a baby over three thousand grams. So if they gain ten to twelve kilos, well. . . . So right from the start they have to [making a gambaru face, laughing]. Japanese women are certainly small—I guess the average is 156 centimeters.

Note that although the relativity of babies' sizes seems a universal issue, Kojima in his narrative finds the specific reproductive anatomy of the Japanese woman wanting. He contends that giving birth to big babies is a difficulty directly connected with the physiology of Japanese women.[5]

Adding to this picture, Hardacre mentions a similar concern in her review of the ritualization of pregnancy in premodern Japan. Then, pregnant women were instructed to bind themselves with a wide belt or belly band, and to keep it tight to prevent the fetus from growing too large (Hardacre 1997, 22–23). Nevertheless, my observations of actual weight-monitoring in Kojima's and other clinics do not show any significant difference in the treatment that taller women receive, which leads me to think that the small Japanese woman is more than a statistical creature: she is situated within the dialectic relationship between the material body and cultural concerns.

I suggest that Kojima's theory echoes a more general Japanese preoccupation with physical dimensions, which was particularly apparent in the writings of Japanese eugenicists (Kowner 2002; Robertson 2002b). Kowner illustrates how, at the beginning of the twentieth century, Japanese obsessions with the dimensions of the body and skin color were formulated as reflecting physical (and mental) incompetence compared with Westerners. Moreover, women's *reproductive* health was marked as an important national goal in the context of improving the Japanese people (Otsubo and Bartholomew 1998; Robertson 2002b).

Returning to the Japanese woman from the obstetrics viewpoint, her *performance* as a bearer of the future generation is at issue. As for the picture of the cooperative and persevering Japanese woman, her physical "smallness" is one more significant feature to bear in mind. While in other contexts feminist writers interpret the medical emphasis on monitoring weight as a way of subordinating pregnant women, turning them into docile Foucauldian-style bodies, here the cooperation and perseverance demanded of Japanese women can be also understood as the way practitioners expect women to "compensate" for their physiological shortcomings to their own benefit.

The image of the cooperative Japanese woman with the small body and diligent spirit makes special sense when situated in the theoretical framework represented by the key concept of *nanzan*, with which Kojima concludes his account. *Nanzan* conveys a range of meanings, far exceeding "difficult delivery." The nuances of *nanzan* are important, because the word is repeatedly used by practitioners to explain their cause, but also because of the *paradigm* that comes along with it. Dr. Kuromaki's narrative provides an example: "The patients who gain too much weight have, of course, more problems with everything. It is a dangerous, slippery slope. Excessive weight gain can lead to a myriad of pregnancy problems. They will have more problems with blood pressure, their probability of getting pregnancy toxemia increases considerably, not to speak of pregnancy diabetes. Pregnancy diabetes can lead to macrosomia, a baby that is too big and therefore too difficult to bear. So the probability of having a cesarean rises. Gaining too much is the way to *nanzan*."

Kuromaki's list of a variety of (familiar) pregnancy complications is thus enfolded in the concept of the problematic birth (*nanzan*). In his narrative, birth is part of the continuum of pregnancy, not a single event. Moreover, the process of pregnancy is not merely indicative of the kind of birth that will take place: excessive weight gain in pregnancy is seen as *leading* to a complicated birth.

Under the regime of this rather deterministic paradigm, not surprisingly *nanzan* has an antonym, *anzan*, literally a good and safe delivery. The idea of a "complicated birth" seems to frighten women and doctors; the "safe birth" is the vividly depicted script and the one to which they aspire. *Anzan* and *nanzan* seldom appear in Japanese obstetrics and gynecology textbooks but practitioners use them freely, especially when communicating with patients and often when they speak and write in the media.

One of the doctors, who edited the pregnancy magazine *Baroon*, defined *anzan* as follows: "What kind of thing is safe birth [*anzan*], for God's sake? Its primary definition is as follows: the baby is mature, it is not a baby that does not cry immediately after emerging from the womb, it is born without a problem [*buji ni*]. From the mother's point of view, a safe birth is one that goes lightly, easily, and then we can call it *koeru anzan* [a birth whose goodness endures postpartum]. This is the birth that everybody would like to have. So what shall we do to bring about such a nonproblematic [*buji*] safe birth?"

By this definition the dichotomous pair *nanzan–anzan* evaluates the mother's and the baby's state of health retrospectively, not just in respect to the relative difficulty of the delivery. The evaluation of the birth starts with the baby's well-being: the first parameter mentioned is the baby being mature. Being mature here should be understood in light of the concern with premature birth, which will be discussed latter. The baby demonstrates its robust health by crying (*oogya*) immediately after emerging from its mother's womb. Only after specifying the baby's condition does the focus shift to how the mother experienced the birth.

A practical question follows. "What can we *do* to bring about such an ideal birth?" The assumption is that obviously something can be done—neither fate nor genetics is responsible, only the pregnant woman. This idea, which has prevailed in most of the narratives explored so far, is stated explicitly and coherently in the narrative of the highly popular Dr. Ootsuma.

There is a saying that goes, "Birth is the borderline between heaven and hell." In ancient times the woman and the baby could lose their lives. Today we are talking about the difference between *anzan* and *nanzan*. The woman is the one who can determine whether it will take this or that direction. Birth is not something that happens suddenly out of the blue. A body that can give a good birth is a body that continuously [*zutto*] piles

up during pregnancy, without [the mother] giving up [*ki ga nukemasen*].
Maternity checkups are not free of charge, so from one visit to another
the mother should check herself, how much she has gained . . . and correct her daily conduct. . . . It's her ordeal, it's a shame [*dame*] to live an
idle life [*bôsuru*].

In my view this quote contains the essence of the orientation to the
frontstage on which Japanese prenatal care is organized. It emphasizes particular
relations of causality as *the* dynamic that is central to the process of pregnancy
and birth; the "inconclusive medical research findings regarding prenatal
recommendations" mentioned by Markens, Browner, and Press, who studied the
messages given to American women (Markens, Browner, and Press 1997, 367), are
barely hinted at. In fact the Japanese medical literature gives evidence of the
connection between weight gain and pregnancy outcomes (see, for example,
Takeda et al. 1992), and the importance of weight-gain supervision is asserted
explicitly in the guidelines of the Japanese association of practicing ob-gyns.
Note that Ootsuma's idea that pregnancy can be *either* heaven *or* hell, depending
on the mother, is expressed by an experienced practitioner, and that such representations are communicated to women unequivocally. This formulation of
gestation is grounded in ideas of continuity and interconnectedness. The process
of pregnancy is connected with birth, and the healthy progression of both is
connected with the woman's conduct of her daily life. The physical dimensions
of the body, the kind of birth this body can give, and the baby that will be born
are all connected. By this theory the woman has a central role as a potent agent
who has the power to determine success or failure in birth outcomes. Her agency
is grounded in the understanding of pregnancy and birth as needing human
assistance for a successful conclusion. Nature needs a helping hand from the
woman. The process of gestation cannot be left to happen "naturally" by itself if
we aim for *anzan* because not every *body* can give a good birth. A body that can
give a good birth is the result of the continuous hard work of "bodybuilding."

Here, too, we encounter a negative version of the pregnant Japanese
patient: the inactive patient who does "nothing" but merely "gaze" at her
pregnancy—an image found in colored illustrations in Japanese pregnancy
guides. One such picture opening a pregnancy guide conveys the "bad pregnant
woman" (as the captions read), who eats and drinks as much as she likes and
spends her time lazily (Utsumi 1996, 4–5). The negative depiction of "doing
nothing" highlights the features of the positive image. It suggests that the
cooperation that marks the positive image is about obedience, but also about
taking action. Secondly, the indifference that is criticized in the "gazing" of the
negative image points even to the scene of women crying, described earlier,
as a subplot enacted by the positive image who (unlike the "gazing" patient)
cares about her pregnancy.[6]

At least some of the texts written for women by doctors explicitly repress explanations that use genetics or disposition-oriented "excuses." For example, in the magazine quoted above readers are divided into twelve different dispositions (*taishitsu*) that might lead to a difficult birth. The writers emphasize that although a disposition is inborn, it can be changed if only the woman would mend her ways. Every disposition is described, and the woman is given detailed directions about precisely how she should change her everyday routine in order to transform herself into a woman who is disposed to giving birth safely (*anzan taishitsu*). For the "nervous type," ways to relax are offered; the "anemic type" should eat more vegetables; the "overtly socially conscious type" should learn to be more assertive and express her personal needs more clearly, etc. This attitude is characteristic of the medical discourse directed at pregnant women: it is very practical in nature, offering "solutions" (*kaiketsu*), advice (*adobaisu*) and strategies (*taisaku*) for each and every uneasiness (*fuan*) and problem (*mondai*)—but no excuses. So the expectation that pregnant patients will be cooperative also arises because in such a causal theory of gestation they are held physically responsible for pregnancy outcomes.

The "Environmental" Theory of Gestation

The Physical Environment

Having gone through some initial concerns of Japanese prenatal care, we must now add a crucial feature to the "portrait" of the pregnant Japanese patient. When ob-gyns speak about their pregnant patients, they alternate between "pregnant" (*ninpusan*) and mother (*okâsan*), an expression that I seldom heard in Israeli obstetrics and gynecology clinics, where doctors refer to pregnant *women*. Moreover, when referring to the body of the pregnant woman (for example, when explaining anatomical aspects of pregnancy), Japanese ob-gyns use the word *botai*, meaning a mother's body. In the same spirit they call the fetus a baby (*akachan*), especially when communicating with patients (when the word fetus [*taiji*] is hardly ever heard). Only in strictly professional contexts is it used.

These expressions, which I found throughout the Japanese prenatal realms, are not unique to the medical sphere but reflect much broader formal and legal discourses. Inasmuch as "the maternal body" (*botai*) is in medical use, the term is applied in legal texts: since 1996 the Japanese abortion law has been called the Maternal Body Protection Law (*Botai Hogo Hô*). The document used to record the medical monitoring of pregnancy is entitled *Mother–Child Health Handbook* [*boshikenkôtechô*]. According to Sato, this title has been in use since 1947 (Sato 1999, 64). Of special interest is the "mother–child" (*boshi*) part of the title. *Boshi* is the *kanji* compound of mother and child that forms a "mother–baby" integrated entity. The formal understanding of a pregnant woman as a mother who for now happens to have her baby inside her reaches its zenith in this concept. Such public and formal terminologies conceptualize the pregnant Japanese woman as a full-fledged mother, not a "mother-to-be" or an "expectant mother." Such conceptualizations are grounded in the physical body: once a woman has conceived, her body is presumably transformed into a mother's body (*botai*), as implied by how the abortion law presents itself as defending "the mother's body."

The *Mother–Child Health Handbook* is an official initial recognition of pregnancy. On her first prenatal visit, once the pregnancy has been "diagnosed," the patient is referred to the municipal national health insurance center to obtain the handbook. It contains recorded details of the pregnancy from the stages before inception through prenatal checkups up until the baby's third year. It registers all the checkups, vaccinations, and examinations of the mother–baby, based on the perceived unity of the bodies of mother and child. From an Israeli perspective, where typically one can never know whether the pregnancy will result in a healthy baby, such a medical file is unthinkable. Instead, Israeli mothers carry a "pregnancy monitoring card" (*cartis ma'akav herayon*) during gestation. Only on her discharge from the hospital, after a successful birth, will an Israeli mother receive a "vaccination card" (*cartis hisunim*) for the newborn baby.

In Japan, the conceptualization of the mother–child continuum is even reflected in the definition of the ob-gyn's domain of practice. If the patient is a "mother–child" entity, and if the role of the ob-gyn is to provide health care for this mother–child continuum, the role of the ob-gyn does not end abruptly once the baby is born. According to this logic, it is still customary in some hospitals for the mother's ob-gyn, not a pediatrician, to perform the routine four-week checkup on her newborn baby. This understanding of the range of practice certainly characterizes older doctors (over sixty) and "old-fashioned" clinics, but I also found it in some clinics run by younger doctors. This situation should not be surprising, considering that the ob-gyn's role is to take care of the mother–baby entity.

That pregnant women are conceived as "mother–baby" entities indeed clarifies the expectation that they will be thoroughly cooperative. However, in my view the most powerful thrust of the Japanese theories of gestation lies in the way they allocate *direct responsibility to the pregnant woman's body*. As will be shown, the mother is not merely "feeding the fetus" (Markens, Browner, and Press 1997): the relationship between her body and the unborn baby is more complex. Let us consider the images and metaphors that Dr. Ooyama, fifty-two, an ob-gyn who practices in a private clinic, uses to explain the mother's body:

> If you want to grow nice flowers, you need good soil—it's a more holistic thinking. . . . The roses at Hibiya Park are so beautiful. You know why? If you feel the earth, you realize that they are planted in very good soil. It is

just like when you plant a seed in the soil, and the seed grows up. . . . pregnancy is the same thing. This is how we see the sexual organs. The earth is the womb. The womb is the mother's body [botai], and therefore if you want to grow good trees, when the earth is not a good earth you cannot. Therefore, in the case of a bad earth you have to till it, to throw the stones out, and the weeds, to water it and nourish it. The mother's body has to be created . . . to create the proper environment for the baby.

"Environment" (kankyô) is a key term in the Japanese theory of gestation. The idea of a "maternal environment" is more complex than the "linear" idea that "anything you put in your mouth . . . will go to the baby" (Markens, Browner, and Press 1997, 358). Environments encapsulate and sustain life. They are ecosystems that provide food, but also shelter and warmth: they are holistic entities that imply the image of an (unborn) baby who is *totally* dependent on every single aspect of the maternal environment.

The "environmental" or ecosystemically oriented approach takes multiple aspects of living into account and sees them as interconnected. This might explain why Japanese obstetrics and gynecology textbooks devote more space to themes such as "postures for physical activity in daily life," which are taken up briefly in American textbooks but are absent entirely from the 1998 Hebrew textbook. In the same spirit, many Japanese textbooks teach that pregnant women should keep their bodies warm at all times, stabilize their bellies and protect them against bumps. Such instructions are absent from the Hebrew textbook, and I have never heard any mention of them in clinical circumstances in Israel. Israeli theories of gestation seem to regard fetuses as "safely insulated" in a womb that supplies constant thermal stability, regardless of environmental conditions outside the uterus. By the Israeli logic, the womb may be an environment but it is "automatically" managed by the body. In contrast, Japanese theories hold that it is the woman who manages it herself.

In the same vein, whereas Israeli doctors often pointed out that healthy babies can develop in the wombs of starved women, and rarely discussed nutrition with their patients, Japanese ob-gyns (those I interviewed, those who answered the questionnaire, and those who allowed me to observe them) all discussed the issue of balanced nutrition with their patients. Significantly the images in the above narrative are drawn from the world of agriculture, where nature is monitored, manipulated, and cultivated through hard work.

That components that make up the environment are all interconnected is obvious from the way that one can ask a question about food and be given an answer about heat. When I asked Dr. Takahashi, fifty-five, if he gave instructions on how to maintain weight, he said,

I used to teach maternity courses. I always emphasize the importance of not cooling the body. I say that this is forbidden, and I use kanpô for that.

Therefore I say, "Don't eat sweets because they cool the body." . . . Among foods that originate in tropical countries there are many fruits that are sweet and juicy, fruit that has a lot of liquid and sugar in it, and they cool a hot body. So people from tropical countries, even if they eat sweet things, the body cools down and it is good for them [chôdo ii]. But people from cold countries like Japan, if they eat the sweet foods typical of tropical countries . . . even during the Japanese summer . . . it is not good.

In this narrative the influence of East Asian medicine is explicit. As Takahashi explained to me, even though he is trained in Western medicine and therefore cannot practice *kanpô* himself, he refers women to its practitioners. As he stated several times, he believes that the "health or disease of a human being all start in what kind of food they consume." Therefore he makes sure to emphasize that counting calories is not enough: one must also eat healthy food like fruit and vegetables. Similarly he frowns on the idea of empty calories being consumed by eating Western sweets (*wagashi*) that are available in convenience stores. In the case of foreign food, even Western natural foods like fruit and vegetables do not necessarily create the proper "environment" for the pregnant Japanese woman, who should ideally consume food from her own "natural" environment, or in other words, Japanese products: "I always say, 'You should eat fruit and vegetables that grew on the same land you grew up on. All these Western sweets in the convenience store do not agree with the disposition of your body.' "

The proper "environment" for a pregnant woman is markedly Japanese. The theory of gestation may only be a specific case of an ecosystemically oriented paradigm of thinking, which sees people in general as being made of their environments. The Japanese are accordingly made of Japanese food, which is made of Japanese soil, air, and sunshine—all interconnected concentric spheres.

To conclude this discussion of the idea of the mother's body as an environment, it is illustrative to consider the word *ohukuro*, used to designate "mother" from the child's point of view. *Ohukuro* literally means a (respectable) bag. The fact that adult men use *ohukuro* when talking nostalgically and sympathetically about their mothers means that grown children still consider their mothers as their environment years later, despite being far removed from her body. Significantly, adult women, who may become somebody else's "bag," do not speak of their mothers as *ohukuro*.

The Mental Environment

The last but not the least aspect of the motherly "environment" that is seriously taken into consideration in the medical discourse is the mother's mental state of mind. I first encountered the idea of a "mental environment" in 1996, when

I participated for the first time as a pregnant woman in a maternity class in a large teaching hospital. At the end of the first lesson the nurses asked the women to introduce themselves. The nurse held up a placard specifying the categories that the participants were required to refer to on introducing themselves to the group. These were name, age, stage of pregnancy in months, and a category which read *shinkyô* but was unfamiliar to me. As it was clearly written on the placard, I could see that *shinkyô* was the *kanji* compound of "heart" and "environment." A quick search in my pocket dictionary seemed to confirm my guess by giving *shinkyô* as "state of mind." To my misfortune, the nurse picked me to be the first speaker. Arriving at the category of *shinkyô*, I just said that I felt fine. However, listening to the way other women elaborated on their *shinkyô* revealed the breadth and complexity of the concept.

Participants gave brief but complex and surprisingly sincere and revealing accounts of the physical conditions and mental quality of their everyday lives. They reported the kind of relationship they had with their husbands, and two said that they were very happy to be pregnant after long years of infertility. The women also stated if they worked out of the house, and if so, for how many hours; and whether they lived with their in-laws, their parents, or alone. They also voiced their worries and uneasiness about pregnancy, and concluded by hoping that the maternity class would provide an opportunity for them to relax from these mental tensions.

Some years later I was more than surprised to discover that the term shinkyô was routinely spoken in the most technical narratives of well-informed ob-gyns. Dr. Satô's statement about what he considered the most important "precept" to keep during pregnancy is one example. At the age of eighty-two, Satô is one of the most distinguished ob-gyns in the Japanese Society of Obstetrics and Gynecology. His favorite story is about how, as a young intern, he was called together with two senior obstetricians to assist the empress in giving birth to the crown prince (now the emperor). After a long, technical conversation, during which he specified his clinical standards, his preference for some prenatal examinations and his dislike of others, I asked him what he stresses the most in the prenatal care directives he gives to women who come to his clinic. Satô answered immediately,

The mother should keep a tranquil heart [*okâsan wa heiseina kokoro o tamotsu yôni*]—this is one thing I always say; the baby hears when you and your husband fight; if the mother is nervous [*iraira*] the baby feels it; and if you smoke it is very bad, so please, always listen to good music and keep a tranquil heart as much as you can. . . . Elevate yourself, be spiritual; even if you are not religious, pray that the baby will be healthy—this is what I emphasize the most. Stroke the baby from time to time, talk to it. . . . At the beginning I emphasize the prevention of infection, I tell them not to get close to people with measles, not to go out to places with bad air. I ask them to be careful about these things. And every time I speak a little bit more, for example, when you can see the heart beat [in ultrasound], when the baby becomes visible. . . . I don't have much time to speak about everything at one time, so every time I say something. I tell them, "Try to bring your husband, come on Saturday with him. Come together and see the baby. If you fight, the baby will not develop" [laughs]. Nutrition is very important, but tranquility of the heart is maybe more important. So, of course, taking walks, and not worrying and being in stress too much. I always used to put on music for the empress, so she had a lot of milk and the prince became a person who is very fond of music.

Satô's narrative illustrates the various techniques he uses to relax the pregnant woman and promote her and her husband's connection with the unborn baby. However, ultrasonography is only one of the techniques used to achieve a goal that actually predates its invention. Satô's theories of connectedness go back to 1933, when Prince Akihito was born, long before obstetrical ultrasound came into routine use. As I saw while sitting in his clinic, Satô is not content with preaching the philosophy of a tranquil heart to his patients, he also makes sure to put on relaxing music in his clinic's waiting room. Since I was already visibly pregnant with my third child when I spoke to him, he insisted on playing a relaxing song to my baby on his organ before I left. I suggest that Satô consciously sees himself and his waiting room as part of the environment with which the pregnant woman is surrounded. Therefore he plays his role in improving "his" part of the environment and contributes to her relaxation as much as he can.

Concern with the "mental environment" is in no way characteristic of older doctors alone: I found different versions of it among younger doctors as well. The clinical style of Professor Tadanori, forty-five, head of a maternity ward, can serve as one example. Tadanori was the only ob-gyn I interviewed who said that he tended not to bother women too much with monitoring their weight. He argued, "Being too strict is counterproductive, since the pregnant woman's mental environment would be damaged." Though he never skips weighing his patients, he rarely discusses their weight with them. His attitude exemplifies the "liberating prospects" that are in store for women in the concept of mental environment. On the other hand, emphasizing mental conditions rather than the physical environment, Tadanori strongly feels that working during gestation should be avoided as much as possible: "If she has a serious career maybe she cannot quit her job, but the stress is not good for her pregnancy. Stress is the worst thing. Or if she lives in economic hardship maybe there is nothing to be done. But if she works only for pocket money, to buy all kinds of accessories for herself, well I think this is unnecessary. In this case I don't see why she shouldn't quit her job. Why does she need all that stress? It's not worth it."

In undermining the value of women's work, Tadanori assesses the positive but mainly the negative aspects of work against the damage it may cause to women's pregnancies. While it is easy to interpret his statement as merely reflecting the patriarchal exclusion of women from the labor market, his insistence on the consequences of work for the state of health of women and fetuses should not be dismissed out of hand. I suggest that had he perceived the fetus as a strictly genetically predetermined being, he might not have formulated his objection to women's work that way. By contrast, pregnant women in Israel, a country where geneticist explanatory models predominate, are expected to work up until the last moment of gestation.

The concern with the mental condition of the pregnant woman adds to her portrait as an all-powerful motherly environment, in the physical and mental sense. The mother is involved in a complex set of physical and mental interactions with environmental factors, which are external to her body and mind, but through which she creates intrauterine environmental conditions. At the center of this "maternal environment" lies the unborn baby, a living creature that is totally dependent on its mother to sustain its health and life. For the sake of this "life," and in the name of causal theories of gestation, pregnant women are held responsible for reorganizing their relationship with the environment by entering a stage of physical and mental discipline.

Preserving Life

My analysis hitherto dealt with the way pregnancy should be "cared for" once achieved. Now I proceed to explore the practices and rhetoric that crystallize around the fear of losing it all together. Since premature babies contribute the most to the rate of perinatal mortality and morbidity worldwide, preventing preterm birth is currently a major concern in Japanese prenatal medicine as it is in Western countries. Despite advances in living standards, health care, and research, and the development of diagnostic and therapeutic technologies, the incidence of preterm birth has not declined; in fact, throughout the postindustrial world the numbers have steadily risen since the 1980s.[7]

In international medical literature premature birth is still considered a puzzle. Although the process of birth and the mechanism of contractions are largely understood, to this day scientists cannot explain what triggers the *onset* of contractions: a fundamental question to understanding both miscarriage and premature birth. Medical research has uncovered an array of problems that can lead to premature birth, which it defines as a "multifactorial phenomenon." Such models have not succeeded in predicting the onset of premature birth.

Moreover, once contractions start prematurely, it is extremely difficult to stop them. (Currently, the medications given to stop contractions are about as effective as the placebo). As one Israeli ob-gyn commented during a conference on the subject in Tel Aviv in 2002: "'Multifactorial' means that we practically don't know the reason and therefore cannot really treat premature birth."

Nevertheless, whereas Israeli ob-gyns tended to be quite skeptical about attempts to "predict" and "prevent" premature birth, many Japanese ob-gyns placed it at the top of their priorities. Five of them said explicitly that the prevention of premature birth is a "national mission." Dr. Yamazaki, mid-sixties, who practices at his home, said: "As you know, Japanese society is going through a process of graying. If Japanese women do not do *us* a favor and have more children, *we* will have a great problem. So we do every single thing that we can to preserve every single pregnancy" (emphasis added).

In Yamazaki's formulation, reproductive relations are explicitly understood as taking place between Japanese women and "us," the Japanese collective. This type of pro-natalism, which is motivated by the graying of society, echoes the statements of Yanagisawa, the minister of health cited in the historical introduction to this chapter, and is reflected in the distribution of research funding in the area of maternal and fetal health. The Japanese health ministry has provided extensive funding for research into premature birth, with the clear expectation that this will yield better practical strategies to lower the rates. At the beginning of the millennium Japan appears to be the best place in the world to give birth prematurely. Perinatal statistics and the Japanese ob-gyns I spoke to affirm that Japan holds a world record for survival of the youngest neonates (born within the twenty-second week of gestation) with the lowest birth weights (less than 500 grams). Morbidity rates of these neonates are claimed to be the lowest in the world (Kaneda 2007).

Professor Aoki was my key informant. He heads the maternity ward at a huge medical center in Saitama prefecture and holds top positions in the Japanese Association of Practicing Ob-Gyns and in the Association for Researchers in Obstetrics and Gynecology; he almost embodies the emphasis on the preservation of "life" in his career. Unlike top Israeli ob-gyns, whose expertise was in either fertility treatments or prenatal diagnosis, Professor Aoki, was an expert on the prediction and prevention of premature births. When I met him in 2000 he had already been directing ongoing research into the causes of preterm birth for the preceding twelve years. That he, too, perceived preterm birth as a "multifactorial phenomenon," like Israeli and other practitioners, had not stopped him from aspiring to prevent it: "We should simply discover all the possible causes and eliminate them one by one. If 60 percent of early miscarriages happen because of chorioamnionitis infections, of which 24.2 percent are intrauterine infections, 33.3 percent are polyp, bacterial vaginosis, and chlamydia, 3.5 percent are amniotic fluid infections, and

25.6 percent are cervical incompetence, something that can be repaired by surgery; so I believe that if we routinely check for them we can detect 60 percent of patients with infections, and if we treat the infections we may prevent at least 50 percent of miscarriages and preterm births."

Since the phenomenon is indeed multifactorial, the project of prevention is based on a strategy of eliminating all possible factors that may cause the problem. Most importantly for the present analysis, the practical implications of this preventive strategy are that routine vaginal examinations should be carried out on all pregnant women. Aoki advocates routine cervical and vaginal examinations, at least until the twentieth week of gestation, to detect dilation of the cervix or infection that might lead to a miscarriage, or later to a premature birth. He told me he sees it as his duty to "educate ob-gyns to do more vaginal examinations."

Currently, the vaginal examination is already performed in Japan as a "pregnancy test," that is, as part of the prenatal routine. Many of the pregnant women whose experiences are analyzed in the next chapter, including those who had seen an ob-gyn before becoming pregnant, encountered the internal examination for the first time only after they conceived. The data I collected show a variation in the number of vaginal examinations performed by different doctors. The minimal standard is once every two to three weeks during the first trimester of pregnancy until the twelfth week, and every week from the thirty-sixth week of gestation. Note that Japanese patients usually attend the first prenatal visit very close to conception, at about the fourth week of gestation. Therefore, a patient may be subjected to a minimum of eight vaginal examinations during a forty-week pregnancy. The maximum standard is to perform vaginal examination on each and every prenatal visit (the number of prenatal visits in an uncomplicated pregnancy is around fourteen).

This practice stands in sharp contrast to the attitudes of Israeli ob-gyns, who seemed to refrain as much as possible from vaginal examinations during pregnancy. Some of them argued that vaginal examinations cannot yield enough information to help the early prediction of preterm birth, and two practitioners even insisted that the test endangers the pregnancy by "pushing vaginal bacteria deeper into the cervix." Others, particularly those who worked with observant Jewish women, said that the potential of the examination to cause bleeding, and thus designate women as ritually impure and sexually inaccessible to their husbands, makes vaginal examinations very undesirable interventions for patients. However, many practitioners commented that they minimize the number of internal examinations to try to conform to the will of their patients, religious or not, who "particularly hate this test." In contrast, Japanese ob-gyns insisted on the high diagnostic and predictive value of the examination and could not see why the sterilized, gloved hand of the ob-gyn could in any way endanger the pregnancy.

The endeavor to prevent preterm birth by the state, with its pro-natal vision, is quite understandable. But what are the assumptions behind the general professional understanding of preterm birth and even miscarriage as *detectable* and *preventable?* These would be difficult to understand without the environmental theories about the "maternal body" and, more importantly, without prevailing assumptions about the docile Japanese pregnant patient.

Miscarriage and Premature Birth as "Environmental" Phenomena

According to the environmental logic explored above, typically problems that occur during pregnancy are (at least in part) due to inadequate management of the relationship between the mother and her environment. In Dr. Ootsuma's narrative, miscarriage and premature birth are no exception:

> Obviously the best thing for the baby is to stay in the womb for forty weeks. If the environment [*kankyô*] inside the womb is good, the baby will stay there. But if it is a bad environment the baby will not want to stay there. . . . The baby is like a parasitic plant on a tree, which takes its nutrition from the tree. But if the tree itself doesn't have anything left . . . when something is wrong with the big tree, it is always the parasite that falls off first. If the maternal body itself is weak for some reason, for example, the mother is working too much, or there is mentally too much stress, then the intrauterine environment becomes bad, and that is when it happens.
>
> When generally the intrauterine environment becomes bad, for example, the mother becomes terribly anemic and cannot nourish the baby (cannot give any more nutrition), when there is some disease in the liver or kidney or heart, when the body itself, the condition of the mother's body itself becomes bad—I think that is when premature birth occurs. The case of pregnancy toxemia is the same. And of course, when there is some infection.

As in the global medical literature, Ootsuma lists multiple factors that may cause premature birth. Yet significantly, her explanatory model is bound up with the concept of the "environment": again, the maternal environment is responsible for failing to "hold" the baby within it. And since the baby's environment is interrelated with multiple aspects of the mother's everyday conduct, her "working too much" may reasonably be suggested as making her womb an inadequate environment for the baby. Again, the mother's conduct can make a difference. So it may not be surprising to realize how far a patient is expected to persevere in order to avoid miscarriage and premature birth. The aforementioned Dr. Satô said so explicitly.

TSIPY: What is the risk you would most be interested in preventing?

SATÔ: Premature birth and premature babies, babies that are born with a very low birth weight. Pregnant women come to my clinic only until the eighth month, and the rest is for the next medical institution to take care of, but still this is what I am most worried about.

You see, there is the problem of traveling abroad; the woman wants to go and I am asked about it. So I tell her, "If for example you live to be eighty, the span of time that you carry a baby out of that is only two years. After the baby is born you may go, but while the baby is in your belly, if, just if, on the plane there was anything. . . . If it's a train you can get off, but you can't get off an airplane. If during the flight something went wrong, even if there was a doctor on the plane, you would have trouble anyway. And if the baby is born small, you will have to suffer until this baby grows bigger.

There are only about two years out of eighty that you will carry a baby, so devote yourself to the baby; the other seventy-eight are your freedom. But if you have to travel, by all means go to a hot spring close by. If you go somewhere close, even if something happens there are hospitals around. I say everything to prevent the baby from being born too early.

At this point, Satô started giving me a detailed account of the importance of cleanliness. One of his major concerns, he said, was infections of the amnion that may result in premature birth. Such infections were caused (among other things) by "impure sex" (*huketsuna sekkusu*). He concluded that the couple should be extremely cautious with hygiene, especially when it comes to sexual intercourse. "In fact," he added, "they should be especially cautious during the last trimester." He summed up his strategies for countering premature births thus: "Anyway, when I say persevere, endure [*gaman shinasai*] two years out of eighty everybody perseveres. In other words, you have only a few times. If you have a miscarriage and lose this baby you will be really sad and miserable. . . . And if they want to go abroad for their honeymoon, I tell them, 'Why don't you get married and go after the baby is born?' "

Satô succeeds in drawing women to what he considers an important cause by his skillful use of the notions of perseverance. He does this by channeling the woman's emotions and arousing her sentiments as a mother. The mother and the couple are expected to exercise perseverance to preserve the life of the child. This new life is conceived as being extremely fragile and needing careful preservation. The woman is supposed to be already thoroughly attached to this life, and to experience deep grief if she loses it. After all, she is having a baby, not just a fetus, and is expected to protect it as a mother. At first I tended to interpret Satô's recommendations as having something to do with his seniority. However, younger doctors had similar phobias about infection. One even suggested rather enviously that the ancient Japanese custom of *satogaeri*, of the wife going back to her natal home once pregnancy had been confirmed, must have prevented the problem of infection due to sexual relations altogether. This made me think that although Satô's recommendations seemed rare, his conception of pregnancy as being extremely fragile and his anxiety about its possible loss were not.

While perceiving the vaginal examination as having an important diagnostic value, doctors are also aware that for women it is still an unpleasantly intrusive procedure.[8] Nevertheless ob-gyns assume that as a mother, the pregnant woman will cooperate in subjecting her body to repeated vaginal examinations for her baby's sake. Dr. Kobayashi, forty-five, a practitioner working in a city hospital, said: "I explain to the patient in simple words [*wakariyasuku*] that this is a very important examination, and that we have to do it in order to rule out the possibility of infections and other problems that can lead to miscarriage and premature birth. And she doesn't want this happening to her, does she? I don't have much time, but I persuade her [*nattoku suru*] and then perform the examination."

Let us keep in mind Kobayashi's verbs of persuasion in his narrative, because none will be found in later sections that discuss the backstage issues of prenatal care. Such authoritative speech is preserved for issues enjoying general consensus: the *shared* understanding between patient and doctor that the patient "does not want a miscarriage (or premature birth) happening to her."

Why do Japanese ob-gyns tend to understand miscarriages and premature births as detectable and preventable? I suggest that first it is because they tend to identify these problems as lying in a maternal environmental frame; secondly, because they assume the mother's cooperation, that is, a "penetrable" and "restrictable" model of the pregnant patient. From a Foucauldian perspective, the treatment of pregnant Japanese women may serve as a classic example of the docile body under the regime of medical power/knowledge. Once women become pregnant, the medical grip on their bodies tightens. This grip is on their size and circumference, but also aims to make sure that their bodies are "sealed" and can keep the baby intact. This grip claims to secure the baby's health while acting on the "maternal environment," transforming it into a site where physical and mental control is legitimately exerted. This "microphysics" of the body cannot be fully understood without the maternal emotional posture that is assumed while the body is being turned into a "measurable," "restrictable" and "penetrable" object of biomedical science.

Negotiating PND

By now the reader will have sensed the gravity of the conceptual tension that PND tests—a set of technologies in which "the embryo and fetus come to be visualized as patient-like entities entirely or largely independent of the woman's body" (Lock 1998, 206)—introduce into a medical system that tends to emphasize the embodied mode of maternal responsibilities for fetal health. PND suggests that "errors" may occur even within the most perfectly nurtured "environment" and that not every "mother" will necessarily consider every "baby" worth nurturing. How PND tests are handled in medical practice, given such tensions, is a question that arises. In this respect, one salient aspect became clear during the early stages of fieldwork: the unequivocal authority with which doctors instructed women about the maintenance of their bodies was quickly replaced with hesitation when it came to PND. Moreover, my observations reveal that PND is practiced in Japanese medical institutions without clear rules and regulations. The most lucid statement on PND technology is the guidelines issued by the health ministry in 1999, saying that an ob-gyn has no obligation to inform the patient of the existence of the triple marker—the maternal blood test whose result is given in probabilities of carrying a child with a genetic or chromosomal abnormality, discussed in the previous chapter. Whereas in the United States and the United Kingdom (as well as in Israel) the triple marker is practiced as a routine second-trimester screening (Browner and Press 1995), in Japan the above guidelines institutionalize an ambiguous state of affairs in which the technology is available in medical institutions but with a formal lack of enthusiasm to use it. In the case of obstetrical ultrasound and amniocentesis, however, no clear guidance comes from the health ministry. Clearly, such guidelines are difficult to produce because, as some ob-gyns said explicitly, aborting a fetus because of an anomaly became illegal in 1996.

The Legal Framework of PND

The Maternal Body Protection Law (*Botai Hogo Hô*) of 1996, like its predecessor, requires the consent of a spouse as a condition (including people who are not registered as married but who are a couple *de facto*) and permits abortion on account of the mother's financial hardship or possible physical or mental damage to the mother due to the pregnancy, or if the mother has been raped. It does not include the list of physical and mental disorders covered by the earlier eugenic protection law. Instead, the introduction to the law states that "The articles of the former Eugenics Protection Law issued in Shôwa 23, which were aimed at preventing the birth of people with inferior heredity along with the protection of motherhood and health, were based on eugenic ideas of preventing the birth of bad descendants. These articles are offensive and discriminatory toward the disabled. Therefore, the regulations that are based on eugenic ideology are canceled, and the Maternal Body Protection Law is enacted instead" (*Kôshû Eisei Hôsoku* IV, 141).

Who is protected by the Maternal Body Protection Law? The law purports to protect the mother's body, but actually the right to life of (previously discriminated against) disabled persons (through protection of the mother's body) is ideologically shielded here. In fact the law ensures the protection of persons with disabilities *from* the "mother." Significantly, the focus on the "maternal" institutionalizes the understanding of pregnant women as mothers. The law puts forward the idea of women as mothers and mothers as bodies rather than women's reproductive choices and women's health. So rather than protecting the "mother's body," the law assigns it the mission of protecting the lives of those who are about to be born. Such expectations of the mother's body certainly fit well into the environmental model that ideally assigns the mother the (nonselective) somatic responsibility of nurturing life. Here, however, it is brought to a powerful climax by being highly politicized and loaded with the historical weight of postwar renunciation.

The prohibition by law since 1996 of abortions due to abnormalities in the fetus is indeed important for understanding the framework of PND.[9] However, also important to bear in mind is one aspect of the 1948 Eugenic Protection Law that was *never* contested in any debate about abortion in Japan. In the 1948 law, as in the Maternal Body Protection Law that replaced it, an abortion is defined as "the artificial discharge of a fetus and its appendages *during the period when the fetus cannot sustain life outside of the mother's body*" (emphasis added), a definition that none of the social actors in the Japanese abortion debates ever questioned.

Thus, gestational age when an abortion may be induced has fallen steadily throughout the postwar years, in keeping with the improvement in the rates of survival of ever younger premature neonates. Whereas until 1994 the law permitted abortion until the twenty-eighth week of gestation, the last version, issued in 1997, limits abortion to twenty-one weeks and six days.

Clearly, the law reflects formal concern with the preservation of life itself rather than with the "quality" of life. As practitioners explained to me, when medical techniques bettered the survival rates of premature neonates, and when they could present convincing statistical evidence that neonates were being saved at twenty-two weeks, the threshold dropped to the new survival frontier. This was regardless of the fact that the statistics also showed considerable rates of morbidity, which the surviving neonates had to live with for the rest of their lives. Sheer survival, that is, success in preserving life itself, was enough to draw the line earlier.

The importance of the maternal protection law for the present discussion lies in the way it practically "frames" clinical practice. Whereas various abnormalities are detectable only well after the twentieth week, the threshold of twenty-one weeks discourages their discovery considerably. So while Israeli practitioners, who are unconstrained by any threshold, pursue new diagnostic enterprises and improve detection rates deep into the third trimester of pregnancy, their Japanese counterparts told me that there is no point in trying to detect abnormalities after the twenty-second week.

Within the frame laid down by the maternal protection law, each medical institution sets its own guidelines. Even so, I found that ob-gyns do not always follow them. In the case of ultrasound, many ob-gyns screen pregnant women with each and every checkup, more often than instructed in the medical compass of their institution. The abundance of screening, I suggest below, is directly connected to the ways in which the diagnostic meaning of the screen is seldom communicated to the patient in any explicit way. Likewise, registration of ultrasound is absent from the mother–child health handbook. This omission is in contrast to the ample space designated for detailed registration of weight gain, height of uterus, circumference of belly (in centimeters), blood pressure, protein in urine (at every checkup), as well as the required blood tests. The ob-gyns whose daily work I observed never skipped one of the above checkups, and registered their measurements diligently in the mother–child health handbook, even though many were not sure about the diagnostic value of measuring the circumference of the belly, for example.

Divergence from the guidelines was also clear in the case of amniocentesis (although in the opposite direction from that of ultrasound). The guidelines of many institutions state that amniocentesis—known in Japan for its 1:300 rate of endangering the pregnancy—should be offered to patients above the age of thirty-five; in practice ob-gyns use a variety of age thresholds that do not always accord with the guidelines. Some practitioners take the age of thirty-five as their threshold and only raise the issue of PND with patients older than that. Some start between thirty-seven and forty, whereas other practitioners do not mention it at all to patients of any age.

This pattern, I suggest below, has to do with the explicit diagnostic purpose of amniocentesis, which is considerably more difficult to hide than ultrasound. Needless to say, no space in the mother–child health handbook is designated for the registration of amniocentesis (unlike in the Israeli medical record). As this brief overview suggests, it is not enough to account for the guidelines of medical practice; understanding the issues underpinning the ambiguity of PND in Japanese medical realms requires an account of the way the possibility of using these technologies is communicated to patients in the clinic.

"Reluctance"

I documented the following scene in January 2000 while in the office of Dr. Hayai, a prominent figure in the outpatient clinic of one university hospital in Tokyo and a key informant in my research. After two weeks of participant-observation in his clinic, I noticed that throughout this period he had not once raised the issue of PND, not even with women older than thirty-five. I took advantage of a three-minute break between patients and asked Dr. Hayai whether he discusses amniocentesis with patients. He bluntly answered: "I am a very direct person. I am not a typical Japanese. I tell the patient everything, directly and precisely, without hiding the facts. I give her the information, and she can decide with her partner by herself." (Then we heard the nurse calling on the loudspeaker to the next patient: "Takeda-san, Takeda Noriko-san.")

Takeda Noriko was a thirty-seven-year-old woman in the twelfth week of her first pregnancy. Dr. Hayai performed the whole sequence of routine tests. After she got dressed following a vaginal ultrasound, Dr. Hayai spoke to her quickly.

HAYAI: The baby is fine, I checked everything. The baby's heartbeat is perfectly clear. It moves its legs and hands vigorously, as you saw on the screen. Now there is one thing that I have to tell you. You are thirty-seven now. After the age of thirty-five there is a somewhat slightly higher probability of Down's syndrome and other chromosomal abnormalities to occur in the baby. Therefore if you are interested, there are some tests that can be done in order to evaluate your baby's chance of being affected. You can, for example, have an amniocentesis. I don't think it is a very complicated test. We insert a needle into your belly, take out a sample of the amniotic fluid, and examine it. If you are interested, the nurses at the desk will give you more information. But the baby is very healthy [genki].

PATIENT: I understand [wakarimashita].

HAYAI: However, your baby is perfectly healthy. Come again in three weeks, please; make an appointment at the nurse's desk. Your baby is perfectly O.K.

PATIENT: Thank you, doctor.

Takeda bowed slightly and stepped out of the room.

Dr. Hayai turned to me with a performer's smile and said decisively, "That's that. Now you saw how I do that." Hayai was clearly performing for me, showing off how tough and direct he is. Nevertheless, even from behind the dramaturgy of directness, he tried to soften the message to his patient by making sure that he told her three times that her baby is healthy, as if to assure her that he is only talking about a "slightly higher probability."[10] If she had been interested, she would have started inquiring about amniocentesis, he explained to me later. Hayai interpreted her response ("I understand") to mean "Thanks, I am not interested in discussing this any further," and that was the end of the discussion. I find this story highly illustrative of the state of mind within which not only amniocentesis but also other prenatal diagnostic technologies are communicated in many Japanese clinics, particularly because it marks the furthermost frontiers to which explicitness and directness can reach.

On the other extreme from Hayai lies the attitude of Dr. Shimazaki, who explained to me that "In Japan there is a serious problem about this—how much one should talk to the patient. What kind of phrasing to use. . . . If the doctor says, 'You'd better do this or other test,' she will probably do it. I think she will decide according to the manner of speech of the doctor. . . . I think that it is enough to communicate with the woman without mentioning it, assuming this is clear."

Shimazaki does not hide behind the nondirective idea that doctors "simply" give information for patients to decide by themselves. She is extremely aware of the effects of the information (even when phrased in terms of probabilities) and the immense influence a practitioner may exert on a patients' decisions by merely mentioning certain possibilities. (Interestingly, some of the pregnant women I interviewed explained that they did not consider PND since the doctor never mentioned it. I return to their accounts in the next chapter.) By contrast, it would be unthinkable for an ob-gyn to avoid weight-gain supervision, as patients are exposed to a wealth of information on that matter.

The attitudes of most of the ob-gyns whose work I observed lie somewhere between the attitudes of Hayai and Shimazaki. I found a range of strategies to raise the subject of PND.

To give another example, Dr. Tanaka, a fifty-year-old ob-gyn who works in a city hospital, stated,

> To women over thirty-five I say that the probability of chromosomal abnormalities rises slightly with age. But I never mention amniocentesis. I ask her whether she is interested in being checked at all. If she says she is, I ask whether she is interested in having a precise test. But usually I don't speak to her at all about the kind of testing that exists.

Dr. Terada, who raises the issue of PND only to patients older than thirty-seven years, makes sure to assure the woman: "You have nothing in you in particular, neither does your husband, to point out that something is wrong, and it is nobody's fault; but such disorders (in the fetus) can occur sometimes."

Whether speaking about probabilities becoming "a bit higher"—one strategy common to all my informants—not mentioning tests by their name, or assuring the woman that discussing PND was not an indication that she did something wrong, these doctors were trying to bring up the possibility of diagnosing fetal anomalies while couching the message in as soft a language as they could. Their strategies suggest that, rather than "pure" medical considerations, minimizing the anxiety of the patient is one of their major concerns. Indeed, when asked directly why they were so cautious, most ob-gyns explained their reluctance as a reaction to their patients' overall tendency to reject PND.

That physicians understand their own style of medical practice as a reaction to their patients' feelings and ideas rather than as a scientific imperative echoes Root and Browner's suggestion that "to some extent, biomedicine relies for its continued hegemony on women's faith in its tenets, both technological and moral" (2001, 209). Thus, if one wishes to understand the social management of these technologies, the important question becomes what doctors expect their patients to feel about PND.

Mother and Baby

One prominent emotion that ob-gyns expected their patients to feel if PND were to be mentioned was guilt. As Dr. Tanaka explained: "To 'commit' amniocentesis toward the baby, and then to abort . . . the mere thought itself is hard to bear. They don't want to think about it. They have guilt feelings towards the child. . . . Let's say they feel the weight of life. . . . That is why they cannot think calmly [reisei ni]."

Significantly, it is a fully fledged child in Tanaka's statement, not a fetus, toward whom the woman would feel guilty to the extent that she would find it hard to even consider PND. The guilt feelings toward the unborn baby echo the discourse that surrounds the cult of the aborted and miscarried fetus (mizuko kuyô).[11] However, rather than a specific consequence of the implied possibility of abortion, I see guilt as lurking everywhere throughout the continuum of childrearing as the negative side effect that comes with embodied maternal responsibilities. That mothers often hold themselves, and are often held, to blame for anything that might be wrong with the child comports with the professional and lay ecosystemic understanding of pregnancy.[12] Of most importance to bear in mind here is that embodied responsibilities are *formally* stretched way back into the most initial stages of pregnancy by the bureaucratic medical and legal discourse of botai and boshi, which defines pregnancy as motherhood as soon as possible. In fact, the idea of pregnant woman as mother seems to "color" prenatal care quite broadly. In the case of ultrasound, it seems almost to push the diagnostic meaning of the screening out of sight. As fifty two-year-old Dr. Ishii said, many doctors do ultrasound, conveying the feeling of "Oh, you have such a cute baby in there."

Taylor, whose research is based in the United States (1998), describes how ultrasound is carried out in the context of contradiction between its diagnostic purpose and its presumed role in enhancing maternal–fetal bonding. This contradictory message is captured in the way ultrasound is presented to women as a test to "reassure" them that the baby is healthy (Taylor 1998). In the Japanese arena, the word "assurance" is almost completely absent. The Japanese doctors whom I observed mainly communicated to their patients the "cuteness" (kawaii) and health (genki) of the baby and avoided giving any clue to their "hidden" intentions. Many doctors said that ultrasound is used by Japanese care providers as "a toy" (omocha) to "show the mother her baby" and has "low diagnostic value." Thus, the diagnostic meaning of ultrasound is often obscured from the patients in a way quite different from what Taylor described for the United States (1998).

That many doctors perform a screening on each and every checkup (this can easily amount to twelve screenings during a pregnancy), that ob-gyns give little albums for ultrasound pictures as presents to pregnant women, and that my pregnant informants were particularly fond of doctors who gave them many ultrasound pictures all suggest that ultrasound might also be used as a tool to gain popularity with mothers of unborn babies. Finally, one powerful aspect of the conception of pregnant women as mothers who are thoroughly bonded to their unborn babies is the way ob-gyns expect these "mothers" to interpret the "numbers"—the medical statistics about the rate of chromosomal anomalies as related to maternal age. Specifically, some doctors suggested that one reason why Japanese seem less enthusiastic about PND tests in general is that they are not as threatened by medical statistics on inborn abnormalities as patients elsewhere.

Probabilities in the Eyes of Pregnant Mothers

To judge by the tremendous prevalence of statistical censuses and their graphic presentations (pie and bar graphs) that overflow from Japanese daily newspapers, the concepts of probability and statistics seem to permeate every aspect of life as in many Western countries (see Hacking 1990); further, one would think that Japanese readers must be very familiar and especially fond of statistical data. Yet, my observations reveal that Japanese ob-gyns are particularly cautious when using this social idiom in communicating with patients.

As the accounts above have shown, Japanese doctors, like their Western counterparts, often mention probabilities when attempting to discuss PND with patients. However, they usually moderate the implications of these probabilities when communicating "risks." Dr. Tanaka suggested that Japanese patients tend to misunderstand the concept of probability, arguing that:

> In Japan the concept of probability is underdeveloped. I think it is normal that people cannot associate these figures with themselves. For example, if you say that there is a probability of 1:300 that the child will have Down syndrome, most people do not think that that has anything to do with them. . . . If you say [to the patients that] something is wrong with the baby, they will become alarmed, but if you say . . . the probability is one percent, then they will think that there is the 99 percent left, and our baby might be O.K. There is a 99 percent chance that the baby will be fine. It does not occur to them [*pin to detekonai*] that this 1 percent could be them.

It should be remembered that rather than conceptual "underdevelopment," there seems to be no contradiction between the interpretations of these patients and widespread theoretical understandings of probability. Indeed, a 1 percent risk means 99 percent nonrisk. In other words, those who tend to focus on the 1 percent chance that an anomaly will be discovered (e.g., my Israeli pregnant informants, who claimed that "even if chances to bear an anomalous child are 1:10,000, if this one is me, then for me it is 100 percent") and the Japanese, who tend to focus on the 99 percent chance that the fetus is healthy, are two equally adequate and complementary perspectives. The tendency to interpret probabilities on their optimistic side might be connected with the way it is presented to them as only "a bit higher." Optimism may be also largely connected with the manifold ways in which routine prenatal care socializes women into understanding fetal health as largely connected with the quality of their own bodily maintenance in terms of nutrition, weight gain, physical activity, and relaxed mental state. Thus, for a woman who does her best to provide top maintenance to her unborn baby, the possibility might seem less threatening.

Nevertheless, the following account by Dr. Wada gives almost an opposite perspective on the attitudes of bonded pregnant "mothers": it reminds us that not only is maternal optimism at play here, but also maternal anxieties. "Let us say that the probability of having a Down's baby is 1 in 300. The probability of having a miscarriage following amniocentesis is 3 in 1,000 patients. So their head spins, they get dizzy from the '3 in 1,000' chance, they say: 'Oh, such a dangerous test?' and consequently they don't do it."

Wada describes a process of weighing probabilities one against another in which the less probable scene tips the scales: for a bonded mother of an unborn child, the 3:1,000 chance of losing the child outweighs a 1:300 probability that this child would be born with Down's. The cognitive processing of information that he describes illustrates how ineffective the concept of probability is as an "objective" aid to decision making: reproductive "risks" are difficult to quantify. When contemplating issues of "risk" it should be born in mind that, unlike Israeli institutions, in many Japanese hospitals, patients who undergo amniocentesis are hospitalized and given antibiotics to prevent infections and undergo ultrasound scans every few hours to assure the vitality of the fetus following the test. Returning to the issue of probabilities, doctors themselves are not quite at ease with this concept either. As Dr. Tanaka pointed out: "In the case of the triple marker, the result is again only a probability, and people who are worried remain worried even if they have it. And therefore, if they are interested [in knowing whether the baby is healthy or not], we do amniocentesis directly."

Tanaka's statement reveals that not being able to give a definitive indication of fetal health situates him in an inconvenient place vis-à-vis the patient. Once the possibility of fetal anomaly surfaces, maternal optimism becomes unbearable worry that no statistics can mitigate. Neither can statistics supply a patient with a basis for taking any sort of decision.

This uneasiness with statistics was made explicit during the three-day discussions between representatives of the two powerful Japanese associations of ob-gyns that predated the issuing of guidance, exempting ob-gyns from the obligation to inform patients of the existence of the triple marker.

The account of Dr. Kojima, a forty-eight-year-old head of a maternity ward in a general city hospital who participated in the 1999 discussions, reveals the kind of issues raised by the participants.

> What the health ministry representatives said was that the producers of the test apply great pressure—they want to sell the test, but they don't provide adequate explanations. As you might know, the test was routinized in the U.S. in order to decrease the number of babies with Down syndrome in the population. . . . However, for the individual patient [the results] always remains at the level of probability. It is not a test that is done for the individual patient. The meaning of this test is not to find out whether the individual patient is carrying a baby with Down's or not, it is to decrease the number of abnormalities in the population at large. And the question is whether you, as an individual patient, are willing to cooperate in this project. . . . In the U.S. they do it as mass screening, but when it comes to the patient, the producer would not take the responsibility. The credibility of this test is very low, with a large false positive. So there was a discussion, and they decided that gynecologists are not obliged to inform patients about this test.

What stands out here, I think, is how carefully the Japanese professionals distinguish between the points of view of the individual patient and society at large in a way that might challenge the stereotypes of Japanese society as collectivist. They explicitly spoke about the concept of probability as an irresponsible and unreliable form of information. When challenging the meaning of "probability" and professional "responsibility," these professionals questioned some of the contemporary building blocks of medical knowledge and practice. Finally, the doctors framed their claims within a politically charged comparison between Japanese medical culture as they saw it and U.S. standards of practice. By viewing the U.S. routine as mass screening to promote selective population policies, these practitioners were formulating a cultural resistance to the triple marker. They were rejecting not only the test itself but also a system of values that they saw as its rationale. This cultural resistance is part of a more general attempt on the part of Japanese ob-gyns to dissociate themselves from ideologies that reigned during the years of World War II. Specifically, ob-gyns are ready to defy anything that echoes eugenics.

The Politics of Disability

In her rich ethnographic account of amniocentesis in the United States, Rayna Rapp shows how the incorporation of amniocentesis into prenatal care took place within two quite opposite and simultaneous streams of social and

scientific development: the move toward improving the rights and circumstances of people with disabilities in society, on the one hand, and the development of prenatal technologies to detect these very disabilities, on the other
(Rapp 1999). Her work encourages researchers to explore technologies of PND in
the interstices between disability politics and the development of the technologies themselves. The Japanese case illustrates the tensions created in this junc-
tion in a particular sociocultural-historical setting.

In fact, issues that touch on people with disabilities became particularly
charged during the second half of the twentieth century because many Japanese
came to identify them with a set of ideologies that led Japan to its historical collective traumas in World War II. These associations became once again vivid in
public awareness when, during a visit to a Fuchu care center in September 1999,
Ishihara Shintaro—the governor of Tokyo and an extreme nationalist—publicly
expressed shock when he encountered the severely mentally and physically
impaired recipients of care. He also implied his doubts concerning state support for people with disabilities (*Asahi Shimbun*, September 18, 1999, morning
edition). His statements prompted a soaring scandal throughout the Japanese
media in which Ishihara was widely condemned. That Ishihara is the same person who openly advocates annulling the postwar constitution to make the
emperor the head of the state and to return to Japan its right to defend itself
with a full-fledged military force once again articulated the association between
nationalist militarism and antagonism toward people with disabilities—in other
words, eugenic thinking.

In contrast to this rare public statement, there are images and narratives in
the Japanese media that generate a call to accept people with disabilities as
meaningful members of society. Oe Kenzaburo, the 1994 Nobel laureate in literature, is well known in Japan for his literary accounts of his relationship with his
mentally impaired son, who grew up to be a fairly successful musician. Oe's
A Personal Matter (1969) reveals a complex mixture of feelings toward his son
that culminates at some point in a (failed) plan to end his son's life.
Nevertheless, his book describes a process of reconciliation with his son's condition, in the course of which he comes to cherish and value his special attributes. Iwamoto Aya is a university graduate in English literature, who discovered
in her second year at university she had Down's syndrome. Her books, written
with her parents, have become best sellers; Hirotada Ototake is a best-selling
author and media star who was born without arms and legs. They and many
more people with disabilities who became public figures participate in the
widening public discourse about the importance of supporting people with disabilities and their meaningful contributions to society. Such public discourse
echoes in the accounts of some ob-gyns who claimed that not a few patients
would knowingly give birth to a baby with Down's syndrome, arguing that they
intend to "raise the baby beautifully." When speaking to these ob-gyns, I also

came across idealized descriptions of children with Down's syndrome as "good kids" who "never get angry."

However, even ob-gyns who saw the birth of a baby with Down's syndrome in less optimistic terms were not overtly active in offering PND. Dr. Kudô, a thirty-nine-year-old ob-gyn who heads a maternity ward in a city general hospital, made a rare claim when he said that "there is a possibility that if this baby is born it will be very unhappy, also the family, including their relatives, and therefore I do think it is important that the ob-gyn tries to find these abnormalities beforehand."

However, Kudô's narrative turned sharply when he explained to me why he himself approaches the subject hesitantly. As he continued: "It might be the same in any country, but there are already people who were born like this, and as an organization, a collective, they are offended by the very existence of these tests. They say, "Is it bad that we were born?" So the state cannot say, "There are inborn abnormalities, so let's approve tests to detect and prevent them." A state cannot make considerations of this kind, therefore they do not approve the tests."

Kudô turned to the considerations of the state at large to explain his own hesitation. This sharp twist illustrates how the Japanese politics of disability restricts medical discourse. Other ob-gyns spoke eloquently about the powerful pressures put on the Japanese government by disability movements that prevent it from subsidizing PND.

Finally, in many of these accounts, the discourse echoing the Japanese politics of disability was tempered by layers of cultural indexes of expression. Dr. Kojima's statement is one example. He said, "If a Down's baby is born, then what can we do about it [shô ganai]? A Down's baby is cute [kawaii], their IQ is relatively high. This way of looking at the situation is more prevalent. There is no general mood of "Let's get rid of the Down's baby. But of course there are things that cannot be said on the frontstage [omote]."

Kojima's use of the word omote indexes the first part of his statement—the discourse of acceptance about babies with Down's syndrome—as belonging to "the frontstage" [omote]. In his choice of words, Kojima is invoking a key organizing principle that is used in Japanese culture to make distinctions of language between social contexts (Bachnik and Quinn 1994). As a host of scholars have shown, Japanese are explicitly socialized into indexing social situations according to a set of distinctions between "inside" (uchi) and "outside" (soto) "front" (omote) and "rear" (ura) and "true feelings" (honne) and "formal expressions" (tatemae) to properly contextualize their gestures, language, content of speech, and display of emotions (Bachnik 1992; Tobin 1992).

What Kojima is attesting to here is a gap between the way people actually feel and what they feel is acceptable to say about people with disabilities. This gap is structured in the conjunction between a cultural indexing system and acceptable discourse shaped by collective historical traumas. Kojima's use of the term *omote* indexes a particular space between discourse and practice, complete with a plethora of cultural common knowledge items about how to maneuver within this space. For one thing, like other arenas in Japanese life in which a frontstage (*omote*) exists, there is always a backstage (*ura*) to complement and supplement it.

Practicing with Tied Hands

Informal statistics indicate that there is more than meets the eye in the Japanese arena of PND. Statistics from Kanagawa prefecture reveal that the overall number of children born with chromosomal abnormalities decreased during the 1980s and 1990s (*Asahi Shinbun* 1996). Indeed, practitioners who hold high positions were courageous enough to explain such statistics, admitting that, in practice, there is another side to Japanese prenatal care. Dr. Takita, the head of a maternity ward in a central city hospital, described the situation as follows: "In reality, prenatal testing exists and is performed to detect inborn abnormalities. And we do them assuming that if we detect something; there will be an abortion. The formally accepted [*tatemae*] reason for having an abortion is not because an abnormality was detected. But, in fact, families who do not want to see abnormalities will have an abortion if an abnormality is detected. For people who would never have an abortion even if an abnormality is detected, prenatal testing has no meaning. Therefore, those who are interested have already decided that if something is detected they will have an abortion."

From both this statement above and the Kanagawa statistics, it is clear that at least some patients are interested in preventing the birth of children with abnormalities and that at least some abortions are induced for these reasons in particular. However, expressing such wishes is constrained by a local politics of disability as well as by ecosystemic paradigms that render fetal health the result of maternal gestational work. Thus, for those who wish to use it, PND and selective abortions must be performed behind other formally acceptable narratives.

After my interview with Dr. Takita, I began asking practitioners: "What do you do when you actually detect an abnormality in the fetus?" I started by referring specifically to ultrasound scans. Younger practitioners or those who practice at their own private clinics typically said that because they are not ultrasound specialists, they would introduce the patient to the nearest university hospital to be diagnosed by such a specialist. However, ob-gyns who practice in university hospitals had no such escape. Their narratives tended to be more emotional and to sympathize with the patient. They spoke about "cooperation with the patient in a moment of distress." Dr. Kojima, for example, formulated the problem as follows: "It is the problem of [the gap between] true feelings [*honne*] and formal display [*tatemae*]. At the level of *tatemae* one cannot induce abortion because of an abnormality in the fetus, but the truth is that some people do it up to the twenty-second week. After that, I think it is extremely rare." Kojima told me how "the doctor has to sign a paper stating that there will be damage to the mother's body [*botai*], and then she can have an abortion, or that there is some mental or physical problem that may occur to the mother, or maybe a financial problem."

Although abortion because of fetal anomaly is forbidden by law, Kojima does not resort to illegality as a reason for his formal management of selective abortions. He understands the problem as lying within the tension between formal expressions and true feeling, conceptions that belong to the realm of emotions and their display. In his formulation, the problem is not whether selective abortion is legal or illegal, or ethically right or wrong; it is not even a question of whether such feelings are legitimate but, rather, one of whether personal feelings of resentment toward abnormal children may be displayed openly. Thus, being empathetic to emotions that cannot be expressed out loud, Kojima acts from behind an acceptable formal front. That the sorting of emotions into the social categories of *tatemae* and *honne* overlap the politically correct legal discourse is no coincidence. In any case, Kojima's account makes it clear that there are ways of avoiding giving birth to a disabled child in Japan. These are illegal and politically incorrect ways, nevertheless, they exist backstage in the prenatal theater.

Interlude: The Bells of Happiness

In November 2007 I went to Japan for the last time before completing this book. My explicit aim was to look for serious new challenges to my previous findings. I was looking for Japanese doctors who are overtly supportive of prenatal diagnosis, and for Japanese patients who were eager to pursue them. Dr. Yamamura's clinic—on whose Web site homepage amniocentesis was clearly recommended to women over forty—sounded like just the person I was looking for. For women over forty, it was clearly stated, the probability of bearing a child with Down's syndrome was higher than the probability of suffering miscarriage following the test, so it was entirely logical to undergo amniocentesis. But while sitting in the clinic's waiting room, painted in hues of pink, and being overwhelmed by the continuous cycle of background music—"Happy Birthday to You" (because someone is about to be born, as Dr. Yamamura explained)—I had second thoughts.

Still, in my first conversation with Yamamura he reiterated the statements on his homepage. Yamamura bluntly explained to me that in his view it was the "mother's right [*okâsama no kenri*] to know [what kind of child she is carrying], and therefore we offer her these tests." After our conversation Yamamura entrusted me to the care of Fujii-san, a woman in her early thirties who worked as an attendant in the clinic. Fujii-san showed me around what turned out to be an all-pink hospital. Not only were the walls painted pink, the sheets on the beds, and even the uniforms of nurses and other staff members were pink. Fujii-san went to great lengths to explain how the nutritionist guided the pregnant women, and how she planned the meals for women who were hospitalized after birth; she insisted that I taste the food to see for myself. When telling me about the different activities held in the hospital she repeatedly stressed how Yamamura emphasized to the pregnant women that pregnancy was childraising. Indeed Yamamura's habit of calling his pregnant patients *okâsama* (honorable mother) attracted my attention. My fascination reached a climax when Fujii invited me to participate in the short greeting ceremony held in the hospital for women a few days after they gave birth. Thus I joined the ten staff members who were gathering quietly near the door to a room on which was pinned a note saying, "Happy chorus." After knocking at the door and asking the new mother's permission, the staff members entered the tiny room and stood in two rows. Then the leader of the chorus read from a special card in a soft voice: "Takahashi-sama, congratulations." "Congratulations," recited the chorus after the leader. "We have a present for you from the staff," continued the leader in her soft voice, "Please listen." Then a tape playing background music was turned on and the whole chorus sang together while swaying from side to side: "Rin don, rin don, the sounds of the bells of happiness are being heard. Rin don, rin don they are carried by the fresh wind. The people of the world are sending words of joy and songs of happiness with these bells to you."

Then the leader read,

> To you who have become a mother.
>
> You, who were granted life by your parents, who grew up within an abundance of love, and who in the spring of life met the man you love, and this love has flourished and now you have become a mother. Until the birth of this child you overcame so many hurdles. We send you our heartfelt congratulations. The baby who has just been born, just like you, feels as if he is beginning to row in a huge ocean. But this is O.K.; the baby has taken the courage and power from this (your) hand that he is gripping, at being born. And like you he will be bringing a lot of happiness to many people. Please take good care of the life that has been entrusted to you. We pray for you and wish you a lot of happiness. From the staff of Yamamura clinic. Congratulations.

"Congratulations," repeated the chorus. The new mother was in tears by now, and the chorus participants, quietly and smilingly left the room, murmuring their fascination with the baby.

Later I gathered the courage to ask Dr. Yamamura how his many practices to encourage pregnant women to think of themselves as mothers accorded with his supportive ideas about prenatal diagnosis. Yamamura looked perplexed. He could not see a contradiction and simply repeated what he had told me about "the mother's right to know." "But if women undergo diagnosis," I insisted, "and learn that the child is seriously ill, don't you think that they might choose to have an abortion? Don't you feel there might be a tension between such choices and notions of motherhood?" "I don't understand" said Yamamura. "Don't mothers raise children with disabilities? What is the contradiction here?"

Ecosystemically Oriented Eugenics and the Embodied Mode of Responsibility

The findings presented here suggest that whereas Japanese pregnancies are at least as medicalized as those in many Western societies, medicalization seems to have taken a different direction, one less reliant on diagnostic technologies to select healthy fetuses (as described by Rapp [1999], Rothman [1986], and others) and more oriented to an ecosystemic understanding of the pregnant body as the creator of fetal health. Put differently, these ideas allocate much responsibility to the maternal body (Ivry 2007b).

Clearly, maternal responsibilities are formulated with local vocabularies of virtuous adulthood (heavily indexed by gender) and present themselves through local paradigms of thinking enmeshed in a specific reproductive politics. The idea of effort (*gambaru*) as a key to achievement and self-cultivation plays a central role in the way doctors perceive the range of influences that pregnant women can exercise over the process of gestation. The particularity of the idea of *gambaru* here is that it renders the body (of both the pregnant woman and of her fetus) as a designable and controllable entity by definition, and the woman herself as a powerful agent who can actively design it. This notion might seem more empowering for women, especially when compared with the limited amount of agency "allowed" them by genetic fatalism or socio-economic determinism. However, precisely this conception of the pregnant woman as a powerful somatic agent "legitimizes" the tightening of medical scrutiny on more aspects of her physical and mental everyday life.

The emphasis on the embodied mode of maternal responsibilities is no less concerned with fetal "quality" than is the geneticized Israeli version of prenatal care, but it echoes a way of eugenic thinking oriented differently. This thinking coincides with the gynocentric-oriented eugenic strategies to improve the environmental conditions of reproduction applied by prewar Japanese governments. Such strategies can be thought of as "ecosystemically oriented eugenics" since their explanatory models emphasize maternal bodies as ecosystems. The potential of these explanatory models to exert pressure on mothers should not be taken lightly.

Nevertheless, the range of prenatal diagnostic technologies that reverberate with genetic ideas in the same medical system cannot be ignored. One might expect that the presence of PND would make patients acutely aware of the contradictions between the notion of fetal health as an achievement of diligent maintenance of the pregnant woman's body and the genetic fatalism that lurks beneath PND. However, the caution with which ob-gyns approach the subject, and the 1996 Maternal Body Protection Law, which forbade abortions on account of fetal anomaly, make the endeavor to detect anomalies *in utero* highly ambiguous (Ivry 2006). Not that postdiagnostic abortions never occur in Japan; but they are done under the veil of secrecy and oblige the ob-gyn to declare an acceptable legal reason for abortion. Local reproductive politics positions PND not so much as a "reproductive choice" but as a politically incorrect backstage ambiguity. Though PND technologies are available in medical institutions, they remain expensive and morally illegitimate options, practiced under a formal lack of enthusiasm to use them, and they hardly affect the ideological prevalence of the ecosystemically oriented *gambaru*.

Whether PND transforms the experiences of Japanese women is to be discussed in the next chapter; however, the Japanese politics of reproduction have clearly transformed medical practice. The medical procedures around amniocentesis in Japanese institutions—hospitalization, the prescription of antibiotics to prevent infections, and ultrasound screening every few hours following the test to affirm fetal health—are considerably "heavier" than the two hours that Israeli women must sit in the waiting room following the same test before they are sent home. Underlying this cautiousness is the image of a pregnant mother without whom it is impossible to comprehend the sensitivities of medical practitioners and their patterns of practice. The exploration now moves to these mothers.

PART TWO

Experiencing Pregnancy

3

The Path of Bonding

The Cult of Domesticity

The official designation of motherhood as a woman's primary life mission, along with the promotion of a meticulous cult of domesticity, as historians point out (Nolte and Hastings 1991; Uno 1991), is a postwar phenomenon. The emphasis on mothering started to intensify at the turn of the nineteenth century along with Japan's efforts at industrialization, modernization, militarization, and colonization, only to solidify well after World War II with the emergence of urban middle-class nuclear families. So the ideal of domesticated motherhood, discussed at length by scholars in the second half of the twentieth century (Allison 1991, Borovoy 2005, Lebra 1984, Vogel 1978, White 1987, to list just a few prominent examples), echoed in the previous chapter and reverberating through this one, results from the continuous molding and rewriting of womanhood, concomitant with a dramatic and often traumatic shift in the gender and family system more generally. As Gail Bernstein states, "From the Tokugawa period and earlier to well into the twentieth century, womanhood was not primarily equated with motherhood, and motherhood was not necessarily defined biologically" (Bernstein 1991, 3).

In the Tokugawa period (1600–1868) prior to the forced opening of Japan, though women were expected to marry and bear children, it was their productive labor, skills of management, care of the elderly, and loyalty to the *ie*—the extended family unit where several generations living under one roof participated in production and reproduction as one economic unit—that were marked as their most significant attributes (Uno 1991).Though sons were necessary for the continuation of the household, adoption of sons-in-law and even married couples was rendered an acceptable solution when no sons or no committed and talented enough sons were available. Kathleen Uno describes a flexible division of labor particularly in rural families, which constituted the majority of the population. Since both productive and reproductive work was carried out in the domains of the household, men, women, and children alike participated in tasks of childrearing as well as production (Uno 1991, 25). Since women's productive work was vital for the maintenance and livelihood of the ordinary farm *ie*, other household members relieved women of child-rearing assignments so that they might engage in strenuous productive work.

In the higher echelons of society the picture was quite similar. Wives of high-ranking warriors employed servants, including full-time nursemaids, to do most of the child-rearing work in their households, while they engaged in the management of the household. Across social class the primary duty of a young wife was *not* child care. According to certain neo-Confucian popular ideas, "Women's extensive moral deficiencies made mothers ill suited for contact with impressionable children; thus childrearing assistance by siblings or in-laws in the lower classes and by servants in the upper classes would enable them to concentrate on other types of productive and reproductive work for the household" (Uno 1991, 30). Such ideas coincided with the "prevailing ethno-embryology, which is best described as male monogenesis, or the notion that the female body serves as a vessel to contain the active life-producing agent supplied by the male alone" (Robertson 2002b, 207).

Only with the eugenic campaigns of the Meiji period did explanations of sexual reproduction start to emphasize the equal contributions of female and male. Moreover, only after the 1868 Meiji Restoration did new political and economic policies create a new vision of Japanese womanhood that included motherhood: *ryôsai kenbô* (good wife–wise mother). Yet as Nolte and Hastings show, the slogan signaled women's compatibility to serve the nation *in part* through rearing loyal and patriotic children and converting the home into a public space, and in no way released them from their productive duties for nation-building. "By 1890 women had become the backbone of the developing Japanese industrial economy. Female workers outnumbered males in light industry, especially in textiles, where a workforce that was 60–90 percent females produced 40 percent of the gross national product and 60 percent of the foreign exchange during the late nineteenth century" (Nolte and Hastings 1991, 153).

The state policy that emerged in Japan between 1890 and 1910 was a "cult of productivity" and not a "cult of domesticity unlike western middle classes of the nineteenth century" (Nolte and Hastings 1991, 154), and governments praised not so much mothers but virtuous wives—women who were dedicated to their families and to the state (Nolte and Hastings 1991, 166). Even during the war years, when the government encouraged women to raise large families, it could not afford to forgo their productive contributions to the war effort (Miyake 1991, 269). These national discourses about the family, the home, and women's roles in society underwent profound change after Japan's defeat and its occupation by the Allied powers.

Japan's rush to rise from its ruins brought forth rapid industrialization which in turn impelled large numbers of citizens to leave the countryside for the cities. This urbanization process was accompanied by the nuclearization of families. Amidst the economic growth in the 1950s a stratum of middle-class families was starting to emerge with its markedly gendered division of roles. The men of the new middle class—called "salarymen" because of their salaries—were required to dedicate themselves fully to their work and were increasingly absent from home (Vogel 1963, 74); their devotion was rewarded by a salary that was enough to support the whole family.

"By the early 1960's," as Amy Borovoy writes, "for the first time in history, large numbers of middle class women could afford to become full-time housewives . . . as women increasingly took over the home and the reproduction of labor and human capital. . . . A cult of domesticity took root" (Borovoy 2005, 74). Yet Japanese notions of domesticity, as Borovoy argues, should not be confused with the notions of women's nonproductive dependency, with which domesticity was associated in the industrializing West at that time. Rather, "The Japanese state promoted the image of the domestic work as public service, and, furthermore, as 'rational,' modern work that is intimately linked to productivity in commercial sectors" (Borovoy 2001, 97).

In this spirit, the state together with the big enterprises actively solicited the "domestication of women; subsidizing women's stay-at-home work" (Borovoy 2005, 74). The Japanese pension and tax system is based on the assumption that the typical family comprises a working husband and a nonworking wife, and thus seeks to institutionalize a situation in which women become eligible for various benefits through their husbands' wages. Under the revised Pension Fund Law of 1986 (only a year after the Equal Employment Opportunity Law was promulgated), housewives became automatically eligible for retirement benefits under their husband's plans (Borovoy 2005, 75). According to the same logic, the taxing system makes it not worthwhile in many cases for married women to earn more than the equivalent of ten thousand dollars per year. In the same spirit, companies of various sizes inundate women with a wealth of incentives to become full-time housewives. Among them are monetary bonuses for those who choose to retire upon marriage or childbirth, as well as temporary unemployment benefits (Ogasawara 1998, 65). Even toward the end of the first decade of 2000 it is still quite safe to argue that the governmental wage and tax policies attempt to preserve the model of male as breadwinner and female as housewife (Molony 2005, 45).

The notions of motherhood as tender, emotional nurturance (rather than the mother as a disciplining agent of the paternalistic state) that emerged under the auspices of state-solicited domesticity described above was also tremendously appealing to the members of a society that was trying to renounce wartime ideologies and build a new democratic pacifist civil society (Borovoy 2005, 76; Yoda 2001).

A host of scholars have illumined the role that policy makers, psychologists, educators, media, and women themselves play in keeping the ideal of maternal domesticity intact, but women's experiences of pregnancy can shed light on the embodied aspects of socialization to ideas of motherhood, a perspective that remains largely uninvestigated. The complex biomedical cosmos that has been explored so far undoubtedly lends its scientific authority to the domestication of mothers, but it constitutes only one segment of the lived experiences of pregnancy. *How women themselves* make sense of their pregnant bodies within their complex life-worlds, saturated with social obligations, has to be grasped.

Prelude: A Contemporary Japanese Vocabulary of Pregnancy

Omedeta: literally, "I have been blessed," that is, "I have conceived."

Kodomo ga dekita: literally, "a child has been created," that is, "I have become pregnant."

Sazukatta inochi: literally, "the life that has been deposited in my care," that is, the fetus.

Taisetsuna karada: literally, "an important body," that is, the body of the pregnant woman.

Onaka no akachan: literally, "the baby in the belly," that is, the fetus.

How does pregnancy feel when it is formulated with such words?

The Woman in the Important Body

Morimura-san and I were sitting behind the counter on squeaky straw chairs in the small and colorful flower shop which she and her husband manage, when she angrily recalled scenes from her first pregnancy, three years before. She was twenty-eight at the time of the interview and pregnant for the second time. Her anger, however, had not subsided.

> When I was pregnant with my first daughter, I worked in a department store in a flower shop. She was born in August so I was carrying her during midsummer. . . . It was so hot I wore sandals and a miniskirt. All the women working at nearby counters were so noisy [*urusai*], they all said the same thing: "This is an important body [*daijina karada*], why aren't you wearing tights or stockings?" even though it was the sticky heat of midsummer!. . . They are not my mother—these ladies were nothing to me and they all said the same thing because they are all Japanese. "This is an important body, it is forbidden to chill it, you mustn't carry heavy

things, it is forbidden [dame]; you mustn't climb up the ladder, you mustn't stretch your body up high like that. . . ." But this was my work! I used to feel a lot of pressure because of this important body thing, and worry a lot.

Becoming pregnant in the everyday life-world of Japanese women means being redefined as an "important body" [taisetsuna/daijina karada]. As we shall see, however, it does not necessarily mean becoming an important somebody. That might be why for Morimura-san, "the rebel" as I called her here, who sees herself as an atypical Japanese, "the important body" symbolizes narrow-minded Japaneseness at work, attempts to "level the nail that is sticking out" [sasu kugi wo utsu] (i.e., herself), to suppress and tame her wild body into Foucauldian-style docility. I suggest, however, that the "important body" is not only about docility and discipline, but also about responsibility and maturity.

The verb daiji ni suru means treating something with caution. "Taking care of" [odaiji ni] is a common phrase that people often say to sick people, meaning "make your body important enough, take good care of it." Although women and doctors insist that pregnancy is not sickness, the importance of the pregnant body implies that at least some connection is made between them. The direct derivative of this importance is a long list of cautions. The moment a pregnancy is announced, people are ready with their unsolicited advice, including endless prohibitions, of which the above quotation represents only a part. That most of these unsolicited advisors do not have formal medical education does not seem to diminish the authority with which they impart their instructions.[1] Among the admonitions periodically encountered are that a pregnant woman should avoid breathing bad air, avoid excessively long journeys, not wear sleeveless clothing, not wear high heels, not eat salty foods, always be sure not to chill her pelvic area, and, therefore, always wear socks or stockings.

This list of dos and don'ts is not specific to any particular stage of pregnancy but is a collection prepared in advance to be "broadcast" to women as soon as they conceive. A pregnant woman is constantly being urged to reevaluate her treatment of her body regularly, and the reasoning often starts with the expression daijina karada. When I asked women to interpret the meaning of this expression, I received two kinds of answer. The first focused on the "content" of the body, as Suzuki-san, twenty-six, in the seventh month of her first pregnancy, said.

In Japanese, there is an expression: "being blessed with treasure-children" [kodakara ni megumareru]. It is generally an expression used by people who have children. "We are blessed with three child-treasures" is one example of how people use it. That is because since time immemorial children have been considered treasures. The bodies of women who are pregnant with a treasure are delicate. But the person herself forgets, and often acts contrarily [*muri suru*]. So the people around her remind her that "this is an important body: take care of it seriously." This is how I interpret it.

By this interpretation the body is important because it contains an important component, namely, the baby within. Suzuki's explanation is reminiscent of ancient Japanese idealized conceptions enfolded in words like *shikyū* (womb). *Shikyū* is the compound of *shi*, the kanji for children, and *kyū*, the kanji for shrine, a reference to the uterus as a children's shrine, thus turning children into little gods. However, Morimura, the rebel, concluded angrily that "it is an important body because it does not belong just to you: you are not the only one in your body."

The second explanation of the importance of the body was oriented to the sensual phenomenology of the pregnant body. Kurashige-san, twenty-seven, a secretary at an architect's office in the fifth month of her first pregnancy, described the pregnant body thus. "A pregnant body is a body which, compared with an ordinary body, cannot tolerate too much [*muri dekinai*]. For example, it is not good for such a body for the belly to harden and have contractions; it is not good if the belly starts to hurt; it is a sensitive body that cannot get along with, cannot get used to, being restricted too much [*muri suru*]."

Kurashige draws a profile of physical performance, a typification of the pregnant body. Using a detailed account of physical sensations she depicts a physically limited pregnant body. She is speaking on behalf of an entity that is *separate* from her, i.e., the body itself: the woman is literally *in* the body, a point that invites a dialogue with Emily Martin's work, to which I shall return later. Her description suggests that she is alert to her physical sensations, but also avails of a rich vocabulary to describe them. Though her experiences draw on later stages of pregnancy, when "the belly" [*onaka*] dominates a woman's sensations and appearance, Kurashige generalizes that the pregnant body is more sensitive and fragile than the "ordinary" nonpregnant body and should not be taken to its limits. The reason is that "the body cannot tolerate it." Other respondents to the question connected the body and the woman, and suggested that when the body cannot bear something, it causes suffering to the woman who dwells within it.

Kurashige-san went on to argue, "This is especially true during the first months, when the belly *doesn't* stick out. . . . It is not that you completely forget that you are pregnant, but rather that your consciousness is lower, and you move your body, you think you can climb up high places "just to get these files," but actually it is dangerous and you have to be careful. So people around you remind you that you are [have] an important body, that you have to be careful." Note the confusing notion of sensitivity in Kurashige's narratives. In her previous statement she concluded that the pregnant body is more sensitive, on the evidence of her detailed account of physical sensations. In the second part of her statement she perceives the sensitivity of the pregnant body as *inherent* to it and independent of what the woman may or may not feel: a state that the body enters at the moment of conception. The nature of this sensitivity may be problematic precisely because it may not necessarily alter the woman's physical sensations (at least not immediately); it lies clandestinely *in* the body. That the pregnant body is put under restriction, she suggests, is not necessarily because of physical inability to perform but because it can be easily damaged. Hayashi-san, thirty-two, a housewife in the sixth month of her second pregnancy, said, "There is the stress that can influence, but that cannot be seen with the eyes. This is the invisible stress that influences the physical condition [of the mother] and the baby."

That the pregnant body can be damaged by invisible causes makes the nature of vulnerability "open-ended." The notions of invisible dangers that one cannot necessarily physically sense or prevent quite naturally widen the range of anxiety. In these anxieties the practical power of the ethno-theories of the important body lie, for (as we shall see) they play a crucial role in shaping women's decisions.

Whereas women's explanations of the importance of the body alternated in different degrees between the vulnerability of the woman's body and the importance of the baby, the sharp conceptual separation of the body from the woman agent cut through the accounts. Significantly this separation occurs in a culture that is often conceptualized in opposition to the Judeo-Christian traditions of separation of mind and body. It is reflected in the way pregnant Japanese women are often asked, "Is your body OK?" [*karada ha daijôbu desuka?*] or "Is your stomach OK?" [*onaka ha daijôbu desuka?*] (which is equally focused on the actual body), rather than the common, "How are you?" [*ogenki desuka?*]. The conceptual separation of the agent from her body, as we shall see, strategically positions the body under her attentive care as she is expected to push away the myriad worst-case scenarios that local ethno-theories of gestation warn against.

Ethno-Theories of the Important Body

The ethno-theories of pregnancy that I shall introduce are not merely a collection of anxieties; they are explanatory models about how damage to the fetus can be caused. They do not rely on statistical evidence or systematic research, but this does not make them in any way less influential. Actually their importance is precisely in how they affect women's daily lives.

The prohibition against excess weight gain, to take one example, is one that enjoys medical support, but ethno-theories have their own explanations for the same dangers of which doctors strictly warn women. Tanaka-san, twenty-eight, mother of a five-month-old baby, explains the dangers of excess weight gain.

I was very careful not to gain too much weight; I supervised my own weight independently. If you gain too much, especially at the end, the cervix, the birth canal, becomes too narrow. It becomes too narrow for the baby to pass through it. I heard about women who pushed and pushed for ten hours, but their birth path was too narrow because they gained too much weight and their cervix became narrowed by the layers of fat. So they made an immense effort and in the end unfortunately there was no other way but to do a cesarean. So that was frightening, and I did my best not to gain too much. Consequently the birth was O.K.

Whereas the medical explanation in the previous chapter focused on babies that were too large to birth or the eruption of pregnancy toxemia, etc., Tanaka's explanation offers the imagery of the woman's internally fattened body, where layers of fat block the birth canal. While Tanaka's explanation and medical theory both associate excessive weight gain with difficult birth, the *dynamics* of how difficult birth occurs due to excessive weight gain are quite different. Significantly, however, these explanations converge.

Not all lay prohibitions have medical parallels. Let us explore a prohibition that doctors seldom mention: against using public transport in general and trains in particular. The following statement was made by Matsuo-san, thirty, mother of an eight-month-old baby. Her words are particularly interesting because she was about to graduate from nursing school when she became pregnant, so she is familiar with medical explanations.

MATSUO: I was already married for half a year . . . so I was glad to be pregnant, even though there were some difficulties. I had to pass the national nursing exam. So I had to commute to school; traveling by train was difficult, and I was worried all the time about having a miscarriage.

TSIPY: What does traveling by train have to do with having a miscarriage?

MATSUO: I read in a book somewhere that it is not good to spend a lot of time on trains, particularly during the first period of pregnancy, because it may cause a miscarriage, so I was really worried all the time. And besides, you hear it all the time, from so many people; it is *common knowledge*. . . But if you think about it there are enough pregnant women who travel by train, so maybe it is O.K. after all. . . I don't know, they say that the jerking movement of the trains is not good, that this is one of the causes of miscarriage.

TSIPY: The jerking movement of the train as a possible cause for miscarriage— is this based on medical knowledge?

MATSUO: I don't know. I guess Japanese doctors haven't really researched it . . . but as you know there are many kinds of books. Books on how to raise children, pregnancy guides, etc. This is the information that comes out of these books. But maybe one had better not pay attention to it. . . .

The "danger of jerking" made enough sense to Matsuo—enough to make her anxious, even though she was trained as a nurse and aware of the lack of medical grounds for this theory. Significantly, she quotes various guidebooks and lay people's warnings as sources of relevant information, just like the American women in Root and Browner's study (Root and Browner 2001). She doubts the importance of being cautious about trains, more because "enough pregnant women travel by train" than because no medical research exists on the subject. Medical explanations here do not seem to enjoy privileged status (as might be expected from hegemonic discourses). Popular materials and lay persons' advice seem to be just as powerful in generating potent anxieties and practical precautions.

The notion of "common knowledge" that Matsuo-san uses echoes Geertz's discussion of common sense. In his comparative study of Islam (1968), Geertz teaches that "common sense is not folk technology, it is not even folk knowledge, it is a frame of mind" (Geertz 1968, 93). In his analysis, science, like religion and ideology, stems from "a perception of the insufficiency of commonsense notions to the very task to which they are dedicated: making sense out of our experience" (Geertz 1968, 94). Matsuo's account suggests that ethno-theories, as well as the science of pregnancy that attempts to surpass them, are all governed by common sense. In her attempt to make sense of her experience and her anxieties, hegemonic and less hegemonic views seem to coexist, all drawing on the notion of the fragile body that must be supported, assisted, and stabilized to maintain a child. This makes medical theories and folk theories almost interchangeable for pregnant women. It also suggests that certain medical theories are acceptable and culturally useful in a certain society precisely because they can make sense of experience in a way that draws on local common sense and at the same time goes beyond it.

The idea that the jolting of a train is dangerous to pregnancy is a private case of a more general precaution against "violent movements and swings" (hageshi undô, hageshi shindô) which pregnancy guides and unsolicited advisors voice in a much more general sense. A humorous account of this idea appears in Tasty Birth (Oishii Shussan), an amusing pregnancy guide for working women that unfolds around the pregnancy experiences of the two writers (or, as they call themselves on the front cover, "child-making working sisters") (Taida and Miyai 1997). Miyai Shiena, one of the writers, illustrated herself walking to work suriashi-style (sliding the feet, without lifting them off the ground) and consequently arriving late. The writer hoped that walking that way would prevent her baby from "falling out" (Taida and Miyai 1997, 39).

Even more prominent are the prohibitions against "violent" sexual relations. In most guides the husband is asked to refrain from "violently" moving his penis inside his wife's body during coitus and to refrain from "deep penetration" (*fukai insato*). Israeli guides treat coitus during pregnancy as a technical problem of improving accessibility of the female sexual organ by "defeating" her protruding belly and accordingly offer technical solutions; Japanese books interpret coitus in pregnancy as dangerous almost by definition, primarily because it involves movement of the pelvis. Therefore Japanese guides include detailed prescriptions of proper positions, as well as meticulous prohibitions against dangerous positions, and other precautions to be taken for every stage of pregnancy. Sexual relations are also considered potentially problematic as they may cause a cooling of the body. Chilling the pelvic area is associated in folk medicine with infertility and miscarriage, and some guidebooks alert the husband to keeping his wife warm during sexual relations.

The *Haraobi* (a belly band which will be elaborated on later) is supposed to solve both problems in one action. Wrapping up the pelvic area with a long sash (*obi*) or a girdle (*hukutai*) is supposed to protect it from violent movements and swings, and to keep it warm. "What would happen if one did not wear a girdle?" I asked Koizumi-san, thirty-three, in the fourth month of her first pregnancy. She explained, "If you don't wear it the baby will not be *stable* enough." Many of my informants said that wrapping up the pelvis made them feel protected and secure (*anshinkan*).

The common denominator in the dangers of violent movements and cold is the assumption that *the body cannot handle the pregnant situation by itself; it needs help*. The body's "natural" capacities cannot keep the baby stable or warm enough. Eli-san, twenty-seven, a mother of two, offered a metaphor for pregnancy that sums up the ideas of the pregnant body discussed so far. "Pregnancy is like nesting eggs. The belly is like a big egg; it should be kept warm and hard. The shell of an egg is hard, but the stomach is soft, so we should protect it."

The image of nesting strikingly captures the ideas of nonmovement, retention of heat, and vulnerability that characterize Japanese ethno-theories of pregnancy; it is quite common in popular media. Eggs are also used as metaphors of "becoming" in Japanese: a mother-to-be is called a *tamago mama* (thus offering a double meaning: a mother who has not yet hatched and still resides in her egg, or a mother whose egg—pregnancy—has not hatched yet). The best-selling maternity magazine of the last decade is entitled *Tamago Kurabu*—literally, "eggs club"; this may well further attest to the importance of the egg metaphor for understanding pregnancy.

Returning to Eli's metaphorical entailment, her image of pregnancy as nesting equates human gestation taking place *inside* the body with a reproductive process that takes place *outside* it. The importance of this distinction is in the notion of vulnerability that it generates: eggs are inherently more vulnerable than in-utero fetuses. In fact Eli's metaphor renders pregnancy extremely vulnerable, as if it were an extra-somatic growth.

Invisible Bodies: Exclusion from the Public Sphere

Why are pregnant women well-nigh invisible in Japan? Or if visible, usually only in suburban neighborhoods? I argue that the invisibility of "important bodies" is a logical and practical derivative of the ethno-theories of pregnancy. This is exactly where the importance of these theories lies: in their far-reaching practical implications for women's lives. The most prominent effect is women's exclusion from the public sphere, in other words, their segregation inside the home.

The urban lower- to upper-middle-class women that I spoke to since 1996 have shown a clear tendency to quit their jobs when they found out that they are pregnant. Some left their jobs much before, even during the stages of *planning* a pregnancy. Women who took time to conceive told me that instead of getting involved in painful and costly fertility treatments they preferred to use a simpler and more efficient technique and to simply quit their job.

Public services for pregnant women in Japan seem to assume that they do not work outside the home. While birth-education courses in Israel are usually conducted during the evening hours (some centers even offer intensive workshops during weekends), in Japan maternity courses usually operate during the morning hours, which makes them difficult for pregnant working mothers, and for most husbands, to attend.

Whenever I would wonder about the connection between pregnancy and quitting their jobs, women would offer me explanations that at least partly located the reason *in* their body. Many mentioned the hardships of using public transportation. Twenty-eight-year-old Umeyama-san, who worked at a publishing company before she became pregnant, told me, "It is terrible to cope with the rush hour when you are nauseous, and the trains are dangerous for pregnancy, you know. Any way you look at it, it is hard [*taihen*] for pregnant women."

We are already familiar with the argument that sees jerky movements as dangerous for pregnancy; Umeyama, however, is more concerned with the physical difficulties of the nauseated mother. Some women simply said the reason for quitting once they had conceived was that their place of work was "too far away." However, even Ueda-san, who commuted to work by bicycle before she became pregnant, commented, "When I became pregnant, it became impossible to ride a bicycle, and therefore I could not get to work."

Other women reported that once *tsuwari* started they became technically unable to work. *Tsuwari* is what would be labeled in English "morning sickness," and the Hebrew expression means the same. However, the concept of *tsuwari* is significant because it is defined as an array of trans-temporal sensations. While the phrase "morning sickness" limits the "legitimate" definition of the sensation to the morning hours, the Japanese cultural image of first-trimester sensations allows a much broader range. *Tsuwari* are felt not only during the morning hours, and it does not just refer to vomiting. It includes headaches, tiredness, a generally unpleasant feeling, being oversensitive to certain smells, being unable to eat properly, and so on. It relates to the woman's *overall feeling* during the first trimester. Thus, while the concept of morning sickness sounds like a temporal sensation that one can overcome toward the afternoon hours (hence be able to get some work done), the concept of *tsuwari*, in its broadness and vagueness, makes sense of "paralysis-like" experiences, as in the following statement by twenty-nine-year-old Fujii-san, who worked as a school teacher: "Once *tsuwari* started I became unable to do anything. I felt so bad that I could not even think of working. I could not handle the physical and mental constraints of working. It was too hard for me physically and mentally."

The narratives of "surrendering" to the body are particularly interesting in the context of the Japanese culture of perseverance (*gambaru*) described in the previous chapter. *Gambaru*, the key concept of doing one's best in whatever one does (Hendry 1986, 83–84), may stand for various kinds of effort, ranging from the mental to the physical, but it is often associated with delaying physical needs. In his ethnography of Japanese preschools, Ben-Ari shows how educators teach children to embody the idea of *gambaru* through daily exercises in overcoming physical pain and mastering physical discomfort. He reminds us that even the "passive" forms of perseverance that are required of children (such as sitting and standing quietly) involve a "struggle with one's body" (Ben-Ari 1997, 85). Set against this background, it seems that pregnancy almost inverts the relationship between the body and the persevering self, and certainly changes the meaning of "trying as hard as possible." Pregnancy-perseverance refers instead to maintaining a disciplined lifestyle that *agrees* with the body. In this sense, quitting one's work to lead a life that agrees with the body is a pregnant version of *gambaru*, not of indulgence, as Israeli women would interpret it.

Returning to the hardships of traveling by public transport and the paralysis caused by *tsuwari*, the latter seem to be relatively "light" compared with arguments saying that work as such is unhealthy. Such was the argument of Sakai-san, twenty-nine, who left a very well-paid job as a personal secretary: "If you have to stand all day or sit all day and not change bodily position, the blood circulation becomes bad, and that is not good for pregnant mothers."

Moreover, women often interpreted their reproductive misfortunes as resulting from their working. As twenty-six-year-old Ooda-san said, "I quit my job because my physical condition was not good. I think that working is not good. The last time I was pregnant it ended up in a miscarriage. I miscarried my *first child*, and that happened because of stress and because I tired my body, which affected my first child badly." (emphasis added)

It is noticeable that Ooda considers her dead fetus her "first child," a point I shall return to later. Ougiuchi-san, thirty-one, mother of two, went still further in conveying the mental crisis that had followed her miscarriage. "The last time I was pregnant I kept on working, and then I had a miscarriage and stopped working. Now when I became pregnant, I thought that if anything happens I don't want to worry about work. I want to rest. I was really shocked by the miscarriage and for a while couldn't do anything."

Like many other interviewees, Ougiuchi and Ooda interpreted miscarriages, as well as other reproductive misfortunes such as premature birth and difficult deliveries, as directly associated with their continuing to work. In both cases, as with other interviewees, these experiences led to "repentant" behavior in subsequent pregnancies—in the form of quitting their jobs. These women explained their decisions by compounding the advice of medical practitioners with widely accepted etiologies and "common knowledge." Some of them formulated their claims against work in a pseudo-medical way. Tanaka-san, for example, thirty-three, mother of a three-month-old baby, put forward a quantitative argument: "There is a higher incidence of breach births among working women," thus pathologizing pregnant working women.

If working is not just hard for women but also the direct cause of various complications in their pregnancies, it might not be surprising that their foremost "prophylactic infertility treatment," should there be any uncertainty as to whether they are fertile or not, is to quit their jobs.

When I first met Nohira-san in 1995, she was a successful coordinator in a large computer company. At that time she expressed tremendous enthusiasm about her work. Six years later, at the age of thirty-seven, she was pregnant with her first child and had not been working for over eighteen months.

TSIPY: I was so surprised to find out that you had quit your job.

NOHIRA: . . . I worked hard until the age of thirty-five, and then. . . I felt I wanted a child. Then I thought that if I had a child in this condition, I would have to put it somewhere to keep on working like that. So there is no point to keep on working. I would quit and *get into my own pace, into the pace of housework, a pace that is proper for children. . .* So I stopped working, and there you are, I conceived [*kodomo ga dekita*]. We were not so sure we would be able to have a child [*kodomo o tsukuru*] so easily because of my age. (emphasis added)

Nohira's strategy "proved" efficient ("There you are: I conceived"), thus moving her into the self-affirmative circle of common knowledge, according to which she decided to quit her job. Her narrative echoes the social arrangements surrounding childcare, yet it is mixed with the idea that conception requires one to enter a totally different "mode of being" that "is proper for children." The very pace of the workplace is hazardous for conception.

So far we have explored the various dangers to the important body that lurk in working outside the home. The following statements suggest that an opposite threat also exists, namely, the one that the important body poses to the orderly management of the public sphere. Tsujioka-san, who became pregnant for the first time at the age of thirty-seven, recorded her body temperature (*kisotaion*) on a day-to-day basis and therefore knew that she was pregnant as soon as the fourth week.

TSIPY: Who did you tell about your pregnancy first?

TSUJIOKA: My colleagues and my boss at work. The moment I knew, I told them. If I became very sleepy and not able to work at the same pace I used to or I didn't feel well, they had to know in advance. They count on me to do the job. When you get morning sickness you become a burden [*meiwaku*] on your colleagues. Actually you become a burden until you enter the stable period [*anteiki*—the fifth month] when the *tsuwari* are supposed to ease off. So I thought that to minimize the inconvenience to the workplace I should tell them immediately. I told my parents only after I entered the stable period.

The criterion for Tsujioka's decision on the timing and order of announcing her pregnancy was the amount of inconvenience that her pregnant body would cause others. Since she saw her colleagues at work as those who would probably suffer the most, they were the first to be informed.

In a similar vein the writers of *Tasty Birth*—the guide for working pregnant women mentioned earlier, one of a number of guides that mark working pregnant women as a special category—suggest that certain steps should be taken by pregnant women before they take their maternity leave, to minimize the nuisance caused to their colleagues while they are absent.

Your body becomes heavy and your movements become sleepy [*nibui*] and slow, and a sweet smile fantasizing about how you are going to spend the precious time of maternity leave until the baby is born spreads on your face[2]. . . but here there is a confirmation to make—did you complete your duties at the office? Did you deal with the things on your desk and in your locker? Did you confirm who will be in charge of your things while you are away? Did you say goodbye to the people that had taken good care of you and helped you [*sewa ni natta*]?. . . If your desk stays as it is during your maternity leave, you should at least make a big note of where you can be reached at your home or parents' home during your leave, the date of your return, everything written very clearly, and stick it there. In addition you should hand a memo of these phone numbers to your colleagues. During your leave they might want to contact you or ask you something. . .

During your maternity leave, they are going to have to give your work to somebody else, aren't they? And that is a burden [*meiwaku*] don't you think? (Taida and Miyai 1997, 100–101)

When I asked Umeyama-san why women tend to leave their jobs on becoming pregnant, she said:

> At the company there are usually very few women who are similarly pregnant, it is a problem of social atmosphere. There is a majority of men, and the pregnant women do not feel very good if these men are careful with them [ki wo tsukau]. It is a problem of how one feels with it [kimochi no mondai]. I hate to become a burden [meiwaku] on my colleagues. It is better to get out of their way when I am in a situation where they have to go out of their way, to be so considerate of me all the time.

Umeyama's narrative embodies what I call the paradox of consideration. On the one hand, the important body (for various reasons) demands consideration. The woman carrying this body must be considerate of its limitations and attend to its special needs, as well as to the people around her. However, ideally she is expected, as general Japanese common sense has it, to be considerate of her colleagues, which means, in the context of the Japanese workplace, that she ought to save them from the burden of "forcing" them to be considerate simply due to her being present. In a way, her presence is too much to bear. Being present at the workplace means that one is fit. Those who are unfit had better relieve others of their presence.

The paradox of consideration is one that women who made the decision to work against all opinion also have to face. These women expressed deep gratitude to their colleagues for their understanding and the acceptance of their condition despite being such a nuisance to them. *Thus, a practical aspect of the important body is that, regardless of the stage of gestation, it is basically a nuisance. In the workplace in particular, it is a body out of context.*

Within the context of a mutual threat, where work is too demanding for the important body and its mere presence is too demanding for the workplace, many women draw the "logical" conclusion and completely abandon the idea of work. Moreover, women I spoke to in 2007 suggested that not all workplaces were at all willing to grant women maternity leave, still less a yearlong child-raising leave, and some refuse to keep their position open for them until after the leave. While few women spoke about explicit conflicts with their employers, a considerable number felt that the social circumstances of child raising forced them to leave their jobs. Umeyama-san sadly complained about the lack of facilities for working mothers. "After giving birth there are very few services for mothers; you really have to be lucky in order to be accepted by the municipal childcare center. Private facilities are so expensive that it is not worth it. . . . There are many women who would like to work but there are not enough facilities."

Umeyama concluded that there was no point in trying to keep working during her pregnancy when she already knew that she would not be able to return to work later. Some women's accounts, however, made me doubt that they really were *giving up* their jobs. Instead they suggested that work was meaningless for them. Sakai-san, twenty-six, who worked at a convenience store, admitted, "I worked just to kill time. Now I want to have an easygoing [*nonbiri*] lifestyle." Maeda-san, aged twenty-eight, who worked as a hairdresser in a beauty salon, said: "I wanted to try doing something other than work." Nohira-san represented the choice of not working as a privilege that comes with age. "When we were young we could not live without two incomes. Now when we are older, it is possible to live on just his income. I have been working hard [*gambaru*] for the last ten years, so I thought it was high time to stop for a while... When you become pregnant, it is not good for your body to be too busy. Now I can really afford not to work.

Moreover, the accounts of the majority of women who could economically afford to quit their jobs gave the impression that "quitting" or abandoning work was not the issue here; it was *replacing* or *changing* one full-time job for another. As Satô-san, a thirty-year-old mother of a new baby, explained, "I wanted to settle down and calmly concentrate on learning housework before I started raising children." Satô is explicit about mothering and housework as roles that require learning and practicing. Morimura-san, the florist, was worse off economically than other interviewees. She worked throughout her pregnancies and consequently faced continuous criticism. She put this critically and eloquently.

TSIPY: Why is it that many women who have no physical problems or morning sickness [*tsuwari*] quit their jobs when they become pregnant?

MORIMURA-SAN: They think that becoming a mother is a kind of a job, the job of raising children.

Morimura describes a social conception of pregnancy as active child raising [*kosodate*]: pregnant women leave their jobs because they become too busy raising their (unborn) children. Morimura's criticism reflects the advent of the "professional housewife" [*sengyô shufu*] (S. H. Vogel 1978) during the mid-1970s, who became the ideal model of the middle-class woman or wife of the middle-class worker [*salariiman*], who devotes herself to "provid[ing] a warm home for husband, children, and elders if necessary" (Rosenberger 2001, 16). Indeed in 1975 the rate of married women staying home as professional housewives reached its peak at 55 percent (Bando in Rosenberger, 2001, 16). Vogel suggests, "A home is defined as too unique and too personal to hire out part of mother's work... The mother is irreplaceable, her major responsibilities indivisible, and her daily schedule inflexible" (E. F. Vogel 1963, 185).

During the last two decades, more and more women have taken jobs outside the home. Nevertheless, the "M curve" of woman's employment, where women start working in their early twenties, stop working once they become married or pregnant, only to return ten years later after their children have completed primary school, is still in place at the beginning of the third millennium. Feminists and writers in the social sciences have elucidated the political meaning of the emergence of the "full-time housewife." As indicated above, the ideal of women as the main care providers is often represented as traditionally Japanese; but the emphasis on it is recent, originating in the early twentieth century, only a few decades after Commodore Perry's black ships forced Japan to open itself up to the West (G. L. Bernstein 1991). Secondly, the image of the full-time housewife providing her unpaid labor to her husband, her children, and other relatives, and thus exempting them from household chores so that they can devote themselves to work and study, was created as the backbone of the Japanese economic miracle (Ohinata 1995). These readings of the "M curve" emphasize the role of postwar governments in directing women into the private sphere of the home, but they do not explain why women themselves (although expressing ideas of gender equality) so often "slip" into total models of domestic mothering and become reluctant to pass responsibilities on to part-time maids and babysitters, or sometimes to their husbands (E. F. Vogel 1963, 185), a tendency that I observed throughout the fieldwork.

The accounts presented here suggest that *embodied* understandings play a role in making women "susceptible" to ideas about the irreplaceability and indivisibility of the mother's role from the initial stages of gestation. In this sense, pregnancy is a transformative experience through which women come to embody the understanding that they become physically unfit to work outside the home and physically and uniquely skilled to work within it. Through this "law of preservation" concerning "physical compatibility," the housewife's chores become indivisible because they are located *in* the constitution of her body.

While women may doubt whether housekeeping is a life that is satisfying or interesting enough to live, it is widely recognized that housekeeping and raising children are time and energy consuming.[3] As we shall see below, being pregnant in Japan has the potential to fill up the expectant mother's days with a myriad things to do.

Pregnancy as Parental Care

How can being pregnant possibly fill up a person's day-to-day life? What is there in it to *do*? The perspective of Israeli women, who tend to see pregnancy as a physical state they can hardly influence, may sharpen the cultural embeddedness of the conception of pregnancy as requiring active "doing." As one of my Israeli informants said, "Pregnancy just happens by itself: I do nothing for it, it just happens." Comparing the daily lives of Japanese and Israeli women, the former seem to be considerably "busier" with their pregnancies.

Just considering the number of times a Japanese woman is expected to see her ob-gyn during the forty weeks of an entirely uncomplicated pregnancy can give an idea how busy pregnancy can be.

According to the Japanese health ministry's regulations, women generally see their ob-gyns fourteen times during an uncomplicated pregnancy, that is, once every two or three weeks on average. This is significantly more than the five times prescribed by the Israeli Ministry of Health for women with similarly uncomplicated pregnancies. Moreover, Japanese women reported one to two hours of waiting before they could see the doctor. Recently, with the decline in the number of ob-gyns, and the closure of maternity services by peripheral hospitals, waiting time has lengthened. To give another example, while Israeli women generally attend one birth-education course, most of my Japanese interviewees attended at least two courses per pregnancy (some even more).

The above examples give an idea of the quantitative dimension of the task of being pregnant. These, however, are only the institutional framework for a large variety of demanding and energy-consuming daily practices through which a pregnant woman attempts to cultivate a moral pregnant self.

The "Bureaucrats" of the Body: Documenting Pregnancy

When I first started interviewing pregnant Japanese women and new mothers, I was impressed by the precision and accuracy of their accounts of their pregnancies. They remembered exact dates and countless tiny details. Most could say exactly when they found out they were pregnant and how much time passed before they went to see an ob-gyn. I soon realized that these crystal-clear memories were aided by written pregnancy "records" that many of the women kept. This happened when one of my first interviewees could not remember the exact date that she experienced *tsuwari* for the first time. She simply reached for a small booklet and browsed through it until she found the exact date. Extremely cooperative interviewees assumed that they were supposed to bring their pregnancy records with them, even without my mentioning it.

After I discovered this very serious and detailed form of documentation, I started asking women during interviews if they were keeping records or diaries of their pregnancies. Most replied, "No, I don't write down anything in particular," but I soon realized that most women actually did do some kind of "pregnancy writing"—they just did not seem to feel that they were doing anything special that deserved the title "pregnancy records." Most women started keeping records very soon after they realized they were pregnant.

Tsujioka-san, a busy Japanese language editor in a publishing company, told me: "I started keeping a record a week after I found out I was pregnant. And of course I summarized everything that happened during that week."

Tsujioka clearly thought that ideally documentation should start at the moment of discovery. Skipping a week was regrettable, and Tsujioka soon made up the omission. Women who could not manage to catch up felt uneasy about "the blank spaces" in their documents. While showing me her notebook, Sugimoto-san, the mother of a four-month-old baby, explained, "Here I felt very bad physically, so here there is a blank space for a while." What do these women record, and why?

The pregnancy records I came across can be generally divided into two categories: "body records" and "reflections." What I call "body records" are exemplified by Uchino-san's approach. "As you know, in the mother–child handbook [boshitechô: the medical record provided by municipalities early in pregnancy] there is space only for basic documentation. There is no place to write what I ate, finer measurements of weight gain, when I had bowel movements. This is what I record. After I eat a meal I quickly write in brief what I ate, just as a memo. I also write down physical exercises, when I went for a walk. It is not that I do any organized physical exercise regularly, I just move my body as much as I can."[4] In the course of our conversation I also discovered that Uchino has kept a record of the gifts she has received from relatives and friends in the same booklet, in order to repay them properly. When I asked her whether she also writes her reflections, or whether she had any plans to use these records after she has given birth, she said, "For me this is just a memo." Uchino, like many Japanese informants I talked to, does not consider her detailed monitoring of her body anything special. Moreover, Uchino's own record-keeping supplements the standard mother–child handbook that she finds insufficient. I find this dissatisfaction with the standard level of documentation highly significant, so I pause here to try to determine the significance of this dissatisfaction by taking a closer look at the handbook before proceeding to examine the wider culture of "reproductive documentation" that it simultaneously reflects and advocates.

The seventy-four-page mother–child handbook (discussed previously as a manifestation of bureaucratic perceptions of the "mother" and unborn "baby" as an integral entity) proves an intricate document that covers a broad array of aspects quite unusual for a medical record. It contains sections on the pregnant woman's medical history and a record of routine prenatal checkups (such as weight, urine, and blood pressure), but also an illustration of the teeth. Each tooth is marked with a number, and the woman is requested to fill in whether there is any decay or infection in any of them. Women are also required to answer questions designed to assess their physical and mental "environmental" conditions (the sections titled explicitly shinkyô—mental environment—and kankyô—physical environment), such as whether the woman works, and if she does, how many hours a day; how long it takes her to commute to work; what type of residence she lives in, and with whom. In the same spirit, the handbook also records the woman's moods. The last part consists of instructions and recommendations of the Ministry of Health on balanced nutrition and general directions on how women should conduct their daily lives in respect to work (including housework) and rest. Prevailing over the entire handbook is the multiplicity of graphs (weight gain during pregnancy, weight loss after delivery, height and weight of the neonate, the baby, and later the child), all of which women are expected to fill in.

By contrast, Israeli mothers first encounter similar practices of marking points on a weight chart only after their child is born. Even then, plotting the graph is part of the professional job of the nurse carried out at the national insurance family health centers (*tipat-halav*). The mothers who come with the babies for immunization manage to get a glimpse of these graphs over the nurse's shoulder, held in a file that is kept at the health center. In Japan, plotting such graphs is not considered the unique job of professionals, but is expected of every pregnant woman. Recording such a wide array of details in the mother–child handbook is consistent with the medical perception described in the previous chapter that sees "environmental" issues as important in the development of the pregnancy. Nevertheless, this specific version of medicalization relies on pregnant women playing a considerably more substantial role than Israeli women. The handbook is a written manifestation and symbol of *the shared responsibility of the mother and medical practitioners*: it is designed for both the mother and the practitioners to complete. That many interviewees felt a need to take even more detailed notes suggests that the enthusiastic participation of women in keeping records goes well beyond the biomedical arena. The way medical records are designed may well reflect a public inclination to document reproductive caretaking. In fact, the mother–child handbook can be seen as an attempt (on the part of health-care providers) to display a commitment to ultimate care.

Some women actually start to monitor their bodies well before conception. It is not rare for women who plan their pregnancies to use a technique called *kisotaion*, which monitors the ovulation cycle through daily measurements compiled on a graph. This is accomplished by recording the basal body temperature, and by charting the amount and quality of vaginal discharge on a graph. Women use a special "ladies' thermometer" that measures body temperature down to the second decimal point. The ladies' thermometer can be purchased from any pharmacy, and it comes with a grid to record daily measurements. *Kisotaion* (or *Ogino*, after the name of its founder) is in wide use in Japan, both in connection with contraception and as a method to identify fertile days in attempts to conceive, as other commentators on Japanese sexual culture have also pointed out (Coleman 1983; Hardacre 1997). In my observations at obstetrics and gynecology outpatient clinics in hospitals, I often saw patients who had come to see the doctor to confirm their pregnancies (because of irregular menstruation or infertility problems) carrying a graph that they had filled in for several months before making an appointment. Such compilations, however, were not demanded by the ob-gyn: the women had initiated the temperature measurements themselves when, for various reasons, they felt a need to monitor their bodies "to see what is happening."

Blank record sheets are considered suitable presents for pregnant women. In the same spirit, doctors often hand out little photo albums for keeping ultrasound printouts. They are typically designed as booklets, with rubrics for writing the date of screening, "the doctor's explanation," "your physical condition," and "reflections." Women who happened not to receive such albums went out and bought one. Pregnancy magazines offer "baby diaries" as little presents for their readers, all replete with daily tables (to specify the timing and amount of feeding, sleep, and diaper change). In sum, "body records" exist throughout Japanese spheres of reproduction, both as private enterprise and as standard medical practice, which only compels one to discover their cultural meaning.

While practices of body monitoring echo Foucault's account of modern mechanisms aimed at producing "docile bodies" (Foucault 1979), women's narrations of their documentations reveal a totally different picture. Awata-san, thirty-five, mother of a five-month-old baby, said, "When you regularly fill in the pages of the mother-child handbook it is really *very enjoyable*, you really *feel* how the baby is gradually being born [*umaretekuru*]. When you look at these records, you say, 'Oh good, Miyachan [the name she gave to the unborn baby] is so and so many grams already.' And then, after she is born and she is a few months old, it is really fun to look at it." (emphasis added)

What might be seen from an Israeli perspective as the burden of keeping records produces pleasant feelings and is perceived by Awata as enjoyable. For her, records of her pregnancy make a nice souvenir. They also make the baby's development more realistic.

Ueda-san, by contrast, felt she had been negligent. At first she said that she kept no record of her pregnancy. But later in our conversation I learnt that she used to stick daily memos of what she had eaten on her refrigerator with a magnet, and I was also shown the two graphs she kept in her handbook. One was the graph of ideal weight gain she had drawn at the beginning of her pregnancy, the other was the graph that she carefully plotted every two weeks throughout it. She told me, "Not everyone has the talent to write a diary, so even people who cannot do it by themselves can write using the mother-child handbook—you just fill in the pages. Not everyone is qualified to document all the details to do with having a baby. I am grateful for having the handbook."

Ueda, who described how excited she was when sent to obtain the handbook from the municipal authorities, sees it as a favor generously granted to her to help her compensate for her lack of skill in this regard. She assumes that ultimately every pregnant woman should aspire to record an account of her pregnancy in as much detail as possible. If "untalented" women "merely" fill in the standard records, then what do the records of "talented" women look like?

In the course of my fieldwork I came across some impressive pregnancy diaries that had been put together very diligently. Most combined body monitoring (weight gain and nutrition) with reflections about particular events. A few characteristics were common to all of the more "diligent" diaries. First, detailed entries were mainly written on the days of a pregnancy checkup. Secondly, ultrasound printouts were carefully attached to the diary with explanations of what were seen in them. Thirdly, little illustrations were often added to enhance the comprehensibility of what had been described in words or could be seen in the ultrasound printout. Fourthly, the theme explored by virtually all the entries was bodily and physical sensations, of the baby's or of the mother's body.

As an example, I quote one typical entry in Kurashige-san's diary. Twenty-seven years old and pregnant for the first time, Kurashige was one of the few women I met who worked until her eighth month and then took a child-raising vacation (*ikujikyūka*):

> This is the eleventh checkup. I usually come on Tuesday, but I am on vacation from work. Last week I felt I was getting edema. The people at work made a farewell birth party for me, so I ate out and the tiredness increased. So over the weekend I let myself rest a while. . . . The result was a great success. The edema disappeared, I had no protein in my urine, and I was even praised about my weight. But lately I haven't had any appetite. The whole area of my stomach is heavy, or should I say it hurts? I do feel sometimes that I am hungry but I feel like eating light meals, say cold things? But thinking that I should eat, I do my best to eat. . . In addition, I have pain where the belly protrudes from the pelvic bone. When I mentioned that to the doctor, she said that the uterus was getting so big that it was hard for the muscles to hold it and therefore they cramp up. I was a bit uneasy, and I thought that the skin would soon begin to "crack," so I have to buy some cream and massage a lot of it into the skin. . . . The baby now weighs 2170 grams and is fine. Today again the doctor said it is a girl. . . . I passed by to say hello to my workmates and they said that Iwada-san gave birth to a baby girl. They said the girl was 3000 grams at birth. It is really lovely that such a girl was born to skinny Iwada-san.
>
> My baby will also be here soon. Let's hold on [*gambare*]. . . . Today I had the fourth blood test. As usual I looked away when they did it. The nurse asked, "Are you all right?" and I was a little shy.

Kurashige-san had inserted a little illustration of her pelvic area to explain where she felt the pain exactly. She had also pasted the ultrasound printouts and interpreted them on the facing page. Kurashige evidently experiences her body through two mediums: her own sensations, and her encounters with the medical management of her body. In both, her body remains at the focal point of the documentation. I was very impressed with Kurashige's diary and tried to grasp what she had in mind as she wrote it. She told me "Some housewives have time on their hands, so they sew clothes for the (unborn) baby, but I do not have time. So this is all I can manage. I collect all the ultrasound pictures I can get. It is something you get for free, and then I write down how I felt and what I was thinking about at that time. When my child is old enough, I'll show it to him or her, and it will be enjoyable [tanoshii] and interesting."

First, Kurashige assures me that what I thought of as her diligent writing "is not enough": she should be doing more for the baby. In any case it is clear from her statement that she is writing the diary to share it with her child when she grows up. However, she did not share it with her husband. Moreover, she thinks that her own minute bodily sensations, not only fetal ultrasound pictures, will be of interest to her future child.

As in Kurashige's diary, in Tsujioka's account the body dominates.

TSIPY: What kind of things do you write in this document?

TSUJIOKA: What I ate; I write very simply, only the facts. Immediately after I found out I was pregnant the tsuwari started. And I. . . . I suffered, but while suffering I also thought, "Oh, how interesting, how interesting. . . ." To say interesting is a bit weird, but it was as if I was conducting an experiment. 'Today I vomited to the extent of vomiting fluids. Today I drank grapefruit juice and I brought it up again . . . Today I didn't eat a thing, only a cracker, and still the tsuwari were strong."

Tsujioka-san sounds like a classic anthropologist taking field notes. The objects of her observations are initially defined (and not as a post-fieldwork reflexive endeavor) as her own body and physical sensations. Tsujioka also experiences a common effect of fieldwork well known amongst anthropologists: estrangement and distance from her object of research. However, the object is her physical being, which imposes a kind of conscious separation between the woman and her body, to the extent that she can be fascinated by the same physical phenomena that are causing her to suffer.

Tsujioka's narration suggests a considerably more positive version of the estrangement of women from their bodies than anthropological accounts to date. In her trailblazing book *The Woman in the Body*, Emily Martin describes the resentful emotional reactions of women who were alienated from their reproductive bodies by medical routines (Martin 1987). By contrast, pregnant Japanese women apparently experience themselves as separate from their bodies but not necessarily in an alienating or negative way. In the Japanese case, separation between a woman and her body is more instrumental and promotes sensitivity to the body.

The culture of documentation of minute bodily sensations and functions can be understood against the background of a literary cultural tradition of

meticulous, snapshot-style documentations.[5] However, the kind of documentation found here is closer to the one described in Ben-Ari's accounts of the
bureaucracy of preschool child care (Ben-Ari 1997). I suggest that the charting of
pregnant bodies can be seen as an introduction to the detailed record keeping
of children in later stages of parenting, when mothers and educators chart
"such matters as eating and sleeping habits" (Ben-Ari 1997, 123). As Ben-Ari
teaches us, charting is an aspect of caregiving. So while the charting practices of
pregnant Japanese women may give the impression that they are the bureau-
crats of pregnancy or the subcontractors of their ob-gyns, to use Ben-Ari's
terminology (Ben-Ari 1990), these same practices define them simultaneously
as care providers.

When asked whether they kept diaries at other stages of life, none of my
informants, not even the most diligent record keepers, said that they did. All of
them said that the first time that they decided to keep proper [*chantô shita*] documentation was when they became pregnant: entering the realm of reproduction triggered the need to keep records of their bodies. Significantly, the
accounts of record keeping presented thus far—to ensure a moderate rate of
weight gain; to experience the gradual development of the child in the womb;
as an enjoyable souvenir that can be shown to the child once he or she is old
enough to understand it—illuminate pregnancy as a process of becoming a care
provider. To bring out this point fully, it is necessary to explore the relationship
between the pregnant "mother" and a powerful protagonist in the drama of
pregnancy: the baby, that is, the being to whom the care is given.

The Baby

During the course of fieldwork, a friend introduced me to a Japanese anthropologist engaged in interviewing pregnant Japanese women. My association with
her developed rapidly, and soon we were exchanging information and ideas. She
was very interested in finding out about what pregnancy was like in Israel. In
one of her e-mails she asked me, "When Israeli women speak to their (unborn)
babies, what kinds of things do they say?" She took it for granted that pregnant
women spoke regularly to their unborn babies; the cultural variation would lie
in what they say. My answer struck her as inconceivable: few of the Israeli
women I interviewed or the many more I met spoke to their "babies" regularly.
From a Japanese point of view, there was nothing she could do but try to explain
this enigma as a problem in my research method.

Indeed, Japanese women seemed to be devoted to daily "communication"
with their (unborn) babies. Many invented a name for their baby and called it
by that name. Most women said that they started soon after they realized they
were pregnant, and that communication became stronger and more "mutual"
as the pregnancy progressed. Or, as Takakura-san concluded while smilingly
embracing her two-month-old son: "I have communicated with him from the

moment I realized he existed to this day." What do women say to their babies? Ueda-san, thirty, mother of a four-month-old baby, said, "I used to say very simple things. I would go out for a walk and tell him what I see. 'Oh, here is a nice tree with green leaves, and this noise comes from the road. Don't be afraid.'"

Rather than merely informative descriptions of the outside world, Ueda's words reflect a developed set of human relations endowed with maternal commitment: she intends to comfort and soothe her baby. By contrast, as I show in the next chapter dealing with pregnant Israeli women, the Israeli fetus remains an ambiguous being throughout gestation. Only after the birth process has come to an end, and the baby has proved itself alive, healthy, and visibly separate from the mother's body, does the mother start communicating with it seriously. Unlike the Israeli fetus, the Japanese baby is communicated with even when the mother has doubts about its health. Satô-san, for example, communicated with her baby under the threat of miscarriage. "At first I had bleeding from a lump outside the womb. This bleeding had nothing to do with the pregnancy, but to begin with I didn't know that. I was afraid it was the beginning of a miscarriage. So I would ask the baby, 'Oh [ara, ara], there was bleeding you know. Are you O.K.? Hold on there [gambatte].' I used to say many things to him, like 'Come out healthy' [genkide dekite]."

Thus Satô talked her baby out of death. Much like the issue of pregnancy documentation, most of the women I met did not feel that they were doing anything special. Women told me that they "just shared their everyday experiences with the baby."

As I slowly realized, women underestimated these forms of behavior, not because they cost them no effort but because they measured them against the "social scripts of ultimate bonding" that are prevalent in popular representations of pregnancy. These representations all share the tendency to go out of their way to construct the fetus as a full-fledged baby by representing it in the most tangible and realistic way possible. A best-selling Japanese pregnancy guide, published in 1998, makes this point explicitly. "The baby's gradual development through the process of ten months from the moment life sprouted in you until birth is presented in life-size illustrations and accompanied by ultrasound pictures.[6] You can understand the size and condition of the baby as if you could hold her in your arms, and therefore as you turn the pages your thoughts of love toward your baby will increase" (Baroon 1998, 6).

Although pregnancy guides form one part of a plethora of popular texts and segments of knowledge about pregnancy (provided by medical practitioners as well as female friends and relatives), the role they play in the life-worlds of pregnant women cannot be underestimated. Since pregnancy has become a "reading assignment" for many women in Japan, as in Western countries, women often make sure to purchase guides or get them from friends, and they read parts or all of them for a range of purposes.

Takahashi-san, a twenty-three-year-old mother of two, explained to me how she sometimes uses guides as substitutes for medical consultation. She said: "The appointment with the doctor is so short, and sometimes there is no time to ask all that you want to ask. So I try the books." All the women I interviewed in their own homes had a little library of pregnancy guides and magazines. Whether pregnancy guides "shape" or "reflect" women's pregnancy conceptions is a difficult question. My analysis tries somehow to bypass this difficult question by focusing only on the parts of best-selling guides that informants mentioned as meaningful to their experiences of pregnancy.

An overall reading of fifteen different Japanese pregnancy guides published over a span of seven years (recommended by interviewees) gave me the impression that these guides can be understood as containing an inherent conceptual tension. They assume the mission of giving practical information to women while contributing to the improvement of their mental environment (*shinkyô*). For example, it is most undesirable to startle a pregnant woman, even a tiny bit. Therefore, guides minimize discussions of the prenatal diagnosis of genetic and chromosomal disorders and try to generate a positive atmosphere. One of the strategies adopted by guides to elevate the mood of their pregnant readers is to emphasize and animate the presence of the "cute" baby.

Just browsing through Japanese pregnancy guidebooks gives a strong visual impression of the baby's presence. Babies peep out of the pages, all pink and cute, as if they have already been born. The purpose of this animation is stated very openly: the writers want to endear the baby to the mother so that (as cited above) "as you turn the pages your thoughts of love toward the baby will increase." In other words, the writers see their role as helping mothers develop prenatal bonding with the (unborn) baby.

To give an idea of the intensity and far reach of this animation project, let us consider how Japanese guides "translate" ultrasound pictures of fetuses for readers. The picture of a fetus sucking his/her thumb is common to most guides in both Israel and Japan. The caption in one Israeli best seller reads: "Already in the womb, a fetus sucking his thumb" (Ber and Rosin 1998, 208). The Japanese caption reads: "I wonder how mommy's breasts taste" (Baroon 1998, 11). Significantly, the Japanese title gives voice to the baby. While the Israeli fetus remains a remote and abstract entity generated by biotechnology, the unborn Japanese baby "jumps out of the picture," his or her voice already fully equipped to express human sensations and awareness of the body within which the baby dwells. This is not an abstract body: the baby recognizes it as the *mother's* body. The baby is depicted as already bonded with the pregnant mother, and, as we shall see, has yearnings for her. The writers did not stop at this: under the above caption the "mother" is quoted as saying: "Is [the baby] already practicing sucking at the breast? Oh I guess [it] is hungry" (Baroon 1998, 11). Clearly the guide features an instance of communication. Petchesky-Pollack, Rothman, and others have noted that obstetrical ultrasound has worked to individualize the fetus while rendering the mother an "outer black space" (Petchesky-Pollack 1987; Rothman 1986), but here the authors find ways to overcome the "blindness" of obstetrical ultrasound and convey the mother through the texts and captions that surround the ultrasound picture.

Interestingly, in Japanese medical institutions women "stay in the room," which is fully illuminated, when receiving ultrasound scans; by contrast Israeli ob-gyns screen in darkened rooms. This reminds one that the symbolic "nullification" of the pregnant woman is not an inevitable feature of the technology of obstetrical ultrasound: sophisticated use of space and props is required to make the darkness in which the fetal image floats on the screen harmonize with the darkness in the room. In the Japanese case, since mother and unborn baby are mutually constituted, the woman's presence is a primary condition for the project of animating the fetus. Put differently, the mother must be available if interconnectedness and communication are to be achieved between her and the unborn baby who "tries" to catch her attention.

The following citations are the captions of a series of ultrasound pictures featuring the development of the baby in the womb during the ten months of gestation.

[First to second months]: "Mama, pay attention, I am already in your belly!" (Baroon 1998, 8)

[Third month]: "*Pukkari puka puka:*[7] What an enjoyable everyday life!" (Baroon 1998, 9)

[Fourth month]: "Hey, look at me, I have become really baby-like!" (Baroon 1998, 10)

[Fifth month]: "I hit *ton ton*;[8] Mommy, do you recognize me?" (Baroon 1998, 11)

[Sixth month]: "How enjoyable; I turn around and kick!" (Baroon 1998, 12)

[Seventh month]: "Speak to me more, I love the voice of my mommy." (Baroon 1998, 13)

[Eighth month]: "I've become chubby, haven't I?" (Baroon 1998, 14)

[Ninth month]: "I sleep and play, there is a pace to my life." (Baroon 1998, 16)

[Tenth month]: "It's narrow here; I want to meet Mom soon." (Baroon 1998, 18)

Note how the baby's animation is oriented to capturing its mother's attention and assuring her that the baby is having fun in her womb. The guide's depiction of the ultimate mother–baby relationship is of a symbiotic couple linked by a positive feedback system, increasing the mother and the baby's mutual and joy-ful bonding. The mother is depicted as providing the baby with a pleasant environment, and the baby as having fun in her womb. Defining the baby as a human being in all respects adds weight to her assessment of the mother's qualifications in nurturing. However, this human baby, far from being a lone individual, is depicted as totally dependent on its mother. The baby "knows" its mother and is seeking communication with her, which in turn pleases the mother and invigorates her attempts to communicate with the baby.

On the other hand, the baby's plea for affectionate communication, which is represented as cute, is also an assertive demand. As a human being, the baby has a powerful voice. It has the power to constrain the mother—it demands that she take the baby's voice into account on all occasions. Mothers who ignore this plea might harm the baby by merely carrying on with their everyday routine "inconsiderately." In an advice column dealing with recommendations for "correct" everyday maternity living, one can find titles like "Put yourself in your baby's place: things like tobacco that relieve mother but make the baby suffer should be given up once pregnancy is realized" (Baroon 1998, 21); "Do physical exercises, while consulting the baby" (Baroon 1998, 22).

Drawing on McVeigh's analysis of "the cult of cuteness" in Japan (2000), I argue that the cuteness with which unborn babies are represented is instrumental in producing "maternal behaviors" in pregnant women. "Cuteness as a human sentiment is so potent," argues McVeigh, "because it communicates power relations and power plays, effectively combining weakness, submissiveness and humility with influence, domination and control" (McVeigh 2000, 135). He maintains that the sociopolitical, operational, and practical applications of "cuteness" are to soften authority.

The cute images of unborn babies convey what McVeigh calls "cuteness authority." Being cute does not make this authority any less authoritative—quite the contrary: it possesses enormous power to evoke and even (gently) enforce nurturing behaviors. The baby's is the voice of a human being, cute though it may be, which must constantly be taken into account.[9] At the same time, we might think of it as the voice of society, as a powerful voice available to any authoritative role player (be it doctor, family member, or even passerby). Indeed, in Cordero's account of delivery in a Japanese hospital, one obstetrician explicitly exploited the authority of the baby when he urged a woman giving birth: "The baby is in pain so move down quickly. Spread your legs open. That's it, that's it" (Cordero-Fiedler 1996, 205).[10]

Gradually surfacing from this examination of women's accounts, pregnancy records, and pregnancy guides is a set of Japanese theories of maternal–fetal bonding that provides a key to understanding gendered power relations and role division in Japanese society. The latter are not simply "enforced" from above, but draw their power from the embodied, day-to-day experiences of women.

Taikyô: A Theory of Maternal–Baby Communication

The notion of the active fostering of maternal–fetal bonding materializes in the concept of *taikyô*. This word (a compound of *tai*, the kanji for "fetal," and *kyô*, the kanji for "education") literally means "fetal education." Magazines cite mothers who interpret taikyô literally as enhancing the baby's intellectual development, but many guides emphasize instead *taikyô's* mental benefits for the baby. I suggest that *taikyô* is in fact a practical theory of communication between the mother and the unborn baby.

All the Japanese magazines and guidebooks on pregnancy that I collected dedicated at least some space to it in varying degrees. The Japanese 1998 best seller mentioned earlier defines *taikyô* as follows: "*Taikyô* is not practiced in order to give birth to a genius. It is practiced in order to deepen the bonds between the mother and the baby, through the mother's recognition of the baby and her acceptance of him. We have summarized here the things that you can do during the months of pregnancy for the baby in your belly to develop healthily. Please refer to this column in order to lead a fruitful everyday life *with* the baby"(Baroon 1998, 145; emphasis added)

Whereas in previous sections I considered the aspects of providing physical care, *taikyô* may be understood as a complementary aspect, namely, providing mental care.

To give some idea of the seriousness with which *taikyô* is perceived, I quote some suggestions as to how and when to speak to the baby. The book actually includes a *taikyô* schedule that accords with the baby's sensory development.

> This is what you should say to your baby: "Don't you hurry, grow slowly and come to meet us.". . ."You are papa and mama's important little one; we all love you." (Baroon 1998, 145)

> "Give mama a sign when it's tasty" (when the pregnant mother is eating). (Baroon 1998, 146)

> "*Yurayura. . . pukapuka*[11]. . . mama and you are like mermaids" (when the pregnant mother is bathing). (Baroon 1998, 147)

> "Good night, in your dreams dance a waltz with mama" (when the pregnant mother goes to sleep). (Baroon 1998, 148)

> "I embrace you inside my body, and therefore be peaceful and come out to me" (when the mother starts experiencing contractions). (Baroon 1998, 148)

Two assumptions underlie the messages that the "mother" is advised to send to her baby: first, that the mother and her (unborn) baby are already bonded through love even before the birth; and secondly, that every experience of the mother is shared with the baby.

The guides and pregnancy magazines expand *taikyô* to greater heights when women are depicted in them as performing elaborate and increasingly creative *taikyô* activities. Takahashi-san was quoted in the Baroon guide "At first I would just talk to the baby, but then during the last stages of pregnancy, I started image training. I would lay my hands on my belly and imagine that I was directing a flow of good light into the baby. The light is my love for the baby, my hopes, joys. . . It relaxed me so" (Baroon 1998, 149).

Similarly, I found in the pregnancy magazine *Tamago Kurabu* an article about a married couple, both music teachers, who gave piano and violin concerts to their unborn baby three times a week. A magazine called *Maternity* had an article about a couple who went on a day trip to Tokyo Disneyland for their unborn baby. The women I interviewed often said that they did not engage in *taikyô* because they did not go as far as its public advocacy indicated. However, some of them seriously read *taikyô* books and followed their advice.

When I interviewed Fujii-san, I noticed that she tapped her belly every now and then. She explained to me that this was a technique she had read about in a *taikyô* book. She communicated with the baby in this way, and the baby would respond to each tap with a kick. She summarized the issue of *taikyô* thus,

> I went to see a friend of mine who gave birth recently. You know how new babies are. She doesn't get much sleep because the baby cries so much and wants to nurse all the time. It is hard. So what I want to say is that *now is the perfect time to bond with the baby, while you are pregnant. Now it is the stage when the baby is at its cutest*—it is not crying, it is not ruining your sleep. . . I believe that women who do not take advantage of their pregnancies and do not bond with the baby have all kinds of problems afterwards. I think that the "child-raising neurosis" [*kosodate noirose*] happens because there has been no bonding during pregnancy. (emphasis added)

In Fujii-san's narrative, not engaging in active *taikyô* is dangerous for future child raising. Paradoxically, the animated baby is much easier to bond with than a real baby. Fujii actually perceives *taikyô* as a necessary preventive measure against mental disorders connected with mothering.

Taikyô was introduced from China during the tenth century and became widespread during the Edo period (1603–1868), first among the wives of *samurai* and later among the general public (Kamata et al. 1990, 100–102). Following the assumption that fetuses experience the same feelings as their mothers, pregnant women were advised to uphold good manners and not to see or hear immoral things (Dingwall, Tanaka, and Minamikata 1991). During the years of the Meiji restoration (1868–1912) and the Taisho democracy (1912–1926), *taikyô* went through a nationalist incarnation as mothers were encouraged to tell the unborn baby tales of heroes to develop its sense of patriotism (Dingwall, Tanaka, and Minamikata 1991, 424).

After the end of World War II *taikyô* was sharply transformed in accordance with anti-war ideologies. In fact, a historical "genealogy" of *taikyô* practices might illuminate the evolution of predominant ideologies in Japanese society from a somewhat new perspective. Such a historical analysis is beyond the scope of this study.

However, for later discussion, note that *taikyô*, as part of a broader understanding of the baby as a living being within an interconnected social environment, predates obstetrical ultrasound. In fact, it echoes animistic intuitions that assign life not only to sentient beings but also to objects and invisible entities. Technologies of imaging may have helped push these notions further, but they are finding fertile ground. The unborn Japanese baby, unlike its American or Israeli counterpart, is not merely a cyborg generated primarily by ultrasound screening—it is a powerful being whose presence predates the invention of ultrasound and transcends the moment of its appearance on the ultrasound screen. With this in mind, let us leave the private rituals of communicating with one's baby and proceed to explore how pregnant women and their unborn babies are constituted in public pregnancy activities.

Maternity Classes as Exercises in Child Care

I shall never forget the first lesson of the first maternity class in which I participated in Japan back in 1996. After the twenty pregnant women present had introduced themselves, the head nurse, all smiles, brought out a baby doll. "This doll is precisely the size and weight of a newborn baby. Have any of you had the experience of holding a baby in your arms recently?" she asked. She then asked the women to pass the doll around, and each woman had to embrace it. I remember how ridiculous I felt holding this doll. Here we have a three-dimensional representation of a baby, coupled with a simulation exercise of a bonded embrace. At that time I had never had the experience of participating in an Israeli maternity class, yet the cultural logic that must have been engraved deep inside me could not tolerate the presence of a baby in the first lesson of what I perceived as a "birth-education class." Eleven years later, in 2007, I was even more bewildered when the doctor heading a private maternity clinic in Southern Honshu invited an education expert to open a "parents' class" for pregnant women and their partners, with exercises of nursery rhymes with playful hand games (*te-asobi*) for toddlers (like "Itsy Bitsy Spider"). An audience of about fifty women and half a dozen male partners in business suits sat in the lecture hall, reciting with the educationalist the rhyme "Falling, falling, what is falling? . . . An apple" (*ochita, ochita, nani ga ochita . . . ringo*) and practicing the parents' part and the child's part alternately (as if catching a round object).

From an Israeli perspective, Japanese maternity classes are organized along a collapsed time axis, of which the presence of "babies" and even toddlers in the first lesson serve as examples. Israeli classes never started with babies, but with fetuses, which only become "babies" after the birth. What are called "birth-education classes" in English-speaking countries and "birth-preparation courses" (*kurs ha'cha'na le'leida*) in Hebrew are very tellingly entitled in Japanese *hahaoya gakkyû*: a course for the mother parent ("maternity class," as it will be called here), or *ryôshin gakkyû*, parents' class, if men are invited to participate at some point.

Generally Japanese women take several maternity courses during one pregnancy, and few women wait until the last stages of pregnancy to join one. The reason is that the information offered by these classes touches on issues like nutrition and weight that are perceived to be relevant to pregnancy from the very earliest stages. Most women I talked to took a course offered by the municipal health administration during the fourth or fifth month, and later a course given by the hospital where they went for pregnancy checkups during the sixth or seventh month. Some women, especially those who gave birth at a hospital near their parents' home (*satogaeri shussan*), participated in a third course given by the hospital where they gave birth.

What may appear as a collapsed time axis is a mere manifestation of the fact that Japanese maternity courses are organized along the axis of prenatal bonding, not the axis of time. Moreover, I suggest that maternity courses take ideas put forward in other media one step further: they offer women an opportunity to *exercise* practical care provision. Women practice embracing and diapering a baby; courses with lessons for fathers have them practicing bathing a baby (which is considered symbolically the role of fathers). Nurses who give maternity courses explain that these practices are meant to create a sense of familiarity (*shitashimi kanji*) with child-raising practices.

Exercising an act physically in order to develop familiarity with it fits well with a social climate that cherishes exercise (*renshû*). More than once, pregnant women in maternity courses reminded me of the *salariiman* practicing golf with an imaginary club while waiting for a train—a frequent sight in day-to-day life in Japan. Returning to pregnancy, it seems that every single act can be practiced to advance familiarity with child raising. Wearing a belly belt (*haraobi*) is a case in point. Up to now I have considered narratives that recommended wearing a belly belt in order to "stabilize the baby," keep the pelvic area warm, and prevent backache. However, according to a text given to participants in a maternity class taught at a large teaching hospital, these are not the primary reasons to wear it. As the textbook explains, "Wearing a *hara obi*, a. Deepens the awareness that you are to become a mother and heightens the understanding of a family. b. Supports the belly, and eases movement and pelvic pains."

The Japanese technique of prenatal breast massage is practiced in the same spirit. The massage is a fixed sequence of movements that medical-care providers claim to be a Japanese invention aimed at preparing the breasts for nursing by "exercising" them. Massaging the breast includes also (among other motions) rolling the nipples between the fingers and pulling them out. Through being massaged, breasts are supposed to "get used" to nursing. The doctor who invented this technique argues that practicing it improves nursing considerably. Ukigaya-san, who told me that she "failed" to nurse "properly" and had problems because of engorged breasts, explained, "I was too lazy during pregnancy and did not practice breast massage. Maybe that is why I did not succeed in nursing"—a typical statement that I heard repeatedly. Breast massage also belongs to the set of ideas discussed in the previous chapter, about the necessity for pregnant women to "build" a proper body. Rolling the nipples and pulling them out is supposed eventually to give them the most suitable shape for nursing.

The paradox, however, is that massaging the breasts has the reputation throughout the medical world of being a catalyst for contractions. In some maternity courses, breast massages are recommended for daily practice as soon as a woman enters the stable period (*anteiki*), from the fifth month. When I wondered aloud about its prospective dangers in the context of a medical community that dreads premature birth, one experienced midwife explained to me: "We do not mean that the mother should violently massage the nipples, just do it few times to get a sense of familiarity" (*shitashimi kanji*). The breast massage did not seem to constitute any sort of paradox for medical practitioners—a point that might illustrate the overall predominance of ideas of prenatal bonding over medical anxieties about premature birth.

While administering an array of care-giving exercises (*akachan no osewa suru renshū*), maternity courses also aspire to prove *scientifically* that the bond is already at work during pregnancy. Such scientifically tinted evidence cuts throughout the variety of videos shown in maternity classes: all of them at some point feature an "experiment."

In one film the picture focuses on a baby in a crib. Electrodes attached to the baby's head are connected to a device measuring its brainwaves, which are relayed on to a screen. A staff of three men dressed in white robes watch the screen. The baby starts crying. The doctors switch on a cassette tape featuring "the mother's heartbeats" and start rocking the crib by means of a mechanically synchronized engine that swings the crib "at *exactly* the same swinging frequency that [the baby] experienced while in the womb." The baby stops crying and falls asleep. Its brainwaves are shown on the screen as having a lower amplitude. "It reminds him of how it used to be in mommy's womb, and even though it has had nothing to eat, it has calmed down," says the authoritative voice of the narrator. Then the frame moves to another experimental apparatus featuring a pregnant woman whose belly is connected to electrodes in one room, while in a neighboring room a person wearing a white robe (i.e., the doctor) monitors a complicated-looking electronic device. The doctor puts on a relaxing piece of classical music and asks the mother to report the intensity of fetal movement. Then he plays some loud rock-and-roll. The mother reports vigorous kicking. The doctor, by looking at the electronic device, confirms the mother's diagnosis and says that the fetus is moving intensively. "The baby is responding to the sounds his mother hears," says the narrator.

Another video shows a baby lying in a crib and a mother with her naked breasts exposed to an infrared scanner. The baby starts crying, and the frame focuses on the screen that images the scan, to show how the mother's breasts fill with milk once the baby starts crying. Then again, in the same experimental spirit, two pieces of white cloth are offered to the baby, one marked with a red heart, the other an unmarked white cloth. "The marked white cloth," the narrator's voiceover tells us, "has the smell of his mother's milk." The baby turns his head to the cloth smelling of "his mother's milk."

What do these experiments prove? Are a mechanical rocker and a representation of brainwaves necessary to know what every nanny knows perfectly well, namely, that babies relax if you rock them? Is an experimental apparatus like an infrared scanner necessary to know what mothers commonly report, namely, that their breasts fill with milk whenever a baby cries (and not necessarily their own baby)? Must a cloth smelling of breast milk be used to know that babies respond to the smell of breast milk?

Moreover, alert audiences may well question such experimental apparatuses. Why was a white cloth with the smell of another woman's breast milk not offered to the hungry baby? How does one know whether the baby is responding to the smell of breast milk in general, or to the smell of *his mother's* breast milk in particular? Does the frequency of swinging in *his mother's* womb differ from the frequency in other women? Will the baby not relax with a slightly different frequency? How do we know whether the baby is responding to the sound of music or to the sounds that *his mother* hears? The video so presents these issues as to encourage the audience to feel that the announcer is simply stating the conclusions of the scientific experiments, but in fact the "experiments" are merely an introduction to the narrator's text. I tend to think of them as music played by a warm-up band. Clearly the videos are "decorated" with "scientific experiments": they use them ritually, and draw on the authority of science to illustrate and support already established truths.

The Virtues of Bonded Motherhood

Pregnancy is not always a romantic and rosy period in a woman's life. Both pregnancies and births alike have a reputation of being (at least part of the time) difficult physical and mental ordeals that materialize into rites of passage (Davis-Floyd 1992). How are the hardships of pregnancy interpreted in a social climate of prenatal bonding?

Women who yield wholly to the idea of prenatal bonding seem able to exploit it in order to ease some of the more difficult moments. Pregnancy guides narrate bodily sensations as a sign language spoken by the baby that should be attentively listened to. To name just two examples, *tsuwari*, or morning sickness, is interpreted as a sign from the baby of its existence. Aches in the lower abdomen toward the end of pregnancy are a sign that "the moment when you *meet* your baby is approaching." The baby is also seen as a companion. In 2001 I carried out fieldwork in Japan during the sixth month of my own pregnancy. The women I interviewed and friends often wondered how I physically managed the hardship of traveling while pregnant. However, many concluded that "at least you are not suffering loneliness: you have the baby with you."

The "baby" also helped women cope with the unpleasant aspects of the medical routine of pregnancy checkups. Most women I met hated the internal examinations that are carried out routinely in many medical institutions. However, many of them explained to me that they were willing to submit to these odious examinations "for the baby's sake." I realized that the majority of women interpret the internal examination as intended to assess the child's development, although it is carried out mainly to check for any possible dilation of the cervix and to rule out premature birth.

However, the most striking case of transcending difficulty by exploiting awareness of the "baby" is how women cope with birth. In Japanese hospitals, pain relief is generally unacceptable: the obstetricians I interviewed insisted that it tends to complicate deliveries. Most women I talked to hoped for a "natural birth" (*shizen bunben*), though in practice this means giving birth in a hospital on a gynecological chair with one's legs strapped in the "traditional" lying down position. This form of delivery is designated "natural," in comparison to the "painless birth" (*mutsûbunben*), in which anesthesia is used from a certain stage of labor. Women who are determined to have an epidural during labor have no choice but to attend one of the private and expensive hospitals that apply them. These "painless deliveries" are therefore rare in contemporary Japan.

In one of the maternity courses I participated in, the nurse bluntly told the pregnant participants, "You must keep it in your mind that birth hurts and that there is nothing to be done about it. That's the way it is." She cited a well-known Japanese proverb: "The child that made one's belly hurt is lovable" (*onaka wo itameta ko ha kawaii*). This proverb attaches a positive value to the pains of birth, and Japanese women, as well as obstetricians, cite it frequently to explain their reluctance to use painkillers during the birth. Dr. Ootsuma, the ob-gyn who is so popular with her patients, told me the following story as an illustration of the truth in this proverb:

I had one patient who gave birth to her first child in a usual natural birth. When she had her second child, she decided that she was going to have a painless birth. Then when she was pregnant with her third child, she came to me and asked me whether we do painless births. I said that all our patients give birth in the natural way. So she said, "Good, I am not having this painless birth again. I decided by all means to give birth naturally." And why do you think that was? She told me that she did not feel the same flow of feelings of love toward the child she had given birth to painlessly. A Japanese proverb says that the child that made one's belly hurt is lovable, and that is why she decided to have natural birth. This is something that came out of her experience, you see. I also hate "painless birth." It has a tendency to get complicated. . . I think this proverb is right. Even if you compare breastfeeding after a natural birth and after a cesarean, you may notice that women who had a cesarean usually do not have enough milk.

Pain is perceived here as a form of bonding, therefore it is logical to allow and even encourage it. Breast milk is the ultimate manifestation of postpartum bonded motherhood, so its lack is understood as an expression of insufficient bonding due to insufficient pain. In a birth entry in her diary close to her due date, Kurashige-san summarized what she had learnt in the different maternity courses she had attended. This entry was titled "The logic of birth."

1. When a contraction comes, pat, rub the waist and the lower back, and the stomach. At this time it is very easy to put a lot of tension in the legs, so I have to keep the legs from becoming stiff. So fold them and move them and take the force out of the body (when you do that, good efficient contractions come).
2. Breathing. Inhale through the nose and exhale a long exhalation while saying "*hu.*" A deep breath. Anyway, try to concentrate on that.
3. *When it hurts, it is because the baby is descending. In my heart, I should say "Baby, hold on, fight [gambare]," and so help cheer it up.*
4. When getting on the birth stool get a towel to wipe off the sweat. (emphasis added)

Kurashige plans how to *cheer the baby up* during labor and delivery. She takes into consideration that the birth is difficult for the baby, not only painful for herself. Therefore, the baby needs cheering up. Note also how this point is casually listed among other technical directions to herself.

In later correspondence, I asked Kurashige if she could elaborate point 3. Here is her answer:

Even when I cheer the baby up and say, "Baby hold on, fight" [my] pain does not go away, but the feeling gets lighter. I am not the only one who is in pain—it is hard on the baby, too. When I think that I am not the only one who is trying hard [*gambaru*], my heart becomes strong; you are welcome to try it yourself.

Matsuo-san's account is oriented similarly:

MATSUO: I really was thinking about it. The baby feels the contractions as well, doesn't he? When they connect you to the monitor, you actually see how his heartbeat changes pace with the contractions.

TSIPY: Are these thoughts you had while in pain?

MATSUO: Yes, I was thinking that there is one more human being here that is making an effort [*gambatteiru*], so I will make an effort too.

The idea of the baby in birth pains totally changes the focal point of birth. Some birth-preparation videos shown in maternity courses actually depict the baby, not the mother, as the "hero" of the birth story. One typical video showed the mother soon after delivery holding the baby in her arms, crying with joy, and saying to her, "You fought hard, didn't you" (*yoku gambatta ne*)?

The Umbilical Cord as a Bonding Fetish

After the long process of prenatal bonding reaches its climax with the suffering of the pains of birth, bonding itself materializes into an object: the umbilical cord. It is customary in most Japanese hospitals to keep a part of the umbilical cord after it dries up and falls off, enclose it in a special little box designed for the purpose, and give it to the mother on the day she leaves the hospital (a week after delivery). The umbilical cord is then treasured by the mother and kept to be shown to the child later when it grows up. Negashi traces the custom of keeping part of the umbilical cord to ancient Japanese traditions, and argues that versions of the custom can be found throughout the Japanese archipelago. Common to them all is the belief that the umbilical cord is connected with the health of the newborn baby and that maltreating it may cause the child disease (Negashi 1991, 338–346).[12]

Women narrated the experience of being shown their own umbilical cord as a happy event. As Tanaka-san told me: "When I reached fifth or fourth grade of elementary school, that was the first time my mother showed me the cord. I have these memories that I was very happy. I thought 'Oh, I am really mommy's child,' and I was really glad. Then I think she told me about the day I was born."

In some households, a ritual is performed around the presentation of the umbilical cord. As Awata-san recalled: "On my birthdays, mother would take the cord out of a chest of drawers and show it to me. 'We were connected through this,' she would say."

Uchino-san told me that in some households, when the child grows up and leaves home, or gets married, the mother customarily gives the cord to the child as a symbol of the latter's separation from the natal unit. Ueda-san told me, with tears of excitement in her eyes, "When I left home to study my mother gave me the cord. It was a disgusting little black object. I was disgusted but at the same time I was very moved."

Some women even cited folk beliefs that attribute nurturing powers to the dry umbilical cord. Morimura-san told me: "When I got married my mother gave me the cord and said that if I were to have health problems or problems of any sort that I should mash the cord and drink it as a tea and it would help. . . . I never tried to find out whether it works or not."

Women, including nurses, who learnt for the first time through my questions that keeping the umbilical cord is not a universal custom were overwhelmed by this notion. I suggest that the attachment to the umbilical cord is grounded in the idea of connectedness that is so easily aroused by it. The umbilical cord is the one organ whose ownership is hard to determine, since it is shared by the mother and her baby. In a culture that emphasizes the somatic continuum between mother and baby, once the baby is born the umbilical cord becomes a fetish of the mystical bond, an object around which private rituals crystallize. The umbilical cord also locates the bonding in the body: if we follow literally the symbolism of the umbilical cord, bonding is made of flesh and blood.

Japanese Male Partners and Pregnancy

If pregnancy is conceived as an enterprise of prenatal bonding, and if bonding is located deep inside the body, made up of a carefully maintained somatic environment and pain, it will not be much of a surprise that men are regarded as basically lacking access to bonding. The understanding of the man as having a "reproductive deficit" since his "knowledge of the fetus is disembodied and therefore more disconnected and abstract than hers" (Draper 2002; Sandelowski 1994, 234) is not specific to Japan. Yet in America, Europe, and Israel an array of medical and semimedical practices aspire to bypass men's disembodied stance vis-à-vis pregnancy, either by giving priority to the visual knowledge of the fetus through the technology of ultrasound (over the embodied knowledge of the woman), or by training men in birthing classes to support their partners in labor (Reed 2005). In the next chapter I devote some space to discussing the experiential implications of such practices, heavily marked with medicalization and technology, on Israeli couples' partnership in pregnancy. Clearly, in the above societies men are coming under increasing pressure to express their commitment to their partners and children-to-be by attending medical rituals. In 2007 I met more (typically younger) Japanese men who aspired to share the experience of pregnancy with their partners, but men's enduring commitment to their workplace, along with the structure of prenatal care services—arenas that have become a primary site for men to attend if they are to express their commitment, made such pressures somewhat less powerful in Japan.

To begin with, women rarely come to pregnancy checkups accompanied by their husbands. When husbands do come, they seldom enter the doctor's office. The nurses I spoke to during my field stint in 2001 said that a couple appearing for a pregnancy checkup is taken as a sign of some kind of trouble. In 2007, again, I saw few fathers-to-be accompanying their partners to maternity clinics, though my informants insisted that men's attitudes were undergoing change. As the previous chapter indicates, if there were any abnormal prenatal diagnoses, the ob-gyn would invite the husband to come along with the wife for a family consultation. Only if a decision is needed is the husband's presence absolutely required.

An informant who finally managed to conceive after six painful years of trying told me how, when she and her husband were on the verge of giving up, the doctor discovered the tiny beating "rice grain" in her womb. Her eyes filled with tears when she reached the crux of the story, which was when the doctor called her husband, who was sitting in the waiting room, to come and witness the miracle on the ultrasound screen.

Ultrasound scans are without doubt understood as the most suitable occasions for male partners to participate. However, as the accounts of the men I spoke to in 2007 revealed, very often, men's working conditions strictly limit their ability to participate in more than one such scan. Maternity courses, to take another case, are also designed in most cases for women only. While Israeli birth-education courses are deliberately conducted during the evening hours or condensed into weekends to enable working people (who are the majority of male and female participants) to attend the class, most Japanese maternity courses are given during the morning hours, the assumption being that pregnant women do not work. This of course thwarts men's attempts to take part, since often they are expected to be primarily committed to their workplace.

A few courses are called *ryôshin gakkyû* or "both-parents' courses." Significantly, unlike Israeli courses (endowed with titles such as "birthing together" [*laledet beyachad*]), Japanese "mothers' classes" (*hahaoya gakkyû*) and "parents' classes" (*ryôshin gakkyû*) are both oriented to the concept of parenting and much less to birth. However, most of the "parents' courses" feature only *one* lesson, out of five or more, in which husbands are actually invited to participate. The special class takes place during the evening hours, to make it possible for husbands to attend, which again reinforces the primacy of their work over their partnership. The content of these lessons varies, but many of them include a practice session of baby bathing for the husbands. As participants explained, bathing the baby is considered the "traditional" role of the father. The reasons they offered were again located in the body: one was that since fathers have "big hands" they are physically best adapted to bathing a baby. Another was that in bathing the baby, fathers will form "skinship" with it. "Skinship" is a Japanese-English term for bonding through the body. Allocating bathing to fathers places bonding in the skin and assumes that fathers lack opportunities to bond precisely because they are not as physically connected to their children as their spouses: they can only begin bonding with their children after they have been born and can be bathed. But in reality many middle-class husbands manage to practice such "skinship" with their children at most once a week at the weekend. Such practices highlight the consensus that place bonding in the body.

Yet men are significantly more visible today in maternity magazines, and more women aspire to share their experiences of pregnancy with their partners. Morimura-san enthusiastically talked about the open and progressive attitudes of the hospital where she attended maternity courses and gave birth. "I liked their attitude. The husband, of course, participates in birth, and also afterwards. It is an attitude that sees birth and the raising of children as the role of both parents."

However, in the course of the interview I found out that her husband never participated in the course. "No, he never came; husbands don't come. They teach the wife, and the husband learns from her at home. They teach you breathing and tell you to teach your husband all that you have learned. So before the birth I tried to teach my husband. We tried to breathe together, but he fell asleep."

Some hospitals teach a mandatory lesson for husbands who wish to participate in the birth. In this lesson the husbands are taught mainly what *not* to do, in order not to become a nuisance to the medical staff. To give one example, in one of my observations husbands were warned not to park their cars in the ambulance parking lot and were asked not to wander round the birthing room, but to stand near their wife's head. Accordingly, the practice of a husband attending a birth is called *tachiai bunben*, a phrase that means "a birth [in] which [the husband] stands by." Unlike the Israeli claim that the parents can ultimately "give birth *together*," a "standing-by birth" does not suggest the illusion of a total sharing of experience between the parents.

The concept of *tachiai bunben* echoes postwar attempts to import American feminist ideologies. In many cases, however, it cannot be realized. First, in some hospitals *tachiai bunben* is not even available "due to lack of space." Secondly, my informants included husbands who asked their wives to excuse them from attending the birth, or wives who preferred their husbands not to be with them during the birth. Kanae-san, thirty, a mother of two who went to give birth accompanied by her mother, could not understand how her husband could possibly help her while in labor. Dr. Ootsuma explained that choices such as Kanae's are more common than one would imagine in a society where new ideas of partnership are on the rise.

The notion of a husband attending the birth opposes the sense of aesthetics [*biishiki*] of Japanese women. Have you heard the ancient Japanese story about Izumi no Mikoto?

Nearing birth, she asked her husband not to look inside the room where she would be giving birth. She told him that she would not be able to be with him any more if he looked. When she went into labor, she entered the room and closed the door. He tried to control himself, but eventually he could not help it and opened the door just a little bit to look.

After she gave birth, she said to him, "I must leave you. Why have you betrayed me?"

Women who practice baby care during pregnancy are supposed to know how to manage babies, but as men do not engage in prenatal bonding they are not meant to "know how to handle" their newborn babies. Books and videos represent the moment of birth as rather embarrassing for fathers. One video shown in maternity courses in a general hospital narrated this moment as follows: "When Yamada met his baby for the first time, he was shy [*tereteiru*]." Then the frame moves to the couple's house, where the mother takes care of the baby while the father is sitting perplexed in the corner. The rather symbolic image of the "husband in the corner" can be found in several other manuals and media (see, for example, Taida and Miyai 1997, 176).

Uchino-san, who narrated her relationship with her husband as especially warm and intimate, was considerate of her husband's not being able to understand her pregnancy. When I asked her whether she shared her experience of pregnancy with him, she answered:

> We talk about all kinds of things, but he is not the person that really goes through it [*honnin*]. Me, I know what my physical condition is, so I know if it's O.K. or not, but him, how can he know? He's not here during the afternoon hours so he's worried. When he comes back, he always asks how it has been. When he's late, he phones me and asks how my physical condition is. When you're not the one who's pregnant, you can get quite nervous [*shinkeishitsu*]. At first he was a little nervous. He would say to me, "You should not eat *ramen*—it has too many calories." When the doctors prescribed bed rest for me because of the bleeding I had, he ordered me to lie down and not go out of the house. They [husbands] don't know; you see, he's not the one most involved [*honnin*].

Uchino's husband emerges from her depiction as a compassionate and committed partner whose anxieties emerge due to his innate limitations: she is quite compassionate to him. As she told me, he wanted the baby to know his voice, so he made sure to speak to the baby often, through a microphone attached to her belly. Given that pregnancy is a time to bond, Uchino's husband had to transcend the physical barrier between his unborn baby and himself, and find a way to communicate with it. However, not being able to feel the same sensations as his wife was a barrier he could not transcend, and he responded by becoming "nervous" about his wife's physical condition. Needless to say, not all male partners feel similarly compelled to make such an effort.

Women reflected their longing to share their experiences with their husbands to differing degrees. Kurashige-san wrote in a fifth-month pregnancy entry:

> Today for the first time I could see a picture of the whole body of the baby. The little heart beating *paku paku*. . . . I said, "Oh, she is really living." I really had a true feeling that she is really living. And I could see in the ultrasound how her little hands grip; without thinking, I said, "Oh, her fingers." That was the first time I saw it so clearly, and I was so excited, that is why I said obvious things. *I wish I could show it to Ichiro. I wish he could see it also.* It was really the first time it felt so real, I was so happy." (emphasis added)

However, when I asked Kurashige whether she showed her husband her detailed pregnancy diary, she said she did not. She added, "I'm sure he knows I'm doing something of the sort." Similarly Umeyama-san, who wrote an equally elaborate diary, did not share it with her husband. Both women apparently assumed that their husbands would not be interested.

One of my informants talked sadly about how lonely she felt during her pregnancy. Her husband was entirely uninterested. He only became involved after the baby was born and "he could see it with his own eyes." After I returned to Israel this informant sent me an e-mail attachment with a birth story she encountered while surfing the internet. She wrote that she deeply identified with the story, which was taken from a midwife's Web site. The subject was "What is a good birth?"

> A good birth is when the baby decides when to be born. A good birth is not necessarily short. I can tell you a story to show this. There was one woman I helped who was hospitalized on Friday night and gave birth after more than forty-eight hours on Sunday. When I came to see her afterwards, I was sure she would say that her birth was terrible, but she told me that it was a very good birth. She told me that throughout her pregnancy she had tried to draw her husband into it, closer to her and to the baby, but without success. He works hard and was totally uninterested. Her labor started on Friday, and she came by herself to the hospital. Then on Saturday he had a day off and came to see her. She was in labor all day and only on Sunday morning was the baby born.

Her husband saw her suffering and that was the first time he became involved. "The baby has waited for his father to come," she said.

This woman exploited the pain of birth to bond with her baby, but also to try to bond her husband to herself and to their baby. How successful she was is unclear, but her "earning" his involvement with so much pain attests to her desperation.

The theories of prenatal bonding designate women as *the* primary creators of their children: with every breath they take, every move they make, women make their children. However, this "godlike" image does not necessarily empower women: the emphasis on bonding through the body helps to segregate women in the private sphere and (together with the primacy of the obligation men are expected to feel toward their jobs) shrinks the idea of a basic family unit into a dyadic mother–child relationship. Navigating within the constraints of their demanding jobs and marginalized by theories of gestation, expectant fathers are squeezed into the roles of sympathetic and supportive spectators, or distant nonparticipants. Women too often find themselves thrust into the demanding vocation of committed child making more or less on their own.

Resistance?

Do women initiate any alternative discourses and/or practices that resist the restrictions prescribed to them by medical doctors and cultural theories of gestation? Clearly, the ideal pregnant woman who emerges from the combination of medical and cultural ideas about gestation is a full-time housewife, who can afford to live on her husband's salary, at least for several years, to engage in time-consuming nurturing and bonding activities. The associations of this ideal image with postwar ideologies about women's citizenship are more than obvious.

Furthermore, women in variously challenging familial and/or personal circumstances might not be able to adhere to these restrictions, even if they subscribe to the ideologies of the important body. Since the Japanese government has exempted itself from subsidizing routine prenatal care, arguing that pregnancy is not sickness, women who are seriously disadvantaged economically may not even be able to afford prenatal care. This became alarmingly obvious when, toward the end of 2007, the media reported an increase in cases of women who showed up for obstetrical care only when in labor. According to surveys, the number of "jump-in" births (*tobikomi shussan*) had quadrupled since 2004, amounting to 148 cases in 2006 (*Yomiuri Shinbun* 21.11.07). Angry hospital officials marked these women, who did not carry a mother–child handbook, as irresponsible and refused to accept them; in one case this led to the death of the mother.

The media reports emphasized that these women (young girls, economically disadvantaged women, and illegal overstayers) said they could not afford prenatal examinations. The fear that surfaced from the women's narratives of the criticism they expected in an encounter with care providers remained almost ignored by media commentators. Yet I suspect that precisely the role that care providers play in a more general social project to "tame" motherhood is a key to understanding why women whose circumstances militate against proper motherly performance wish to avoid encounters with health-care institutions as much as possible. The cases of economically disadvantaged women deserve special study. In the present context they mark the farthest divergence from proper motherly behavior. But what about women who face relatively less challenging circumstances?

These women, some of whom could be safely categorized as "middle class," manifest a range of resistant behaviors from discursive to practical (cf. Root and Browner 2001). Let us begin with the "initial" level, which I call "discursive criticism." These are cases in which informants' narratives contradict common theories, though their actions remain unaffected. Women with no "ideological" tendency to resist often criticized and doubted some of the restricting aspects of the important body theories. Fuji-san said:

> My neighbor is a very dedicated woman. She is dedicated to managing her house and taking care of her husband. She is the one person I know who took special care of her body [*daiji ni shita*] every time she became pregnant. And what happened? She took care of it so seriously she hardly left the house and rested a lot, and in the end she had a miscarriage. I know many women like this. It seems to me that it is the reverse. The more one takes care [*daiji ni suru*] of one's body, the more the person is in danger of miscarriage. All the women I know who had miscarriages were the women who were most careful. So I think maybe it is better not to take care too much.

Since Fuji's criticism is based on observation of close acquaintances, it seems to hold a liberating potential. Yet she, too, spent her own pregnancy at home, though she did go out of her house to meet friends, go shopping, etc. Fuji's narrative represents a latent level of resistance, the level that challenges existing consensus without far-reaching practical implications.

Another level of resistance is what I call the "discursive normalization of pregnancy," that is, pretending to proceed with a "normal" life despite the pregnancy. This level is characterized by indirect and rather mild criticism combined with an amendment of the restriction at issue. Take for example the major restriction zone of eating habits. When I inquired about these, some of my informants said they did nothing special and just kept on living their lives as usual. Matsuo-san's answer was typical: "I ate whatever I wanted and did not limit myself in anything." In the context of the theories of the important body, which advocate general changes such as leaving work, withdrawing to the private sphere, and starting a healthy diet, merely leading one's life as usual is already a sort of resistance. However, in the course of the interviews, I realized that women who responded like Matsuo were far from being as negligent as one might conclude from such statements. Matsuo indeed ate *whatever* she wanted, but not *as much* as she wanted. She recorded every bite she ate and stuck a memo on the refrigerator. If she thought she had eaten too much, she went out for a walk to expend some calories. In Matsuo's case, eating whatever she wanted did not mean indifference to weight gain: she regulated her weight gain by offsetting it with physical exercise. I found out that Matsuo's strategy was common among women who narrated their conduct in terms of nonchange. I call this type of resistance the "*discursive* normalization of pregnancy," because "normalizing" pregnancy occurs at the level of discourse only. From her actions, Matsuo clearly assumes that keeping moderate weight gain throughout her pregnancy is highly important. On the practical level, she makes sure to maintain her weight using a slightly altered technique. Only at the discursive level does she narrate herself as carefree.

The third level of resistance is of women who knowingly transgress strict prohibitions. I call this level "practical resistance." I found two kinds of practical resistors: "secret resistors," who resisted without engaging in a rhetoric that would legitimize their deeds; and "*shinkyô* resistors," who legitimized their practices with an acceptable rhetoric about the importance of the mental environment.

One "secret resistor" told me that she felt a strong urge to travel during pregnancy. When she at last succumbed to it, she took the train from Tokyo to Kyoto for a week's trip, and *slowly* strolled among Kyoto's shrines. She made sure not to tell anybody about her trip, but she clearly made sure to conform to the norms of moderate body movements while she was away.

The informants who did not feel they had to hide when transgressing prohibitions had a typical rhetoric to justify their deeds. Ueda-san, mother of a six-month-old baby, said: "I wasn't careful at all with meals and I even drank coffee. Even now I drink coffee and I have a lot of breast milk. There is no end to these restrictions, so I rather think that if I don't drink coffee, my child will be more nervous because I will become increasingly nervous, so I guess it is better to drink coffee and relax *for the sake of my child*." (emphasis added)

Ueda uses the *shinkyô* or mental-environment aspect of the theory of prenatal bonding to justify her transgressions. As we saw in previous sections, the mother is considered the baby's physical environment, but also its mental environment. Ueda's rhetoric helps her to resist practically and openly, though this rhetoric is still "trapped" in the same prenatal bonding assumptions of pregnancy; she merely emphasizes the aspect of mental "environment" and exploits it for her needs.

This style of reasoning was mainly used by women who decided to keep their jobs while they were pregnant. Umeyama-san was one of them. In the following statement she offers her interpretation of *taikyô* as connected to the issue of work during pregnancy: "After I found out that I was pregnant, I worked for three months. I think that for me it is much better mentally to work. For my mental condition it is much better to go out for a while than to stay at home. And things that make me feel good are good for the baby. I think that for me, going out to work is like *taikyô*. I did not put on special relaxing music for the baby or read to the baby from children's picture books, as I saw some pregnant women doing on the train. I made sure to do the things that made *me* feel good."

It seemed easier for women in practice to overstep the red lines drawn by common ethno-theories when their actions were backed up by a rhetoric, slightly modified, of existing terminologies and arguments. Also typical of this rhetoric was its wrapping of contemporary horror stories of corrupted Japanese motherhood. I heard stories about the misconduct of immature and uncommitted mothers who were not bonded enough. One such typical story was about a teenage couple who wanted to go out and eat *ramen*, "but since a baby is a nuisance in a ramen bar," as thirty-six-year-old pregnant Katô-san explained, they left it in a coin locker at the train station. Though such stories involved couples, the informants who told them held the mother responsible: "She still wants to play and is not responsible enough to take care of a child" was an explanation I heard numerous times. Significantly, in these stories the baby was basically understood as a nuisance (*meiwaku*) in public, which reinforced the idea that babies belong in the private sphere of the home under the care of their mothers.[13] Such stories must have made informants who transgressed some restrictions feel mature and sufficiently committed mothers.

On the other hand, informants tell horror stories about overly bonded mothers. One such story was about a woman who murdered her friend's five-year-old son after she came to pick him up from kindergarten at the request of his mother (her friend). The boy had passed his entrance exams and was accepted by a reputable elementary school, which had rejected her own son. This boy's mother lured her friend's son into a nearby public toilet and strangled him to death with her scarf.

Morimura-san explains this incident as follows:

Nowadays incidents like this are reported every day in the newspapers. There are more and more mothers like this today. It happens because these mothers enter a world in which every day is just the same as the previous day. They are totally devoted to taking care of the children and the house—cooking, sending their kids to kindergarten and then coming to pick them up, and thinking only about the welfare of the kids. So their head "hardens," they become increasingly neurotic, and that is how very serious people commit suicide or kill their children or both.

Their world becomes narrower and narrower. They have no existence except for the child; it is like a soup that is overcooked and becomes a sticky lump. . . . They are alone in all this—the men do not participate; they don't understand how many things a mother has to cope with. . . . That's how it happens.

This mother, who killed her friend's child, was a very diligent woman; her husband is a priest. It is just that her head was filled only with the entrance exam—that is how it happened. *The danger of becoming like this exists for every mother.* That is why I make sure to do some things for the sake of my own mental relaxation. (emphasis added)

Morimura, the twenty-eight-year-old florist who is quoted in the beginning of this chapter, told me about incidents like these to support her decision to keep her work during pregnancy for the sake of her baby's *shinkyô*. The incident she cited basically involved an overbonded mother, who devoted herself wholly to her child, to the extent of becoming murderously jealous. Note also how this story reiterates the idea that children cannot be left to the care of non-mothers, since the child would not have been murdered had his own mother come to pick him up from kindergarten. Such stories represented for Morimura, and for many other informants, frightening examples of how obsessive adherence to the model of totally bonded motherhood can ruin a mother's mental condition and lead to disastrous results.

Returning to Morimura, (or "Morimura the rebel," as I came to think of her), she represents the fourth level of resistance that I found. My first interview with her was characterized by her boundless anger whenever the conversation turned to her encounters with the common ideas about pregnancy expressed by customers who came to buy flowers at her shop or just neighbors and passers-by. She openly flouted all the rules. As we saw in her previous quotation, she did not bother to wear tights or to warm up her belly with a belly belt. She not only drank coffee during her pregnancy, she also went as far as smoking cigarettes and drinking *sake*. Morimura-san used the familiar *shinkyô* rhetoric to justify her deeds.

I don't believe so much in *taikyô*—this business about having to listen to good music and read nice stories. . . The problem is with stress, when your heart beats very fast and your blood pressure goes up. Your physical condition becomes bad because of that stress, which is not good in general, not only when you are pregnant. This is not good for the child in the belly either. When I was pregnant with my first child, I was so nervous

I could explode because of a lid that was not in its place. So it's better to smoke a cigarette and relax.

If the relationship between the couple is not good the child will not develop properly—no matter whether it is inside or outside [the womb].

It is noticeable how, in her seemingly unconventional narrative, Morimura gives credence to all the basic assumptions of prenatal bonding, including the idea that there is no real difference between an unborn baby and a baby.

However, at the time of my second stint of fieldwork I felt that "the rebel" represented the resistance I was searching for. She hid nothing, despite people's continuous criticism. Although pregnant, she flew with her husband to Hokkaido, rode horses, snorkeled, smoked, drank *sake*—all before the eyes of scandalized friends, family, in-laws, neighbors, and customers. Her narratives often sounded as if she was ready to dissociate herself from cultural constraints. "All these aunties telling me what to do: 'Don't do this, don't do that; this is an important body, don't chill it.' And what about me? What do they think about me? Japanese are people of rules and regulations, they manage to think only inside the frames of rules; that is why they cannot understand people like me, who are exceptions to the rule."

Morimura grew up in a poor family that could not afford to send her to university, although she was considered very talented at high school. She was married to a man twenty years older than herself, and together they struggled to survive financially while managing their flower shop. Morimura maintained an outsider's view of society, primarily from a disadvantaged economic situation. This was not all. Morimura dreamed about America, which seemed the ideal place to be for individualists like her. She looked forward to interactions with Americans and told me that several times in her life she had tried to save some money to go to America but could never afford it.

Shortly after her first child was born she returned to work at the florist's with her baby. Now she had to cope with even harsher criticism. Although her conduct was still informed by the assumptions that render the mother–child dyad inseparable, child raising belongs to the private sphere. Her customers could not understand how she could raise her "poor" (*kawaisô*) daughter in a flower shop that was "dirty" with soil, its air filled with pollen. People's criticisms made Morimura increasingly "disobedient" and angry.

My third field trip to Japan marked a turning point in my thinking about resistance. This time I was visibly six-months pregnant. The trip was arranged for February, the coldest month of the year. When I contacted former informants through e-mail, all of them, including those who were critical of common ethno-theories, expressed their worries about my physical condition and doubted my ability to survive the trip. The following responses are all from women who expressed, in their narratives and practices, one of the levels of resistance listed above. When I tried to arrange a meeting at the entrance to a café with an informant introduced to me by Uchino-san, she e-mailed me, "It's very cold and you're pregnant; you should not stand and wait in the cold outside." Tsuchiya-san, who kept working throughout her pregnancy, wrote, "I really want to invite you to my house to interview my friends, but the problem is that my flat is on the fifth floor. Will you be able to climb up? I'm a little worried." However, I could not believe my eyes when I received the following e-mail, from "Morimura the rebel." She wrote: "I was very surprised to hear that you are pregnant. Is your body O.K.? The month you are coming is the coldest in Japan; will your belly be all right?"

Bonded Anxieties

The accounts of adherents and resistors alike attest to the predominance of a "well-written dramatic script" or "dramaturgy" (in Goffman's terms) of pregnancy: one that depicts highly committed pregnant mothers in the process of responsibly making the babies, to whom they are tightly bonded. This script predominates in multiple arenas of pregnancy, which makes it readily available to Japanese pregnant mothers: women who wish to bond have a wealth of images and information to work with.

What happens, however, when the script is disrupted by another set of ideas—those that do not agree with the "ecosystemic" model of gestation and lead to thoughts of prenatal diagnosis? Once thrown into this realm, Japanese women have to improvise their way out. The accounts below remind me of Goffman's metaphor of the embarrassing moment when the actors are on stage ready to play their roles, but somebody has put the wrong cassette on. How do women cope with being told an unexpected problematic diagnosis by their doctors? Morimura-san told me about a friend of hers.

> A friend of mine gave birth in the same hospital that I did. She had a miscarriage with her first child, and with the second child. . . well she gave birth to the second child, but from the very first stages of pregnancy my doctor told her that the baby was not developing properly in the womb, and that maybe, if this child was born, it would have some sort of disorder. He suggested that maybe she should give up this time [*konkai wa akirametara*].
>
> My friend got very furious; she left this doctor and changed to another ob-gyn. She said she hated the idea of abortion so much.

Morimura's friend chose to reject the doctor's diagnosis. She pretended not to have been confronted by the possibility of having a defective child by "changing the cassette" and going to another doctor who would put on the right cassette, with all the texts of bonding.

Note that Morimura describes her friend as having two children: she did not "have a miscarriage." Rather, she "miscarried a child" (*kodomo wo oroshita*). The child that she eventually gave birth to was her *second* child. This echoes LaFleur's (1992) study of the conceptions that surround abortions in contemporary Japan. Observing Japanese cemeteries for children, he points out that although the overwhelming majority of the children memorialized there are "fetuses whose progress in the womb was terminated," the word used is "child" (LaFleur 1992, 10). Pointing out the "relatively 'happy' mood" that characterizes such cemeteries, he suggests that the setting and the rituals that take place there are modeled on "reunion rather than separation": in many ways the child, even though dead, is assumed to be still "alive," and the cemetery is where the family comes to communicate with it (LaFleur 1992, 9–10). In this vein, Morimura's friend's son is his mother's second son in a rather literal way. In contrast, Israeli women and men talked about the first and second *pregnancy* in similar contexts.

I interviewed Kurashige-san when she was in the fifth month of pregnancy. At that time, I was determined not to mention fears of genetic and chromosomal disorders to pregnant informants or to discuss them directly unless they raised the issue. Kurashige was especially friendly to me, and we continued our correspondence. After her daughter was born, I approached her with the questions I had feared to ask while she was pregnant. Did she experience any fear of having a baby with a genetic or chromosomal disorder? And did she ever consider amniocentesis? Her answer was, "I did not worry much about chromosomal and genetic disorders; to be precise, I did not think about them at all. And I think that there is hardly any woman who submits to amniocentesis. Isn't that the way? I think there are many pregnant Japanese women who are worried about allergies and atopy. Some women even cut milk and eggs out of their diet. I have no allergies and therefore I ate everything."

Like Kurashige, women I interviewed seldom mentioned anxieties about genetic or chromosomal disorders—they seemed too busy with other anxieties. Many were anxious about having overly large babies that they would not be able to deliver vaginally, so they engaged in a weight-gain control regimen. Others were anxious about transmitting their allergies to the child. When I asked informants directly whether they had thought about genetic and chromosomal disorders, many, like Kurashige, said that they had never given it any serious thought "because we have no genetic or chromosomal disorders in our families."

Asked whether they had ever considered amniocentesis, some women said there was no point to such a test if one was not prepared to have an abortion. Many said that since they believed that the baby was a life that had been entrusted to them (*sazukatta inochi*) and they planned to give birth to any child, they would never consider such a test. In 2000 and in 2001 a number of women were not sure what amniocentesis diagnosed exactly. One of the interviewees, who initially said that she would have had amniocentesis had it not been so expensive, asked me at a later stage of our conversation what Down's syndrome was.

In 2007, though more Japanese women I spoke to were aware of PND, they were still considerably less informed than Israeli women about the disorders themselves and the biotechnology available to diagnose them. The reason may simply be that Japanese women are less exposed to information of this sort. Japanese pregnancy guides, which dedicate many pages to healthy diets, physical exercises for pregnancy, and advice for efficient weight control, and come complete with large, colorful illustrations, dedicate minimal space to the discussion of genetic and chromosomal abnormalities and their prenatal diagnosis. Guides one hundred and fifty to two hundred pages long would on average dedicate one paragraph to the subject. However, even when the subject is elaborated at relatively greater length, the message conveyed is less alarming than the messages conveyed in the Israeli pregnancy guides discussed in the next chapter.

One example is an explanatory brochure on the subject of the alpha-feto-protein blood test routinely given to patients at a private clinic in Tokyo. At first sight, the pink brochure featuring a mother embracing a baby could have been a guide to breastfeeding. Only on reading the title does one discover that the booklet is about prenatal testing or, as the title goes, "A prenatal test that uses the mother's blood: about the triple marker." One of the detailed explanations in the brochure deals with Down's syndrome as one of the disorders that the test screens for:

> With what types of problems are children with Down's syndrome born?
>
> Babies with Down's syndrome show a delay in development and various complications (having other diseases simultaneously). However, there are individual differences in the extent of problems, and there are people who grow up and lead (normal) everyday lives that are no different from those of normal children, and there are plenty of people who participate in social life thanks to early detection and early treatment.
>
> At present there is still no medical treatment that can "heal" Down's syndrome.

Unlike Israeli narratives, this one does not express a sense of tragedy. Rather it emphasizes the existence of individual cases under the general term "Down's syndrome." Women who have had no opportunity to encounter Down's children directly might read such an explanation and conclude that raising a Down's baby is not beyond their power.

Matsuo-san, who directly encountered disabled children in the course of her training as a nurse and was pregnant at the time of this encounter, is a case in point.

TSIPY: Did you worry that your baby would have a chromosomal abnormality?

MATSUO: First of all, when you think about the probability. . . . I was thirty-two when I became pregnant, and high risk is defined from thirty-five, so I thought, "Wow, that's close," but when I thought, "What would I do if such a child was born?" I thought, well it's this life that was entrusted, treasured in my hands [*sazukatta inochi*], so first let's give birth, and then we'll see. I talked to my husband about this, and this is what we said to each other.

TSIPY: This is what you said before conception?

MATSUO: It was after I became pregnant. Before I became pregnant I had all kinds of thoughts about how I would go through all kinds of testing to diagnose inborn chromosomal abnormalities, but when I really became pregnant, all of a sudden I started thinking about it again. . . . And there was another thing. When I was pregnant we visited an institution for handicapped children. There were all kinds of children there: children with physical deformations, with all kinds of chromosomal abnormalities, children with no lips, children that from whatever angle you look at them are somewhat far from being human beings. It was terrible [*sugoi*]. But when I met these children and their mothers, I thought that these children could grow up and develop because they live in Japan, which has facilities for that. . . . And then I thought that this must have some kind of meaning. . . . I also talked about it with my husband.

Matsuo's account of her encounters with children with disabilities is imbued with a kind of national pride that reminds one of the ob-gyn in the previous chapter who stated that the IQ of children with Down's syndrome is higher in Japan than in other places. To give another example, Sakamoto-san, thirty-seven, mother of two boys aged three and two, whom I met in 2007, decided to undergo the triple marker during her second pregnancy. Her reason, she explained, was that she and her husband were in the process of buying a house at the time; otherwise she would not have undergone the triple marker. Had any indication of a child with a disability appeared, she said, they would have considered a house accordingly: "For example, if the child could not walk, we would buy an apartment on the ground floor." Throughout the process her mother, a special-education expert, encouraged her not to worry; based on her close acquaintance with children with disabilities, she promised her daughter that they would manage with any child. It is interesting to compare such reasoning styles with the conclusions of a thirty-nine-year-old Israeli psychologist I interviewed during her pregnancy. She used her in-depth information and familiarity with abnormal children to say that it was terrible to bring a child like that into the world. The fact that she knew such children well, from her point of view, added authoritative weight to her statement.

So far I have considered women who either do not take into consideration the question of anomalous children or who are prepared, at least theoretically, to cope with raising a child with special needs. However, in Japan women are also clearly to be found who are anxious about having children with genetic and chromosomal disorders, and who have enough information about the available prenatal diagnosis. How do these women manage to live through pregnancy in a social climate of prenatal bonding?

Yasuda-san's story is an example of perseverance in the face of anxiety. I was introduced to Yasuda-san by a friend, a former informant I knew from my first fieldwork session in Japan. Yasuda and my friend had babies of about the same age. We met at my friend's house, and while she looked after both babies, Yasuda and I spoke in the hall. Yasuda was a tiny woman with delicate gestures and an eternal smile. Trying to retain her smile, she told me how she went through long and costly fertility treatments to become pregnant. Bearing this in mind, her attitude to prenatal diagnosis surprised me at first. She remarked, "There are many people who would give birth even to a disabled child. Some people even go through prenatal diagnosis, believing from the bottom of their heart that everything will be O.K. And what do I think of that? I think it is better to do *all* the possible prenatal diagnoses. Whether the child is healthy or not can influence my life after birth a lot—that is why I would have liked to have all the tests."

It is noticeable how Yasuda clearly expresses "mainstream ideology" and juxtaposes it to her own. I was very surprised by her answer. It was revolutionary compared with the attitudes I had met till then. Although she had long anticipated her pregnancy, her attitude resembled the views expressed by many Israeli women. So I continued.

TSIPY: Have you had any tests?

YASUDA: Yes.

TSIPY: Amniocentesis?

YASUDA: *I did not go as far as having such a dangerous test as amniocentesis.*

TSIPY: Did you have the triple marker [alpha-feto-protein]?

YASUDA. Yes, I had the triple marker.

TSIPY: Anything else?

YASUDA: I had three-dimensional ultrasound screening. There are only a few places in Tokyo. There you can see clearly if there are fingers missing or a leg missing.

TSIPY: What do you think you would have done if you had discovered that there was a finger missing?

YASUDA: If there was only one finger missing, this would be still O.K., but if there was a leg missing I think I would have had an abortion. [Yasuda whispers her answers.]

TSIPY: What would you do if the baby had Down's syndrome?

YASUDA: I would have had an abortion [whispering even lower].

TSIPY: Even though you made such an effort to become pregnant?

YASUDA: Yes.

Except for describing amniocentesis as going too far, Yasuda-san's narrative was reminiscent of Israeli narratives. However, she gave these answers in a very low whisper, choked with tears. We were silent for a few seconds, then I went on:

TSIPY: This is rare, isn't it?

YASUDA: Really?

TSIPY: In Japan it is rare, but in Israel it is quite common.

[At this point, tears break through Yasuda's eternal smile, and she whispers and cries, while looking round intently to make sure that my friend does not hear her from the living room.]

YASUDA: My husband cannot walk on his legs. He is disabled, he has a heredi- tary disease. I felt that if they found something. . . I would have an abor- tion. . . even though my husband leads a normal life, he works and we are very happy, and even though I think he would have been very sad if I had had an abortion. . .

TSIPY: So all through the pregnancy you carried these worries in your heart?

YASUDA: Yes [crying]. I feel so bad about the whole thing, as if it is unfair to my husband. He lives a normal life and I love him a lot, so I felt much uneasi- ness about the pregnancy. It was very frightening, it was a real challenge to go through with it.

TSIPY: What have you done to get over these fears?

YASUDA: In my case, the thing I was most frightened of was that the baby would be like my husband, so I had three-dimensional ultrasound screen- ing, where you can see the baby very, very well. This was my greatest relief [kokorosasae].

TSIPY: Didn't your ob-gyn talk to you about prenatal diagnosis at all?

YASUDA: No. I didn't say that I wanted to have anything, and for her part she didn't say that I should do anything.

TSIPY: And she knew about your husband?

YASUDA: Yes, but she said nothing. She made a diagnosis using ultrasound, and everything seemed fine to her.

TSIPY: I suppose that you managed to cast off the fear only after he was born?

YASUDA: According to the results of the triple test, amniocentesis wasn't nec- essary, but I was still worried.

TSIPY: I think that if you had been pregnant in Israel, your experience of pregnancy would have been different.

YASUDA: Yes, I guess I would have been able to get rid of my worries: ten months is a long time to be anxious.

TSIPY: Yes it is too long. . . .

TSIPY: [after a long silence]: Are you thinking about another pregnancy?

YASUDA: I really want another child, but I'm so frightened of going through another ten months of anxiety. . . . I'm not sure I have the strength for another ten months like these.

Yasuda has substantial reason to be frightened. Her daily encounters are with her disabled husband. She knows how to recite the common argument of "caring for any child," but she has a different view. Note how experiencing anxiety raises unbearable guilt feelings toward her husband, whom she loves. Merely speculating about possible abnormalities in the baby makes her feel guilty. Yasuda "did not go as far as having amniocentesis," but her decision not to engage in "such a dangerous test" resulted in ten months of "living in hell." However, even when she thinks of having a second pregnancy, it does not occur to her that her suffering could be shortened from ten to five months of anxiety by having amniocentesis. She is ashamed of her fears, although they are understandable in her circumstances. Yasuda told me that although all the tests she had gone through indicated that the baby was completely healthy, she never talked to him. She only started to do so after he was born healthy.

Awata-san was the only informant (out of fifty-three women) who had undergone amniocentesis. She is a talkative, vibrant, and open woman, aged thirty-seven when she first became pregnant. She told me: "In Japan from the age of thirty-five you are allowed to do amniocentesis. If one doesn't want to do it, that's fine. *To tell the truth*, I did do amniocentesis." (emphasis added)

Awata's narrative notably takes the form of a confession about amniocentesis: "to tell the truth" [*jitsu wa*]. She continues, "As expected [*yappari*], I was worried. I was certainly worried, but amniocentesis costs a hundred thousand yen [about a thousand U.S. dollars], and at my hospital it was ninety thousand. . . so expensive, but it is still cheaper than a car. What shall I do? I guess if it had been a million yen, I would not have taken it, but I thought if it's ninety thousand, let's have this test."

Worried though she was, Awata still intimates that financial considerations could in theory have prevented her from taking the test (For the Israeli women I interviewed, financial considerations were not to be measured against their anxieties.) Awata continued,

> But it is really not at all a very good test. It was already the sixteenth week
> of pregnancy, it is the nineteenth week by the time you get the result. The

baby is already fairly big, and your belly is already quite protruding [*detekiteiru*], and in spite of all that, if they tell you, "Oh, your child has Down's syndrome; do you want to have an abortion?". . . I would be at a loss, I would not know what to do. My hospital is a Catholic hospital. They don't do abortions there. They send you to another hospital. I think it is hypocritical but anyway. . . I was really anxious about what I would do if they told me there was a problem, but I had already done the test, so there was nothing to do but sit and wait patiently [*jitto gaman shiyô*] for the result.

I think that even if a baby with an abnormality is born, it is certainly cute [*kawaii*] and you have to care for it, but it is no surprise [*yappari*] that both parent and child would be grateful [*arigatai*] if there were no abnormality. So every day I prayed in my heart. We are not religious people, and that is why we pray in the heart. "Miya-chan . . . baby, please be healthy."

Awata, like Yasuda, can recite the formal frontstage (*tatemae*) version, the socially accepted and culturally correct attitude to inborn abnormalities, by saying that "every baby is cute and has to be taken care of and raised." This sounds as if on a theoretical level she does not dispute the formal ideology. Interestingly, she prays to the baby "under suspicion," not to God. Nor does she distinguish Miya-chan, her present baby, from "the baby" within.

AWATA: Therefore I didn't tell any of my friends that I was having a baby [*akachan ga dekita*].

TSIPY: Until what point?

AWATA: Until the nineteenth week [when she got the result]. I think it is so strange that I told nobody. I did tell my husband, my parents, and my parents-in-law, because they congratulate you and they are very happy, but I told none of my friends.

TSIPY: Until you got the result.

AWATA: That's right; I was waiting for the result. By having this amniocentesis, one can know for sure whether there is Down's syndrome. . . When I think now of aborting Miya-chan, the baby, I get scared myself. . . Anyway, as you can see, I am such a talkative person [*oshaberi*], and for me it is real suffering to shut my mouth and not to say anything. So I thought, "If I only persevere at this [*gaman suru*], there will be a good result. If I make myself suffer [*tsurai me ni atte*]. . ." and I decided to be silent. However, that was really hard, wasn't it, Miya-chan?

Often I asked informants for their explanations of why Japanese women are so reluctant to have amniocentesis, given that a growing percentage of mothers-to-be are over thirty-five (officially the age that doctors should start mentioning the possibility of diagnosing fetal anomalies). Are these women not worried about the consequences of having a child with serious disorders? Moreover, in a culture that emphasizes the total responsibility of mothers to their children, such a child would deeply affect its mother's life. Though rhetoric in support of disability rights is clearly on the rise in Japan, parents of children with Down's syndrome, to take one example, are not eligible for any sizable financial support from the state. In such cases, the mother will often be expected to be absolutely dedicated and to leave everything to be at the side of the disabled child. Yet according to Awata, older mothers are usually those who tend to be reluctant to undergo prenatal diagnosis. I close this section with Awata's elaborate interpretation of the paradox of access to amniocentesis:

> The young people who graduate from high school, immediately go to work, and quickly get married are not likely to have amniocentesis: this is not the age at which doctors usually offer this possibility. And anyway, at this age the rate of having children with disorders is low, so they have no right to have amniocentesis. And the older women, who have graduated from university and have their own careers, these women are educated and therefore believe that every child, regardless of whether it is disabled or not, should be raised lovingly. So these women are entitled to have amniocentesis, but they are precisely those who would not have an abortion on principle, precisely because they are so educated and think that there should not be any discrimination against the disabled.

Awata's explanation connects age and education with reluctance to or enthusiasm for amniocentesis. Interestingly, the women with the highest risk of bearing anomalous children are those who oppose PND on moral grounds, in striking contrast to older, educated Israeli women, who often see it as their duty.

Bonding as a Social Script of Pregnancy

Japanese ethno-theories of gestation seem to have come a long way since the heyday of male monogenesis during the Tokugawa period. In fact, the idea of gestational mothers as merely vessels of the life forces emanating solely from the male "seed" proved particularly intolerable when the Osaka municipality refused to register a pair of twins, born in California through a surrogacy agreement, as the sons of their commissioning parents. In the Tokugawa period it might have been sufficient to indicate that they were conceived from the husband's "seed." However, in May 2005 the mayor insisted that only by giving birth can a woman become a mother. Far from male monogenesis, Japanese ethno-theories of gestation evolved almost in the opposite direction, perhaps best captured as "female monogenesis." This echoes official versions of domesticated motherhood; it might even be understood as the ethno-biological version of an official cult of domesticity. But as the data presented here show, it emanates from personal experiences of pregnancy at least as much as from official ideologies and population policies.

Japanese women negotiate a broad array of bodily sensations, social and biomedical dictates, and folk and personal explanatory models in making sense of their pregnancies. Significantly, there is little clash between medical knowledge and the knowledge that women draw from their bodily sensations (or "haptic knowledge," as Root and Browner (2001) would call it). The reason, I suggest, is that both the medical and the haptic forms of knowledge draw on a common cultural script, according to which pregnancy is a project of maternal caregiving and a process of prenatal bonding with the unborn child. In other words, the scheme on which pregnant women draw to interpret their bodily sensations is quite similar to the environmental scheme on which medical doctors rely for their directions. Indeed, as Root and Browner observe, it is "difficult to isolate the biomedical within pregnant women's practices and reasoning" (Root and Browner 2001, 205). Clearly, in the Japanese case, medical and nonmedical knowledge systems evince many affinities: often, even where the processes of reasoning differ, the conclusions and the practical implications agree. Interestingly, even the most explicitly resistant behavior in pregnant women was deeply informed by the dominant social script of prenatal bonding.

This script singles out the key metaphors and key ideas that become *available* to pregnant women to think with; it narrows the range of meanings that can be attached to pregnancy. Yet as we have seen, women also use it creatively, somewhat to minimize the constraints that gestation brings into their lives.

But even more important than the key metaphors is the "grammar" that "holds them together." When a Japanese woman writes a pregnancy diary she "weaves" her experience into the core idea that is conveyed by the very existence of such a script, namely, that a "plot" along which pregnancy develops *does* exist, that it is basically positive, and it can be told. It is precisely this story of the development of bonding that is documented in detail in pregnancy diaries, promoted in daily *taikyô* sessions, and ultimately materializes in the umbilical cord.

The Role of Reproductive Technologies

Clearly, population policies and national ideologies of motherhood echo in Japanese women's experiences of pregnancy. But what about reproductive technologies? How do they contribute to the experiences of pregnancy? To consider this question one should recall that different technologies point at quite divergent directions: obstetrical ultrasonography has been understood by scholars in western countries as working to enhance maternal fetal attachment (while the diagnostic elements of this technology are played down by practitioners), but more explicit diagnostic technologies such as the triple marker and amniocentesis have been understood as threatening such a bond, thereby turning pregnancy into a tentative endeavor.

As for the transformative powers of explicitly diagnostic technologies, I suggest that the conceptual frame of pregnancy as a process of maternal fetal bonding robs them of much of their power to generate an overall transformation in public conceptions of pregnancy. As the experiences of Yasuda and Awata attest, within a general understanding of pregnancy as an early stage of child raising, women who dread fetal abnormality face tremendous difficulties in managing their anxieties, and their anxieties might not necessarily lead them to undergo diagnostic tests such as amniocentesis: as Yasuda said, she did not "go as far as having such a dangerous test." Women who seriously consider diagnosis are tortured by self-assessments as insufficiently committed wives (clearly in Yasuda's case) and mothers, rather than possessors of an agency to "choose" whether they would like to continue or terminate the pregnancy. They ashamedly silence their unbearable experiences: they avail of no social script to interpret their personal experience in a way that it can be openly talked about.

At the same time I am also doubtful about the extent to which obstetrical ultrasound transforms the experiences of pregnant Japanese women. At first sight the "message" carried by ultrasound seems to agree with the range of contemporary Japanese ethno-theories of gestation, and indeed this technology is used openly and quite liberally. Yet the reader is reminded that many pregnant Japanese women do not rely on ultrasonography alone to sense their unborn babies. Rather, ultrasonography has become one more technique among a rich array that have been available to Japanese women for at least the last hundred years. Whether the vivid image of the unborn baby predates obstetrical ultrasound in Japan is a point I raise in the final discussion of the book, but the contemporary Japanese mother may already be quite well "acquainted" with her unborn baby (through other techniques of daily communication such as *taikyô*) when she comes for an ultrasound scan. Watching their babies on the ultrasound screen might *echo* the feelings that mothers cultivate through other techniques.

Moreover, while ultrasonic devices might indeed work to heighten the mother's sense of the baby's reality, significantly Japanese unborn babies (just like newborn babies) seem to lack both the individuality and rights that scholars working in the U.S. report. Nor can one feel that mothers are "bypassed" or made transparent in public or medical discourse, as Petchesky-Pollack (1987) claims (or that mothers belittle their own contribution to fetal health in any way). To this effect, in Japan I have never seen ultrasound scans performed in darkness (as I often have in Israel). Japanese mothers do not "merge" into the surrounding darkness dominated by the ultrasound screen but are visibly present in a brightly lit room on the occasion of seeing their unborn babies on the screen. Neither are they absent when ultrasound pictures of fetuses are shown in the media: when pregnancy guides feature ultrasound images of fetuses, they often make sure to convey the presence of the mother through the texts that "narrate" the pictures. The captions to such ultrasound pictures have the unborn baby "speaking" to its mother, and the mother is cited responding to the baby's "words."

The key to understanding the meaning of such different uses of ultrasonography, compared with the uses one finds in American or Israeli clinics and media, is paying attention to the lack of conceptual *separation* between mother and baby, the element that Barbara Katz Rothman claims lies at the heart of the transformation that reproductive technologies have brought about in the West. She is quoted in Davis-Floyd and Davis as follows:

> Diagnostic technologies, from the most mundane and routine ultrasound to the most exotic embryo transplant, have in common that they work toward the construction of the fetus as a separate being—they verify, they make real, the fetus. They make the fetus a visible, audible presence among us, and they do that by doing two other things. They medicalize pregnancy, and they render invisible and inaudible, women.
>
> The history of western obstetrics is the history of technologies of separation. We've separated milk from breasts, mothers from babies, fetuses from pregnancies, sexuality from procreation, pregnancy from motherhood. And finally we are left with the image of the fetus as a free-floating being alone, analogous to man in space, with the umbilical cord tethering the placental ship, and the mother reduced to the empty space that surrounds it.
>
> It is very very hard to conceptually put back together that which medicine has rendered asunder. . . . As I speak to different groups, from social scientists to birth practitioners, what I find is that I have a harder and harder time trying to make the meaning of connection, let alone the value of connection, understood. (Barbara Katz Rothman, in Davis-Floyd and Davis 1997, 315)

In the data presented here the fetus can never be imagined as a free-floating being alone, and mothers can never be reduced to black outer space. Babies can be imagined only *as part* of a maternal–child interactive bond, without which the child could not have won life in the first place. If anything, ultrasonography has provided another set of illustrations for notions of maternal–fetal connectedness, notions much favored by the political promotion of the cult of domesticity.

The Nurturant Maternal Body

The source of the persisting power of domesticated nurturant motherhood in Japan is becoming increasingly puzzling in what seems to be a changing society where a generation of vibrant well-educated women aspire to develop their own careers, often far away from home. The Japanese labor market is undoubtedly changing, as more women of childbearing age are becoming part of the workforce (as the slightly higher M curve of women's employment shows). However, I suspect that this does not reflect so much the growing numbers of working mothers, but the decreasing birth rates, and the growing numbers of women whose commitments to career tracks have made them give up the option of bearing children.[14] Women who do become mothers, on the other hand, seem to "slip" into the domesticated model of mothering, and as the ethnography reveals, they often withdraw from the workplace much earlier, while pregnant. Childbearing and career making remain pretty much an either/or option, which returns us to the question of whence the model of domesticated motherhood draws its power. Do women simply adhere to official ideologies of virtuous motherhood—or better still, become disenchanted with working because of the lack of accessible and affordable childcare?

The lack of affordable childcare arrangements for working mothers influences their choices profoundly. But the ethnography presented here illuminates an additional and crucial element that underlies the organization of child care in a way that deters mothers from using it, namely, their socialization into an embodied understanding of nurturance as biologically located in their own bodies. In other words, pregnancy is revealed as a powerful locus of embodied experiences, through which women are indoctrinated into a meticulous style of nurturing their (unborn) babies. Apparently Japanese society offers ample opportunities for women to learn and practice nurturant behaviors, but through pregnancy women come to understand nurturance as an exclusively maternal biological attribute. Through bodily practices supported and augmented by authoritative medical instructions, and solicited and unsolicited advice from relatives and friends, women are physically socialized into maternal nurturant behaviors while they are pregnant. Some pregnant women indeed challenge notions of parenting skills as embodied, yet they, too, end up continuously negotiating with them. Other pregnant women come to understand themselves truly as the ecosystems and "makers" of their babies. This feeling of exclusiveness might turn against them when, sometime later, they may find themselves segregated. Nevertheless, women themselves might find the assumption of their own exclusiveness difficult to challenge, since their own understanding of it is embodied.

The literature about Japanese women is abundant with accounts of women who years later are still engaged in the powerful dynamics of nurturance that keeps them so busy as to prevent them from assuming serious commitments outside the home. Mothers are described as busy preparing carefully calculated nutritiously balanced and perfectly decorated lunch boxes for their nursery school children (Allison 1991), or preparing midnight snacks for their elementary or high school children; they will sharpen pencils, make sure the school uniform is clean, and attend periodic PTA meetings; they will be expected to make themselves available to support any educational enterprise at school, the assumption being that, as mothers, they should be available for any activity connected to their children's academic advancement.

As in the process of gestation, women will be given numerous instructions, will be supervised and tested by schoolteachers and other authority figures, and will be evaluated on their achievements. Allison writes: "If the child succeeds, a mother is complimented; if the child fails, a mother is blamed" (Allison 1991, 203; see also Fujita 1987).[15] The ethnography presented here reveals pregnancy as a key site to understanding the persistent power of the ideal of domesticated motherhood. Women emerge from the process of gestation—as it is cared for and narrated in Japanese medical spheres, in the public media, and within circles of family friends and other acquaintances—touched by an embodied experience of nurturing, complete with its potential for pleasure as well as the guilt of those who embody responsibilities.

4

The Path of Ambiguity

Motherhood and Other National Missions

Since the time of the pre-state Jewish settlement (*yishuv*) at the end of the nineteenth century, mothers have been eulogized in Israeli public culture and official discourse at least as much as in Japan. Motherhood, a host of scholars claim, is an entry ticket into the Israeli collective for Jewish women, and has been constituted as a "national mission": the most important contribution a woman can make to society (Berkovitch 1997). To fully understand how the national aspect is engraved into the institution of motherhood, recall that Israel is defined as a Zionist-Jewish state, in which non-Jewish women's fertility is perceived as part of the demographic threat with its direct association with the Israeli–Arab conflict.

In fact, Jewish motherhood was endowed with national meaning long before the constitution of the state of Israel and even before Zionism emerged as a national movement. Rabbinic law grants mothers the sole power to define their children's national-religious affiliation: only individuals who are born to Jewish mothers are considered Jewish according to the Halacha (though the traditional Jewish family has always been essentially patriarchal and patrilineal: see Leissner 2000).

However, official Israeli ideology has developed in a profoundly different direction from the Japanese advocacy of "good wives and wise mothers." First, at no stage in the evolution of the Israeli gender ideology has it promoted a cult of domesticity. The discourse about womanhood has instead been immersed in an *ethos* of gender equality since as early as the pre-state Jewish settlement. The Zionist movement, fed on "socialist-egalitarian notions," sought "to create a new, modern, and advanced society" (Rapoport and El-Or 1997, 574). This does not mean that the first female Zionist settlers in Palestine did not have to fight for their labor rights (Bernstein, D. 1992) as well as for suffrage (Herzog 1994); neither does it mean that actual gender equality has ever been realized in the new state (Azmon and Izraeli 1993; Swirski and Safir 1991). But significantly, especially in the context of a cultural comparison, one must acknowledge that the politics of gender in Israel has evolved under a *rhetoric* of commitment to equality.

To take military service as an example, Israeli law, which mandates conscription of both women and men, is one major symbol of equality. In a state entangled in continuous military conflict, participating in the security effort is conceived as a right and symbolizes participation in society. True, men serve in compulsory service longer, and only women may be excused from military service on the grounds of conscience or religious belief.[1] They may also be exempt from military service due to motherhood or marriage, which all but explicitly declares the prioritizing of their mothering roles or potential mothering over soldiering (Izraeli 1997; Leissner 2000). Nonetheless, it is necessary for the comparison here to note that Japanese women of any age or marital status were never admitted to soldiery, even at the height of World War II.

The state of Israel, then, has encouraged fertility, and also nurtured "a consensus regarding parenting and with it a discriminatory and sometimes debilitating stereotype . . . as first and foremost the function of women" (Raday 1995), but ideologically women have never been impelled into the home. Instead, the state assigns many familial functions to the public sphere while channeling women to participate in society through and along with their familial roles. Accordingly, child-care institutions in Israel are subsidized by the government, on the clear assumption that mothers work. Providing working mothers with maternity benefits has been officially dubbed as serving "a function of national importance," parallel to the state benefits granted to soldiers (Raday 1995). Moreover, the taxation system provides tax relief "points" only to working mothers (and not to their male partners) regardless of the number of children in the family. So, contrary to the Japanese M curve, Israeli-Jewish women experience no significant change in their rate of working on reaching childbearing age; Israeli society has managed to cultivate a cult of fertility and motherhood without giving rise to a cult of domesticity. Where is pregnancy positioned in such set of simultaneously converging and diverging trajectories of childbearing and child raising?

Prelude: Ordering Baby Supplies

In Israel, chain stores selling baby furniture and clothing customarily invite expectant couples to choose prior to birth whatever they need for their future baby—that is, to make a "birth order," without paying for it immediately. Peculiar to Israel, however, is that the parents do not take the goods home: the store keeps the order until the baby is born. Israeli parents-to-be (particularly first-time ones) are expected to be completely disorganized in awaiting the new baby. This highly impractical custom, practiced by Israeli Jews from a broad array of ethnic origins, is compensated by the "birth order" strategy of preparing while adhering to unpreparedness. Such marketing strategies, I suggest, tune in to a broad and common perception of pregnancy that acknowledges it as a fertile enterprise only retrospectively, after a healthy baby has been born. This chapter endeavors to illuminate the socio-cultural schemes that underlie the lived experiences that constitute "birth orders" as attractive, logical, and convenient arrangements.

This chapter partly covers issues quite similar to those raised in the previous chapter on Japanese women's experiences, but with significant departures. As in that chapter, it opens with an assessment of the location of pregnancy vis-à-vis the public sphere of work, but then goes on to explicate an important characteristic of the Israeli context of pregnancy: the expectation that male partners will participate in it. Next, unlike the Japanese chapter, which explores prenatal practices of child raising, this chapter probes Israeli women's quest for medical information about prenatal diagnostic technologies. Parallel to the Japanese accounts, I trace the kind of relationships forged between women and their fetuses, this time within a general understanding of pregnancy as tentative, augmented by the dominance of PND. Finally, as in the Japanese chapter, I look for experiences of pregnancy that offer an alternative to the dominant perceptions.

Pregnancy as a "Nonissue"

Unlike Japan, where the pregnant body is conceived as out of place in the public sphere, in Israel pregnant women are highly visible. While the Japanese public sphere tends to ignore pregnancy, in Israel a pregnant woman getting on a crowded bus will usually be offered a seat. On the other hand, women are expected to carry on with their usual tasks. Women themselves are often keen to resume their regular responsibilities as if nothing has changed. Pregnancy does not prevent them doing their jobs or performing any of their other daily activities right up to term, that is, the birth itself.

On a practical level, few pregnant women expect people in the public sphere to be considerate of their condition. Miriam, a thirty-three-year-old social worker, mother of a three-year-old child and pregnant for the second time, told me laughingly, "I was standing in line for the cash dispenser and suddenly the lady standing in front of me stepped aside and let me in before her—I was so surprised. Wow, she let me in before her, what a thing."

For Miriam this was an unexpected event, since she did not consider herself eligible for any special consideration. As she explained to me, "Here [in Israel] nobody so much as looks at you—you're just like everybody else. You have to stand in line for the cash dispenser, just like everybody else. Here, half the country is pregnant, so being pregnant is nothing special."

Miriam echoes the phenomenon that I call "the trivialization of pregnancy," in reference to the idea of its being a common occurrence in Israeli life. She accepts the "common sense" that links pregnancy's statistical frequency to its trivialization. However, as she told me later, "Although you feel as if you are carrying out your life's mission, people think, 'Well, here's another one.'" Clearly Miriam senses a gap between her perception of her own pregnancy as important and unique (somewhat reminiscent of Berkovitch's conceptualization of motherhood as a national mission) and the way her pregnancy is perceived by others.

Some women ideologically cooperate in the trivialization of their own pregnancies. Oshrat, a secretary, had one two-year-old child already and was now pregnant for the second time; she told me that she was slightly offended when an elderly man got up to let her sit down. "I told him, 'I am fine, I am fine,' but he insisted. What does he think of me? I'm not a cripple, I'm just pregnant. So what if I have a big belly? It doesn't mean I can't stand for ten minutes." Oshrat insisted that she was *just* pregnant. For her, accepting the man's offer connoted being physically disabled. Often women consider themselves privileged to live in an environment that does not "make a fuss" of pregnancy and birth.

Yael, a social worker, described the satisfaction she got from her workplace. "I work in a place with many women colleagues, so all the time women give birth and come back to work, and then again give birth and come back to work after three months. The boss is also a woman, so generally there is *tolerance* in my workplace" (emphasis added).

Tolerance echoes the benevolence extended by the workplace to the troublesome otherness of pregnancy and birth, but it also signifies a quality of relationship different from consideration (encountered in a similar context in Japanese women's narratives). Being considerate is an *active* state of mind, directed to recognizing another person's legitimate *needs*. Tolerance in this specific context is a *passive* state of mind, directed to *putting up with* the other person's difference and even incompetence. Unlike some Japanese working women, Yael is not greatly concerned by the possibility that she might become a burden. The workplace is not going to be considerate as such, it is merely going to tolerate her. Moreover, the women in the workplace minimize possible frictions. They are pictured as moving easily in and out of work in a smooth cyclic motion. So, unlike many Japanese women, who will withdraw from the workplace in order not to become a nuisance (especially if they can afford it financially), Yael kept her job and felt grateful for the tolerance others displayed of her condition. Note that in Yael's narrative the "effortless" motion of women in and out of the workplace remains unproblematized.

Pregnant Israeli women, across the lower, middle and higher-middle class, usually work until they give birth. By law, women who have worked one year prior to conception can take maternity leave up to forty-nine days before the due date (as designated by a doctor), but they rarely consider this possibility. Israeli law allows fourteen weeks of maternity leave (paid at 100 percent of wages by the national insurance) beginning from the first day of leave. If a woman chooses to take this leave prior to birth she will have to return to work fourteen weeks later, regardless of the actual date of delivery. As many interviewees explained to me, they preferred to spend these precious weeks with the newborn baby. Women would only take their maternity leave prior to birth if an emergency arose. Otherwise, they would work as usual until the very end of the pregnancy.

Not all Israeli women feel so grateful to their workplaces. I met Leah, twenty-six, a mother of two in the last month of her third pregnancy, in a noisy bazaar, where she had worked for the previous year. Unlike women who held well-paid and high-status jobs, she did not feel grateful to the workplace for tolerating her. She told me, "I am so tired I would go to my mother to be spoiled if I only had the chance, but I must work to get the national insurance to pay for my maternity leave." Before I left the bazaar, Leah's superior caught me on the way out and, looking sternly at Leah, complained that "the women these days are so spoiled, they take advantage of the law and leave work so many times to see their doctors, or just to stay at home and nap, things that women in my day had no time for." Interestingly, both Leah and her boss equated not working with indulgence.[2]

Work and Postponing Discomfort and Pain

The tendency to "not make a fuss" of pregnancy may have far-reaching implications for Israeli women's alertness to emergency medical situations, a point that deserved further research. Some of my interviewees told me how they continued working in spite of unexpected complications with their pregnancies. Carmit, a twenty-eight-year-old secretary in her second pregnancy, experienced preterm labor contractions in her seventh month. It took her a few days of pain and self-prescribed attempts to relieve it until she eventually decided to see a doctor. She was hospitalized immediately and was prescribed four weeks of bed rest.

> They said I should be at home for at least four weeks. But if I had stayed home I would not have had a salary, because at that time National Insurance [*Bituah Leumi*] did not define rest in bed [*shmirat herayon*] as an illness. So if it isn't an illness they don't pay anything. And I wanted to get my salary, so I stayed at home for two weeks and then went back to work. I was deeply offended. What kind of thing is it to say that preterm contractions are not an illness? What is it then, a picnic? Am I sitting at home amusing myself? So getting the flu is better. You get more respect getting hepatitis than being in bed resting when it comes to your rights. I cannot understand why pregnancy cannot be considered an illness in this case—it's much more frightening than illness.

Only when a pregnancy complication occurs does Carmit challenge the idea of "pregnancy as a nonillness": she redefines preterm contractions as an illness. The expression *shmirat herayon*, which designates bed rest in Hebrew, is noteworthy: while the English expression "to rest in bed" is almost a phenomenological description, *shmirat herayon*, literally "guarding pregnancy," indicates special protection. It also implies that most pregnancies do not require such special protection.

Why was Carmit so offended by the legal definition of *shmirat herayon* as a nonillness? Not because she would prefer to define herself as ill but because such definitions do not acknowledge her suffering but reduce and silence her pain and discomfort, defining her as spoiled and indulgent. She interprets the law as if it "suspects" her of spending her time leisurely at home. Carmit insists that resting in bed is a serious business. Moreover, it is important for her to assert herself as a loyal worker who would not miss days off work "just because of a minor discomfort."

Here an axis is revealed, along which pregnant women position themselves; it is oriented quite differently from the Japanese axis, which extends from "too bonded" mothers to "immature and insufficiently bonded" mothers. First, the social scripts that constitute the Israeli frame of reference are not about mothers at all: they are about women and their physical competence to continue performing their roles in the public sphere; they range from the key image of the spoiled woman to a particularly Israeli version of "superwoman." The power of these images lies in their continuous use by women to negotiate the "location" of their own pregnancies. Carmit, for example, would not permit any implication of herself as a spoiled, lazy woman and worker.

Since Carmit had a medical certificate confirming the necessity of a full bed rest, she could have resorted to the authoritative medical definition of her condition. However, at some point Carmit decided to go back to work. Interestingly, here the authority of medical prescription seems to lose its force in the face of the more powerful cultural image of the spoiled woman that lurks behind it.

Why did Carmit return to work? Certainly she wanted to continue to draw her salary. However, if she had believed that resting in bed was crucial for her pregnancy, she would not have endangered it. Later, she told me: " 'Well,' I thought, 'What can happen if I go in for a few hours every day?' I had a feeling that everything would be all right." She explained her decision by saying, "They didn't give me much medication, *only* bed rest . . . so what could happen if I went back for a few hours?" [emphasis added]

Carmit's use of "feeling" echoes Browner and Press's (1997) suggestion that women take medical knowledge into account only when it accords with their experiential bodily knowledge (Browner and Press 1997). However, it seems to me that we have an additional effect here. The image of the spoiled woman haunted Carmit to the extent that it prevented her from understanding bed rest as "serious" medical treatment, perhaps even in spite of her bodily sensations. When I talked with Carmit, she was at the end of her last trimester, still working, and still annoyed by the idea that resting in bed could not be perceived seriously. "I am now in the thirty-seventh week of pregnancy. Do you think I'm interested in my work? Do you think I'm interested in anything? Not even a tiny little bit! If I could, I would gladly go home, sit, read books, rest a lot, and make myself comfortable. I have already said goodbye to everybody, so there will be no unexpected surprises. I go to work, but my mind is elsewhere."

Carmit admitted that working through to the end of the third trimester was not at all easy. Yet she never considered taking her maternity leave before her due date. Although she seemed fed up with working, she looked puzzled when I told her about the working habits of pregnant women in Japan:

TSIPY: Japanese women tend to leave their jobs when they find out they are pregnant. Even if they continue working, they would certainly leave six weeks before the due date.

CARMIT: Oh, but what on earth do they do all day long at home?

Carmit's response was typical of the expression of surprise with which most of my interviewees greeted the idea of giving up work at some stage in their pregnancy. In my view their bewilderment emphasizes their perception of pregnancy as a "nonlegitimate excuse" to alter their working conditions. Women are apparently prepared to pay with their health to continue participating in the public sphere. The implications of women's cooperation in the trivialization of pregnancy are far-reaching because, through the process of their daily suffering, women trivialize the meaning of bodily sensations to the extent of disregarding pain, sometimes to the point where it becomes unbearable. In a number of cases, women's disregard of pain clearly delayed the identification of conditions that require medical help according to criteria of health-care providers. The story of Mira, a twenty-seven-year-old graphic designer, was a case in point.

The ordeal she told me about started in her fourth month of pregnancy, when her doctor prescribed iron pills. With hindsight, it became clear to her that these pills gradually caused her to dehydrate, which eventually led to preterm labor. This complication happened slowly, developing over as long as a month of suffering, during which Mira complained of not being able to eat and drink and of continuous diarrhea. She went to seek the advice of her doctor, who merely told her that her symptoms were "natural effects that happen during pregnancy." Although she felt strongly that something was clearly wrong, her family, and her female relatives in particular, all of whom had experienced pregnancy and birth, discouraged her from becoming alarmed at her sensations. As Mira told me, her mother, grandmother, and aunts said that "This is natural; it's because of the pregnancy. You'll see, you'll suffer from these symptoms until the end of your pregnancy."

Over many weeks it never occurred to anybody that Mira was in serious need of medical attention, and Mira herself tried to delay hospitalization to the very last moment when painkillers could no longer help her overcome what turned out to be frequent contractions of preterm labor.

Whereas Mira's story shows that disregarding pain may lead to dramatic consequences, other less dramatic stories seem to have "taught" the women who told them that pain and discomfort are part and parcel of pregnancy, and that, as Rachel, a thirty-five-year-old high school teacher, explained to me, "It is impossible to call the doctor for every little twinge your body gets."

Pregnant Heroines

Interestingly, not even women who persevered with pain considered themselves "special," since they compared their own image with "real heroines." In the course of the interviews, women often measured themselves against mythic images of pregnant Israeli heroines whom they mentioned, for whom pregnancy or pain seemed to be nonissues. The fact that all these stories were based on rumors did not diminish their glamour.

Women tell stories that they have heard about "a friend of a friend" who drove herself to the hospital while in active labor; another mythological woman, a medical student, sat a difficult university examination while suffering both severe backache (due to scoliosis worsened by pregnancy) and contraction pains; several other stories dealt with women who arrived at the hospital "with the baby's head popping out" or gave birth in the cab, just because "they waited until it was too late."

My interviewees clearly differentiated themselves from the brave images they spoke of. In their own eyes they were never as brave and unspoiled as the women in the stories. The tendency to underestimate the potential hardships of pregnancy in the women's everyday lives should be understood in the context of such stories, which make any human discomfort look pale. These stories are part and parcel of the trivialization mentality. They build an impossible model of the endurance of pain and discomfort that most women simply cannot meet.

Carmela, a thirty-three-year-old graphic designer, compared herself to the image of the religious Zionist settler: "You see pregnant women all the time and everywhere, even in places that I would not imagine going to. . . . All these religious women, all these 'fighter women' [faiteriot] in the territories—you see them, with their big belly and five kids scattered around them, and she goes around in the street with an Uzi. . . . You see her and you feel like, 'Who am I anyway, while she is such a hero?' . . . It is a different style of being, you know, but still there is some general consideration of your self against that."

Carmela has nearly nothing in common with the image she describes. She lives in a small house surrounded by a nice little garden in a middle-class neighborhood on the outskirts of Jerusalem. She defines herself as secular and is politically oriented to the left. She has one child and is pregnant for the second time. Nonetheless, the image of the vigorous, brave, religious pregnant settler is in her head. Although this image clearly belongs to a social group that is different from her own, Carmela measures her own "pregnancy competence" against it. The mere presence of such an image is enough to diminish Carmela's own "bravery" in juggling her demanding work with caring for her child while pregnant, with almost no help from her partner or parents.

Such images, whether they concern actual women or are fabricated myths, signal to women that the expression "pregnancy is not an illness" should be understood as "pregnancy is nothing." This becomes clearer when compared with the range of Japanese perceptions of pregnancy: like Israelis, Japanese insist that pregnancy is not an illness, but this does not deprive the pregnant body of its *importance.*

Still, what we have seen trivialized so far is the womanly aspects of pregnancy. As we shall see, the "fetal" parts of pregnancy are taken seriously: trivialization, I argue, is permitted through a conceptual separation of pregnancy from "pregnancy outcomes." To comprehend the trivialization of pregnancy fully, it is necessary to consider how fetuses are perceived (a point I return to later). But before that, one more element is important in clarifying the social setting in which pregnancy is experienced in Israel: the expectation that men will participate in it.

Men's Contributions to the Trivialization of Pregnancy

The idea of sharing pregnancy and birth with one's partner is, of course, not an original Israeli idea. Since the establishment of the discourse of "new fatherhood" in the 1960s, men in many western countries have been increasingly encouraged and expected to be more active participants in child rearing and more intensely involved in their partners' pregnancy, labor, and birth (Draper 2003; Mitchell 2001). Pregnant partnership is heralded in psycho-social scholarship as highly beneficial for both partners and for their relationship. It has been suggested that increasing involvement of fathers during childbirth can reduce the pain suffered by women (Henneborn and Cogan 1975) and help couples negotiate the transition to parenthood while preserving their relationship as a couple (Diemer 1997).

Biomedical technologies play a major role in the attempt to "draw men closer" by functioning as "proxies" of embodiment for male partners who are often conceptualized as lacking access to the direct embodied experience of pregnancy (Draper 2002, 779). Ultrasound, Draper claims, creates for the British father "the potential . . . to have the same visual access to the baby as his partner, thus *equalizing* their respective positions as knowers of the baby" (Draper 2002, 782; emphasis added). She also claims that "ultrasound is an example of a range of contemporary rituals, helping men make and mark their transition to Western fatherhood" (Draper 2002, 790). Nevertheless, other accounts by anthropologists and feminist writers call into question the "equality" advocated by reproductive technologies. Sandelowski argues that while men are indeed becoming involved more than ever before in pregnancy thanks to the development of obstetrical ultrasound, ultrasound itself is making the woman more and more invisible. While the doctor provides information to the husband, the woman herself is often left out (Sandelowski 1994). In the same vein, Van der Ploeg argues that women are pushed out of the metaphorical status of "pregnant patient" by their husbands and fetuses (Van der Ploeg 1995). Even *Spiritual Midwifery*, the highly popular book among advocates of the American natural-birth movement that emphasizes participation by husbands as crucial to successful deliveries, warns in various places throughout the book that some husbands lack the knowledge or the emotional and spiritual ability to help their partners (Gaskin 1977, 321–322, 344, 440–441). These accounts exemplify some of the tensions that arise in making husbands equal and full participants in pregnancy and birth.

During the last two decades Israeli men have become frequent visitors at maternity clinics. As will become apparent in the following sections of this chapter, significantly more Israeli men are found today accompanying their partners, especially to ultrasound scans but also to various medical checkups and consultations, amniocentesis, birthing classes, and the birth event itself: nearly all Israeli hospitals allow expectant fathers to be present at the birth of their children. Men's experiences of pregnancy and birth have only recently become a focus of studies in the anthropology of reproduction, and they certainly deserve analysis in themselves (Ivry and Teman 2008).

Here, however, I consider not so much men's experiences of pregnancy as the effects of their participation in medical rituals on the overall social atmosphere of pregnancy, in particular the couple's partnership. The Israeli endeavor to share pregnancy, I suggest, has acquired a particular flavor that ought to be taken into account, if we are to understand Israeli women's experiences of pregnancy.

Dragging Men In

I met Lior when he and his wife attended a birth-education course in the midst of the second Lebanon war during the summer of 2006. Lior, who had missed the previous class because of military-reserve duty, smiled at the birth educator as he entered and said. "See what a dedicated partner [*mashkian*] I am? I came straight here from reserve duty [*miluim*]. My father—all of his children were born when he was away in the army. He received a letter saying, 'Mazal Tov, you have a boy, you have a girl.' And here am I, coming directly from *miluim*."

The birth-education teacher responded with a warm "Well done [*kol hakavod*]," and Lior's wife looked at him proudly.

Whereas Lior was applauded for overcoming the fatigue of military service to participate, other men I met in birth-education classes and elsewhere were applauded for significantly less heroic acts of devotion, such as giving up a football game on TV or missing a meeting with friends (Ivry 2009a). These cases illustrate a situation whereby men are expected to participate, but their participation is never taken for granted and is often applauded by wives, birth educators, relatives, and friends. Clearly, participating in all medical activities was collectively understood as the ultimate expression of commitment to one's pregnant female partner. Still, my findings show that men often negotiated their participation with their pregnant partners. The negotiations varied in content and emotional intensity, but they were always present. The urgency expressed by female partners played a major part in men's motivation to participate. Individual pregnant women expected different degrees of participation from their male partner and exerted different amounts of pressure on him to take part (Ivry and Teman 2008.)

It was not rare for men to express feeling unnecessarily "forced" into a medical activity by their female partner. Sometimes men reported being angrily reproached by their partner for not attending a prenatal test. Shaul, thirty, an accountant, described these tensions: "She comes complaining to me that I am not as excited as she is. She says: 'I feel that I'm going through this alone.' For example, there was some test that I could not attend because I had a lot of work, and I also was not overly upset about missing it. I said to her: 'I came to the ultrasound scans, but I don't feel the need to come to a routine checkup.' So she got really upset [*hitkomema*]. She said, 'Don't you feel the need to come? Aren't you excited to hear the pulse . . . ?' I told her: 'I've already been with you to the important tests.' "

Shaul's words illustrate how emotionally charged the issue of men's attendance of medical tests can become for some couples. Moreover, it reveals an unwritten hierarchy of importance between different biomedical activities that might feed into men's considerations. The order of priority reflected in Shaul's narrative echoes that of other male partners I spoke to, as well as comparable cases in the anthropological literature (Draper 2002; 2003). Top priority goes to ultrasound scans, which seem to bring even the most resentful of men into the clinic. However, as Shaul's story illustrates, female partners do not always accept such hierarchies as legitimate excuses for nonparticipation. For later discussion, it should be borne in mind that in the process of such continuous negotiations, medical rituals become indexes of commitment, through which expectant fathers can be "measured" and graded. (Ivry and Teman 2008)

Whereas ultrasound scans were indeed top on the list, birth-education classes were perceived as "mandatory." So whereas I briefly consider men's responses to ultrasound scans later, birth-education classes offer a unique opportunity to witness how men negotiate pregnancy in a public space that is explicitly meant for them as well as their partners, and to explore the kind of atmosphere they bring into the shared pregnancy.

Kursei hachana leleida, meaning literally "birth-preparation courses," are oriented specifically to birthing and not to parenting (as we saw with Japanese classes). Unlike Japanese maternity classes (*hahaoya gakkyû*), which are also aimed at improving women's daily lives and therefore are given much earlier, Israeli classes are given during the last months of pregnancy. The issue of nutrition, for example, which is central to *hahaoya gakkyû*, is rarely raised in Israeli birth-education classes.

Classes for the secular and religious populations in Israel assume almost axiomatically that pregnant women will attend the classes accompanied by their husbands.[3] Therefore, classes are oriented to meet "male tastes" as much as the needs of women.

Experienced birth educators, however, are aware of the presence of disenchanted men and try to cater to their needs. The pamphlet advertising a course entitled *Giving Birth Together* quotes an anonymous husband: "My wife dragged [*garera oti*] me. I was afraid that it was going to be too 'feminine' and boring for me. But on the contrary, I was really into it [*hayiti bainyanim*]. The course is not only for women. It is basic training [*tironut*] for fathers. A must [*hova*]."—Eitan, an Israeli army officer

What message did the birth educators who had designed the pamphlet want to get across by citing Eitan? First, they "formally" recognized as legitimate the fears and unwillingness that some men might feel. Secondly, while "femininity" is equated with boredom in the officer's narrative, the birth educators apparently wished to assure the pamphlet's readers that even the most "manly" of men, that is, army officers, found their class relevant. The equation of femininity with boredom remains unchallenged, but it is subtly implied that the classes use a language that is common to men as well as women. When asked about the problem of a husband participating unwillingly, Paula, a fifty-year-old experienced birth educator, explained to me that her classes merited his presence because "I am teaching him a language that is easy for him to learn."

Paula supposes that the highly medicalized language she uses in her classes will suit a "natural disposition" in men, thereby echoing the traditional categorization of men as "rational" and more comfortable with technologies (cf. Reed 2005). Ruth, another birth educator, expressed this view clearly on the occasion of the "guided tour through birthing rooms" that she offered the couples on her course. As soon as all the couples in her class had entered the birth room, she started to explain the medical equipment in the room. As part of a particularly detailed explanation of the monitor, she said: "You can see in this monitor the fetus's pulse. A fetus's pulse usually is between 120 and 170. I am saying this for the men because they like numbers and machines. The first thing they look at when they move into the birth room is the monitor."

However, although birth educators do their best to draw men in, men complain about various aspects of the course. It is assumed that both partners work and therefore classes usually take place in the evening. At the end of a long day of work, some men complain of tiredness. In one of the classes, Yoni, a thirty-year-old lawyer, yawned repeatedly. At one point Ruth, the birth educator, told him slightly angrily, "Do me a favor: go and make yourself the thickest black coffee you can and come back."

Yoni went obediently and did as he was told. However, in the elevator, on their way down to the first floor, I recorded the following conversation between Yoni and his wife, Tali.

TALI (gently): You see, you should have taken a nap in the afternoon.

YONI (cynically): I should have slept the whole day, shouldn't I?

TALI: But this way you can't concentrate and don't learn anything.

YONI: There you are: you [pointing at me] are yawning now, and Ruth also yawned at some point, but I'm the only one she picks on [nitpelet].

Tali assumes that there is a lot to learn. For Tali, who is studying for a master's degree and defines herself as a feminist, Yoni's physical presence is not enough. She wants him to participate fully, which means getting to *know* about pregnancy. Yoni, for his part, feels that though he is trying his best, he is just being picked on.

When classes end slightly late, some of the husbands mutter their dismay. Moreover, although classes are usually abundant with visual aids, many husbands still complain of boredom. From the above account, a considerable amount of the implicit and explicit friction between husband and wife during pregnancy clearly arises from the expectation that husbands should participate. Significantly, the partner's negotiations about the husband's participation in medical rituals, which I found in relation to earlier ultrasounds, checkups and other medical consultations, continue right up to the last months of pregnancy.

Making Sense of Pregnancy

Since men participate in medical and semimedical events during pregnancy, they often find themselves negotiating these particular meanings of pregnancy with notions taken from their own life-worlds, and they bring these images into the common life-worlds in which women experience their pregnancies. What kinds of images arise from their attempts to understand pregnancy, and how is pregnancy seen from their perspective? Let us return to Ruth's class. In the first lesson she started with an elaborate presentation of the anatomy of pregnancy, using an impressive collection of visual props. At one point Ruth turned to one of the women and asked,

RUTH: How much amniotic fluid do you have, Miriam?

MIRIAM'S HUSBAND: Three liters.

RUTH: If your wife had three liters of water in her belly, she would have walked like this [mimics a heavy backward-bending type of walking].

MIRIAM'S HUSBAND: When I was in the army, I carried fifty liters on my back regularly, and I walked straight.

RUTH: But this isn't the same thing! This goes in front, in the belly [laughter from couples taking part].

As Ruth told me later, through her elaborate anatomical description she aimed to explain why women "complain so much" during pregnancy. Doing this, she felt, might do women an important service. However, we should pay attention to the technique she used. Ruth cited numbers and utilized her huge anatomical charts to illustrate as vividly as possible the amount of strain that pregnancy places on a woman's body. Hearing her detailed anatomical explanations, I could not help thinking that in more ways than one medicalization was a way out of trivializing the burdens of pregnancy. Only authoritative knowledge was capable of turning mere "griping" [kuteriut] into legitimate complaint that deserved attention.

In deciding to empower her women clients, Ruth used medicalization as a form of agency, a pattern that is seen in other contexts as well. For example, Sargent and Stark, as well as Davis-Floyd, show how women empower themselves in the birth setting and gain more control over their births through the appropriation and consumption of more rather than fewer medical interventions (Davis-Floyd 1994; Sargent and Stark 1989). Teman also shows how, by "medicalizing" their pregnancies, Israeli surrogate mothers empower themselves and acquire a sense of control and distance from their pregnancies (Teman 2001; 2010). Nevertheless, the role that Ruth takes upon herself is particularly difficult since, by military standards, carrying the burdens of pregnancy seems to be nothing to fuss about, to say the least. Although she (as an authoritative birth educator) challenged the husband's comparison in terms of pregnancy's position in the body, none of the participants offered any other challenges. No one mentioned that pregnancy is not a load that one can drop at the end of the day, or questioned the exaggerated weight the husband said represented the normal pack that any soldier carries.

The above example shows vividly how the aspiration to include men in all the most intimate details of reproduction creates an inner tension. In part, this tension stems from the paradox of the ideal of sharing between men and women in a society with a strong tendency to draw on military images. Nonetheless, measuring pregnancy against military standards is still only one way in which pregnancy can be trivialized.

In this respect, one of the characteristics of male narratives that I noticed throughout the classes was humor, a dimension almost absent from "woman's talk" about pregnancy. The following are typical examples of jokes told by men. The first scene happened when Daniela, a midwife teaching birthing classes in a hospital, stood in the doorway to welcome the couples coming into her class.

DANIELA (smiling): A belly is the entrance ticket to this class. [Daliya enters the room. Daniela strokes Daliya's belly and says to her,] "What a nice belly! What do you have in there? A developing fetus?"

AMOS (Daliya's husband): "She's just fat."

On another occasion I recorded the following joking exchange.

PAULA (mimics end of third trimester heavy walking and says to Ayelet): You are walking with spread legs—pay attention to the position of your spine.

CHAIM (Ayelet's husband, laughing): This is her normal walk.

The transfer of meaning common to these jokes is the nullification of the fertile aspects of pregnancy. When the quality of pregnancy as represented and symbolized by the baby is de-emphasized, pregnancy comes to be seen as a sheer physical oddity, from which it follows merely that pregnancy is like carrying some type of baggage. The above jokes take the nullification of pregnancy to an extreme, which is exactly what makes them humorous. However, as I will suggest later, these jokes merely use existing notions that separate the somatic continuum of mother and unborn baby.

Time and again I heard men expressing their puzzlement or resorting to cynicism; they felt that too much medical fuss was made about pregnancy and birth, these being natural processes that needed little intervention. During one of the breaks, Noam told me, smiling,

NOAM: I told my wife, "What do we need this course for? In the past people gave birth in caves, near the fireplace . . . what's the big fuss?"

TSIPY: But babies and mothers died much more often in those caves.

NOAM: Yeah, that's what my wife told me.

Noam's wife (and I) represented pregnancy and birth to him as events that might turn out to be dangerous; both of us used medicalization to counter his trivialization of birth. It is notable how Noam draws his image of birth from the domain of the primitive: how did uneducated Neanderthal women, he was wondering, manage to give birth without learning and without medical intervention, which is now assumed to be basic information for parents-to-be?

In the same spirit, Shachar, a thirty-five-year-old accountant, told me: "During my military service we worked with Bedouins. Once I saw a Bedouin woman giving birth—she had no problem giving birth. And we have to study and go through courses."

Yoav, forty, a father-to-be, told me about a birth event he claimed to have witnessed on one of his journeys to Thailand. "I saw, in Thailand, a woman—she gave birth squatting on a banana leaf and then kept on working."

While I doubt the truth of stories about foreign men being admitted to witness Bedouin and Thai women giving birth, the importance of these stories, in my view, is in the way they are used by the men who tell them to reflect on their own wives' pregnancies and birth-giving.

When measured against women in "nonmedicalized" contexts, Israeli women end up being portrayed again as spoiled, as requiring excessive care that unspoiled women living in less modernized areas of the world can do without. All the above images depict birth as belonging to the natural or primitive realm of being. However, this is not nature in its grandeur, but rather nature at its most simple and banal. It is no surprise that the Israeli women quoted in the previous section feel the need to keep on working when confronted with implicit and explicit expectations such as these from their husbands and probably from their friends as well.

These ideas, culminating in outright cynicism, peaked in the following scene that took place in a birthing room in the maternity ward of one Jerusalem hospital during Ruth's "birthing rooms guided tour." Ruth justified these tours to me on the grounds that she wanted her clients to be very well acquainted with the arena in which the birth would be taking place. Consequently, one bright Friday morning I joined Ruth and eight pregnant couples in the reception hall of the hospital.

After going over the details of the hospital registration we headed toward the birthing rooms. As Ruth explained to me later, she wanted to show the couples how they could alter the atmosphere inside the birthing room and manage to create a more intimate feeling, in spite of all the medical equipment around the place. The following is what I wrote in my field notes at the time.

Ruth went and with a whoosh sat herself down on the obstetrical chair. "Even if they are going to let you wander around while having contractions, you are most likely to end up here," she said, pointing to the obstetrical chair. "So we [had] better learn how to manage this chair. This is how you lift the back . . . to assist the woman in pushing the baby out. You see, this chair may be used in creative ways." Ruth squatted on the chair, then went down on all fours, saying: "This is a favorite birthing position for many women, who says you cannot perform it on an obstetrical chair."

Then she remembered that she wanted to show us the "traditional" birthing position as well. Sitting on the chair, she tried to lift the stirrups and fasten the screws. However, the moment she lay down on the chair and put her legs in the stirrups they collapsed, making a loud metallic sound (clang). On her first trial, the audience burst out laughing. Ruth tried again and again, but could not manage to get the screws fastened. She tried again and again, going on and off the chair. At some point the couples started to talk quietly among themselves. And then Uri said to Arik,

URI: Arik, did you see on TV last night about the flood in Mozambique?

ARIK: Oh, yeah.

URI: Did you see that woman?

ARIK: She gave birth on a tree.

TSIPY: What?

ARIK: Didn't you see? There was a hurricane and she got stuck on a tall coconut tree. She gave birth there and stayed there for two more days until they got her off the tree when the flood started going down.

[Zzzong, the sound of the stirrups collapsing again]

URI: We spoil the girls too much. Nurses, massages, beds, tranquilizers, rub their backs. . . . This woman gave birth on a tree.

[Zzong, the stirrups collapsing again]

URI (to Ruth, the birth educator): It's better in a tree.

I argue that the men here are challenging not only the relevance of the specific pieces of knowledge taught to them in the birth-education classes, but the whole (medicalized) conception of childbirth that underlies and organizes the practices of pregnancy and birth. Note that their criticism of medicalization differs profoundly from the feminist rage against medicalization as the cause of the alienation of women from their bodies in medical-birth settings. Quite the contrary—*in these narratives the medical organization of childbirth is seen as acting in the best interests of spoiled women.* I suggest that the above statement of antimedicalization can be seen as another technique of trivialization, not necessarily as a critical response to the authority of medicine as a privileged cult of authoritative knowledge.

Given this all-encompassing climate of trivialization, it becomes easier to understand why women might fantasize about strategies to make their pregnancies better appreciated, as did Tsila, cited below. I recorded Tsila's statement during Ruth's guided tour, when Ruth took her couples to see how premature babies are treated.

RUTH: A day in the NICU ward [neonatal intensive care unit] costs twenty thousand dollars. It is better to have national health insurance."

TSILA: Can you imagine the state paying us twenty thousand dollars for every day of gestation?

If women are to lend their bodies "voluntarily" to the state of Israel, the state should pay them for every day of gestation. The implication here is that in practice women serve as incubators for the future citizens of Israel. However, being "employed" on an unwritten contract by the state means that women are giving their services for free, almost exemplifying the classic Marxist paradox of workers being distanced and estranged from the commodities they have created. Tsila's fantasy is a reflection on the banality and trivialization of pregnancy from an inverted point of view, namely, that of the state.

From the above, it seems logical for women to be more than interested in their men "learning" what there is to learn in birth-education classes, not so much to memorize the information in the tiniest detail but to internalize the atmosphere of importance that accompanies the medical management of pregnancy and birth; in other words, to combat trivialization. So what happens when husbands do get involved and learn the "relevant" language that birth educators try to teach them?

The case of Tali and Yoni, quoted above, is an interesting example of the kind of relationship that can be created when the husband decides to assume a greater role in the pregnancy. Tali, who defines herself as a feminist, was quoted earlier urging Yoni to take a nap in the afternoon so that he could concentrate on what was being taught in the birth-education class. However, when Yoni does become more deeply involved, she withdraws to a different position. As she told me:

> Yoni wanted a child for a long time. I took more time. And we said for a long time beforehand that he was going to share it with me. He even managed to take half the maternity leave so that I could get back to work earlier. Yoni is the kind of husband that makes my girlfriends die of envy.
>
> But on the other hand, when they [men] participate, they also think they are entitled to have a say. But with all due respect, I'm the one who's going through this. For example, we said that we weren't going to tell anybody that I was in the birthing room. So Yoni asked, "What if your labor becomes longer, and I get tired? What shall we do?" So I said we might call my mother. So Yoni said, "What about *my* mother?" I said, "No way, this is me giving birth, absolutely not!" He thinks that since he knows what dilation means, he's entitled to take decisions for me.

Yoni is seriously prepared to participate, but this suddenly seems to threaten Tali. When Yoni can cite authoritative medical terms, this very knowledge is turned against him. Now Tali seems to have adopted a new criterion for eligibility to decide, one that has to do with the body and with experience, rather than with understanding medical terminology.

Birth educators are aware of the "dangers" of involving men. Paula warned the husbands: "Never tell your woman: 'But you vowed not to take any tranquilizers; you wanted a natural birth, didn't you?' She's the one who's in pain."

Men are expected to participate in pregnancy and birth, but it is not at all clear *how* exactly they are supposed to participate. What should they actually do? In other words, men's social role in pregnancy is anything but well scripted. That they are usually "invited" to participate in spheres with many professional care providers and technologies makes their role even more ambiguous.

Tami and Benny had come for a "refresher birth-education course." This was their second pregnancy. When Ruth asked them why they had come, Benny explained: "With our first son, I tried to use the massages we had learned at the birth-education classes on Tami. But at some point Tami bluntly told me: 'Just leave me alone, don't touch me.' So we figured out that this time I should learn how to do it properly."

Benny seems to have accepted the idea that massages are necessary for his birthing wife. He also accepted the role of massager that was offered to him as the "husband's role" in the recent course. His problem was that he did not massage her properly. When I interviewed Tami after the birth of their second son, she was still seeking a role for her husband. She told me: "Birth is not for him. He doesn't like the sight of blood and doesn't know what to do, so he videotaped the birth. If he videotapes, that's something for him. Maybe it's my problem that I don't know how to *activate* him" (emphasis added).

Benny was present in the birthing room, but even after the "refresher course" he remained typically a spectator. Tami admits that Benny is not necessarily the person most suitable to help her while she is in labor. "I have a wonderful sister who could help me," she said. However, the idea that Benny can be excused and not be in the room when she gives birth does not even occur to her. She found techniques to keep him physically present in the room but not too involved. The video camera keeps Benny far away, but still in the room to witness the birth of his son, mediated by the lens.

Tami's solution is quite common, to judge by Ruth's advice to her couples:

RUTH: Don't forget to take a picture of mommy and daddy coming out of the hospital with the baby. This is a standard picture in every family, for the kid as well, so that when Mommy goes to give birth to the next child. . .

NOA: Hanan already sleeps with his camera.

RUTH: Take care; some fathers realize in the birthing room that they have left the film at home.

The role of a spectator who is responsible for documenting the event, rather than a "coach," seems typically assigned to men. This promotes men to the position of deciding what "deserves" documentation and what does not, what is socially acceptable to show later to family and friends and what is not. In a way, women are left with the "physical labor" of giving birth, while men are again given roles that have to do with managing and manufacturing external representations.

The above account suggests that the inclusion of men in the process of pregnancy and birth might actually heighten rather than relieve the tensions in women's and men's respective experiences of pregnancy. First, men do not always participate willingly: rather, they often have to be "tempted" or "pushed" into the arenas of pregnancy and birth. Secondly, when they do try to make sense of it, they import images taken from their own, very different, life-worlds (military life, nonmedicalized forms of sociality), which can in some cases have the overall effect of trivializing pregnancy. From the perspective of Israeli men's life-worlds, pregnancy may be seen as a grotesque fattening of women, who thereby become figures of fun. Once inside the arenas that mark pregnancy, some men contest the necessity and importance of the social schemes that organize pregnancy, namely, its medicalization. As Sandelowski (1994) and Van der Ploeg describe (1995), men are expected to associate themselves with pregnancy via technology and medical knowledge. Paradoxically, while many Israeli men tend to criticize the medicalization of childbirth, women seem to embrace it in part as a means of countering trivialization. But pregnant life-worlds being saturated with medical knowledge carries additional and often far more striking effects.

The Quest for Medical Information

The Israeli bestseller *The Israeli Guide to Pregnancy and Birth* states in its introduction, "We believe in women in general and in a woman's right over her own body in particular. Therefore it was important for us to speak to you looking you straight in the eye. To treat you as an intelligent, thinking human being who can understand the process of pregnancy and take part in medical monitoring. Knowledge is power, and we have done our best to supply you with both. The various processes that happen during pregnancy and birth are reviewed in detail for you to know more, and consequently fear less, and for you to be able to express your opinion when possible" (Ber and Rosin 1998:20).

The way in which Ber and Rosin make use of Foucault's concepts reflects the tension within which pregnant Israeli women consume medical knowledge. On the one hand, they are marketing "knowledge" as empowerment. On the other hand, they imply that the woman can make only limited use of the knowledge that she will acquire by reading their book. First, Ber and Rosin predict that the knowledgeable woman will fear *less* (thus constituting fear as essential to pregnancy). Secondly, whereas "knowledge" seems to be a prerequisite for expressing her opinions, even a knowledgeable woman is only permitted to express her opinion "when possible." Interestingly, the concept of "choice" is missing from their account of why knowledge is so absolutely necessary. Ber and Rosin's statement explicitly situates the pregnant woman within a locus of power in which medical-care providers maintain their hegemonic status.

The fact that sixteen of my twenty interviewees had read *The Israeli Guide to Pregnancy and Birth*—a 570-page book complete with an appendix on "How to read test results" and a glossary of medical terminology—and that five women explicitly called it "the pregnancy bible" suggests that the writers had correctly identified the readers' thirst for "heavy" medical knowledge. Indeed, the women I interviewed, regardless of their level of education, socio-economic status or ethnic origin, described themselves as being in constant pursuit of more and more information, from their care providers or social networks or by surfing various Internet sites.[4] Concurrently, these women tried continuously to interpret and make sense of the different kinds of knowledge they collected and to make practical decisions.

This quest raises a series of questions about the effects and uses of medical knowledge by pregnant women. What kind of "knowledge" do women receive? How do they interpret and negotiate this "knowledge"? Can their practical decisions be understood as derived from the information they have collected? Does the information that they accumulate indeed empower them or lessen their fears, as Ber and Rosin suggest? Empirically, I focus on information about different kinds of prenatal diagnostic tests—the largest volume of information that circulates in medical and popular arenas in Israel and the type in which most women show the utmost interest. By contrast, relatively little information circulates on nutrition and physical activity.

But note first that, significantly, women of every ethnic origin and diverse ethnic marital combinations were concerned about inborn genetic and chromosomal anomalies. Although a number of congenital diseases common among Ashkenazi Jews have captured much attention in the media, Oriental and Sephardic Jews are afflicted by as many congenital diseases. But even more important, most women, as we shall see, are primarily worried about their prospects of carrying a baby with Down's syndrome, the iconic chromosomal anomaly (in the majority of cases) of which distribution does not vary across ethic origin.

Returning to the accumulation and use of medical knowledge, my informants (like the American women in Browner and Press's study, 1997) did not accept medical authority uncritically. For Israeli women, contesting the accuracy of the information and challenging the medical indications based on it were inseparable parts of consuming the information.

Noa, thirty-four, a history teacher (of Polish origin), and her husband, a business consultant (of Moroccan descent), were advised by the ob-gyn to undergo amniocentesis following a 1:400 result in the AFP test. This was Noa's first pregnancy, and she was clearly reluctant to endanger it. She explained to me: "I know that they tell you to get an amniocentesis if you are over thirty-five, and I am only thirty-four. But he [the doctor] said that it has nothing to do with age, just the result of the AFP is suspicious and why should I take the chance? But when you think about it, the risk of losing a healthy fetus is 1:200—much larger than the probability that the fetus is really sick. So we are really at a loss [over what to do]."

Noa told her doctor that she was frightened of losing the fetus and that she could not make up her mind. The doctor insisted that Noa and her husband would have to decide for themselves: he could not help them make the decision. He suggested that she and her husband attend an explanatory class for those interested in undergoing amniocentesis. Typically, acquiring more information is offered here as a solution to the problem of making a decision. Noa and her husband did not challenge the idea that more information was indeed what they needed in order to make "the right decision." Noa invited me to take the explanatory class with her, so one gray winter morning, we headed off to the hospital where the class was taking place.

Explanatory classes for those interested in amniocentesis can be seen as the practical solution that care providers have devised to deal with the large volume of work. The routinization of AFP no doubt contributes to this workload, since the proportion of women with "suspicious results" who are referred for amniocentesis is constant. This figure, of course, is in addition to the number of most pregnant women over thirty-five who apply for state-subsidized amniocentesis, as well as the number of women with no prior indications of any fetal problem. The explanatory class is thus a convenient way for busy staff to "give patients all the information they need to make difficult decisions," as Elinor, the nurse in charge of the class, told me.

Since Noa invited me to join her, I witnessed five more explanatory classes, all of which were structured as follows. The couples were shown a video with an introduction on inborn abnormalities and a detailed explanation of the medical procedure of amniocentesis. Then a nurse answered patients' questions. There was no time limit, and participants could ask as many questions as they wished. After the questions, participants had to sign official papers, mostly stating that they had attended the class and had understood the explanation. The nurse invited couples to consult her privately in her room afterward.

Often the atmosphere in the classes was charged with tension. At various points during the showing of the film people sighed and stirred uneasily in their seats, especially when the needle was shown penetrating the belly of the pregnant woman. In the following account I focus on the question-and-answer session after the film. Such classes, I contend, provide an opportunity to observe the negotiations that occur between consumers and providers of medical information. One aspect that repeatedly concerned participants was how to interpret the statistical data that were presented to them. Soon after the video machine had been turned off, Noa jumped up to ask Elinor the same question that she had mentioned in her conversation with me.

NOA: What if our chances [of having a Down's syndrome baby] are 1:400 [according to triple test results] and our chances for miscarriage due to amniocentesis is 1:150? What then?

ELINOR: The question is whether we are looking at it numerically. For some people a 1:400 risk of having a Down's syndrome child is a lot, and they are prepared to take the risk of miscarriage. For others Down's is not so bad . . . and for yet others . . . well, it's all a question of chances against risks. Everyone decides according to their own reflections, their culture, and their values. You've got a lot of information and you're upset now; go home, relax, and think. Can you live with a Down's child or not?

Elinor's reaction to Noa's question sharpens the issue of how relevant are the numbers and statistics, which so characterize medical information, for actual decision making. When pressed, Elinor actually admits that numbers are almost irrelevant to practical decisions; she stresses cultural values more. Nevertheless, Elinor makes sure to remind participants that they have "got a lot of information" and now should go home to reconsider the nonnumerical question of whether they can "live with a Down's syndrome child or not."

Another problem often raised relates to a slightly different set of figures, namely, the age thresholds set by the Ministry of Health as criteria for a woman's eligibility for subsidized testing. This problem concerns the confrontation between medical statistics, state regulation, and costs.

Ruchama, a thirty-five-year-old secretary, was referred to the class "because of my age." She was clearly reluctant to go through amniocentesis, claiming that she was "only looking for an escape."

RUCHAMA: If I became pregnant before the age of thirty-five and I will be giving birth after thirty-five, what is my risk of having a Down's syndrome baby?

ELINOR: It's all a matter of the health ministry's recommendations. Until a few years ago, it was recommended that women over thirty-seven should undergo amniocentesis. If you had to give birth a few years ago, what would you have said then? Why should I do amniocentesis? I'm only thirty-five.

RUCHAMA: I'm only looking for an escape [petah milut], a way out of this.

While the age threshold for eligibility to subsidized amniocentesis set by the health ministry is often presented as guided by medical criteria, Elinor's answer exposes its arbitrariness. Ruchama, however, does not recognize this, but feels that there is no escape from the verdict. In fact, nobody at the sessions I attended ever challenged the logic behind the health ministry's regulations.[5]

Esther, twenty-seven, a special-education teacher in her first pregnancy, came to the explanatory class with no prior indications of any fetal abnormality. She had decided to take the test well before becoming pregnant and therefore chose not to undergo AFP. Before the class started I overheard Esther saying to Elinor: "I have seen these children, I have worked with such children, and maybe because of that I am determined not to have such a child." Nevertheless, the video showing the medical procedure aroused Esther's anxiety. At some point Elinor seems to have felt the difficulty Esther was experiencing, through her questions, and suggested that maybe she should undergo AFP so that the results would give her an "indication" of her risk and thus help her decide. Esther reacted strongly to Elinor's suggestion, and countered the idea with her own experience. "A friend of mine did the triple test; the result was not good. She did amniocentesis; it showed a normal result and she gave birth to a healthy child. My neighbor did an AFP test; it was normal, and she gave birth to a Down's child."

Esther is expressing her distrust of a test that is routinely prescribed to all pregnant women. Her experience shows that this statistical test cannot serve as a reliable indicator. Esther's explicit expression of distrust raised a spate of questions, as if the participants suddenly recognized "an escape." Noa asked: "What about diagnostic mistakes? We hear all kinds of stories about women who were told to terminate the pregnancy, and in the end it became clear that the child was healthy."

Noa draws on a whole "genre" of salvation stories that some women offer to resist medical authority. In response, Elinor raised her voice and explained that

In chromosomes there are defects in number and in structure. Defects in the number of chromosomes can be discovered with absolute certainty [*beofen chad mashmai*]. As for deformations in structure, some results are less clear. But I cannot accept the notion of a "wrong" screening test at all. With screening tests we never know completely. It is all a matter of chances and risks. Let's say that if there's a 10 percent risk of the child being affected, then there's a 90 percent chance that it will be nice and healthy and normal. . . . Nobody is going to tell you after any test that your child is 100 percent healthy.

Elinor makes a sharp distinction between statistical tests and tests that yield results that are "absolutely certain" [*beofen chad mashmai*]. She tries to point out a conceptual misunderstanding of statistical results, stressing the inapplicability of the concept "wrong" to probabilities. However, from her defense of such tests they clearly can never be "right" either.[6] Although she offers an alternative view of statistics, showing how they can also be interpreted more optimistically, her answer is most revealing. *Nobody* who is given the results of *any* test can be sure that the child is completely healthy.

It is therefore hardly surprising that despite care providers' attempts to "explain" the meaning of statistics, medical indications of risk, and test results, for many patients this information remains a confusing mass of facts and figures that still needs to be made sense of (cf. Rapp 1999, 66–73, 175, 177). Even after they have taken the decision to undergo a certain test, many patients do not cease to search for explanations. This pattern was especially prominent in my observations of the actual procedure of amniocentesis. Ayala, thirty-two, was of Egyptian descent and her husband was of Iraqi descent. In her fourth pregnancy, she was recommended by her doctor to undergo amniocentesis following a suspect AFP result. She was very quiet throughout the procedure. However, after the sample of amniotic fluid had already been taken, and the doctor remarked while screening the fetus, "I guess the AFP was wrong," the following exchange ensued:

AYALA: With the two previous girls it was also like that, but with my son it didn't happen. If it's a girl I'll be more relaxed.

DOCTOR: You should be relaxed anyway [looking attentively at the ultrasound screen]. It's a girl.

AYALA: (smiling) So this might be the reason. Thank you, doctor.

Here Ayala is trying to construct an explanatory model (in Kleinman's idiom, 1988) connecting the AFP results with the sex of the baby. When the doctor assures her that the fetus is female, she relaxes considerably because the sex fits her own explanatory model, which predicts good results. As Browner and Press show (1997) for American women, here, too, the woman's relaxation is directly linked to the coincidence of her own explanatory model, based on her own experience, with the medical version.

So the next question is how far women act on the information they have collected. I met Noa a week later in the waiting room for amniocentesis. She told me, "We went back home and we thought, can we live with a Down's syndrome baby or not? And we arrived at the conclusion that we can't. It was just as Elinor said."

Figures were absent from Noa's considerations. The figures appear to illustrate the authority of the information given, but in no way the relevant and important aspects required for a decision. In the same spirit Batya, twenty-nine, a participant in the same class, whom I met in the waiting room, explained to me: "The person it happens to [a person who gives birth to an affected child] is not interested in statistics. For them it's a hundred percent, and I'm not willing to take the risk. I was determined from the very beginning of pregnancy to have an amniocentesis." Batya's narrative expresses explicitly the irrelevance of statistics altogether as a meaningful criterion in decision making. The class merely confirmed a decision she had already made.

Ora, a thirty-four-year-old homemaker of Turkish descent (husband of Bulgarian descent) in the sixth month of her second pregnancy, decided to undergo amniocentesis well before she heard the test explained, and even though she was not eligible for reimbursement. Ora had divorced her first husband shortly after her first son was born. Now, seven years later and happily remarried, she was hoping to build a new life for herself. Ora, her son, and her new husband live in a tiny two-bedroom apartment on the seventh floor of an old building. Ora was fired from her job as a secretary soon after she conceived, and the three of them then lived off the modest income of her husband, who worked as a gardener.

ORA: This pregnancy is a bit more frightening.

TSIPY: Why?

ORA: Because of my age and all that can happen.

TSIPY: But you aren't thirty-five yet, are you?

ORA: So what? It's close, so there is not a single test that I skipped: fragile x, and cystic fibrosis, and AFP, and amniocentesis. I told myself that I'm building a new home and I don't want to bring an unhealthy child into it; that is like asking for trouble. And I'm entering a second relationship that needs to be strengthened, it doesn't need any extra tensions and pressures. I don't want to be in a war for the rest of my life. . . . Life here is so hard anyway, so we are trying to do our best to prevent anything that would make it even more difficult.

Ora views an unhealthy child as a threat to the stability of her new marriage. Although previously in our conversation she cited the statistics of how the risk of having a baby with Down's syndrome rises with age, this does not seem to be the major reason why she decided to undergo amniocentesis. Nevertheless, Ora was afraid. "I was not afraid of the pain or the fee—I was afraid of losing the pregnancy. So I took the best professor [sic], and I didn't mind paying a lot of money. . . . I look up to him, and for me he's like God. I chose the best, he's the head of a maternity ward, and he's done amniocentesis to forty or so people, who recommended him. I did my best: I took the best doctor, the most sterile hospital, paid a lot of money . . . I did all I could."

Ora devised a strategy to have her cake and eat it, extracting the most reliable medical information about the health of her fetus while minimizing the dangers that the procedure entails. Interestingly, her attitude shifted considerably when we discussed environmental factors that may risk fetal health. Although she is a heavy smoker who is aware of the statistical correlation between smoking mothers and babies with a low birth weight, she defends her heavy smoking furiously: "I apologize in advance to him [the fetus], not to you [the interviewer]. . . . I assume full responsibility for his being small . . . There's nothing I can do; I know it's not healthy for me or for the fetus. It's not that I don't understand, but you're speaking to an addict . . . There are so few joys in this life, really few moments of bliss in this difficult life, and I enjoy my cigarettes so much, so I hope he forgives me; I really hope that he won't be too small because of the cigarettes. All other factors—I've done everything I could to avoid them, and that's it."

In a similar vein, Ora made a face when I asked whether she had altered her nutrition at all for the sake of fetal health. She had collected a wealth of information, but she attributed different importance to medical knowledge about different kinds of risk. Still, even her practical decisions concerning the genetic and chromosomal risks that she considers most threatening cannot be understood as simply resulting from the information. She is impelled by a pragmatism that goes beyond mere statistics (Lock and Kaufert 1998), seeking to eliminate any threat to her new marriage, any new difficulty in her life, which she perceives as difficult anyway.

Nevertheless, even women who reached their decisions "rationally" from the information they had collected seemed unable to stick to them. To take one example, Limor, thirty, an educational consultant of Romanian descent, whose husband was of German-Polish descent, told me about a long process of decision making, at the end of which she had a number of genetic tests that she thought were "worth doing." But when she actually went to the hospital, "I gathered a lot of information and really thought about it. I consulted my sister [an MD] and we came to the conclusion that given my and my husband's [ethnic] background, I would do only the genetic tests for Canavan disease and for CF and that's all. But when I got there the nurse told me, 'You can pay just two hundred shekels more and also do the Gaucher.' So I thought, 'Why not? Two hundred shekels won't break me,' and I did."

Although Limor was determined to act on the information she had collected, her informed choice was implicitly reduced to a matter of costs, and she was easily persuaded to take an additional test that, according to her informed considerations, was irrelevant.

Some women spoke expressly about the monetary aspects of the proliferation of testing and stated their uncertainty and distrust about the practitioners they consulted. Hanna, twenty-nine, a ballet teacher of Polish descent, her husband of Moroccan descent, told me about her second pregnancy:

This time I did genetic tests for fragile x and for CT. It is a painful issue, all these private tests that people who have money do. . . . It has become a financial business. . . . First of all the doctors who do it make sure to advertise it and spread the information, because this is in their interest; they make a lot of money from it. . . . You know, it's not that we're rolling in money, but you know . . . someone who is middle class and can somehow afford it does it, and those that can't afford it don't.

I don't know what exactly we must do and what we needn't do. I went to my doctor. I think he doesn't have any personal interest. There are six tests that you do: fragile x, CT, Gaucher's, Canavan—*I don't remember the rest*, and he advised us to do CT and fragile x, because my husband is of oriental ancestry. Later we spoke to my sister-in-law's father, who is a doctor, about the CT, and he said that . . . well, what did he say? He said that if God wants, even a broom can shoot [a humorous modern Hebrew proverb implying that impossible things can happen], but as for the chances that we two may have a child affected with CT . . . In short, he thought that the test was not necessary. So what I wanted to say is, it might be that the doctors themselves are not 100 percent sure which tests should be done. . . . There's something strange here . . . and it costs a lot of money. . . . *I don't know.*

And the things that can be tested and discovered increase all the time. There are all kinds of tests that for my first child were nonexistent. *I really don't know.*" (emphasis added)

The abundance of "I don't know's" in Hanna's account attests to the uncertainty and doubts that the proliferating information evokes. Hanna has gathered a lot of information but she doubts whether those who provide the knowledge are 100 percent sure whether a test should be done. That every additional test costs money makes practitioners even more suspect. However when it came to the actual decision, Hanna did the test. Like her, other women I talked to indeed confirmed that in their later pregnancies they underwent more testing than in their earlier ones, despite their often being more critical of prenatal testing than women with first pregnancies. From my conversations with women, as well as from the interviews with men that I conducted in 2006, it is clear that many disagreements between partners occur in connection with privately paid additional diagnoses. Men tend to be far more critical of the nature of medical knowledge, and ever more conscious of the financial aspects of testing. Typically, male partners relent and agree to pay for testing, just to make their pregnant partners feel better. (Ivry and Teman 2008)

Finally, does medical information help women reduce their fears? On the one hand, many interviewees acknowledged the receipt of a negative amniocentesis result as a positive turning point in their pregnancies. Ora commented, "Only after I got the result did I start spoiling myself. I went to a nice shop and bought myself something nice to wear. Only after they said that he was healthy, did I start enjoying his kicks and start waiting for them. The peace of mind I got after this test was worth every penny. I couldn't let myself go through a whole pregnancy worrying whether he was healthy."

Nevertheless, later in our conversation, Ora remarked, "Even after amniocentesis comes out fine there's nothing like complete relaxation. . . . One has to be stupid or too young or mindless or irresponsible to be relaxed. Pregnancy is not a relaxing thing. . . . Even those women who pretend to be relaxed on the outside, I don't believe them."

Fervently collecting information about prenatal diagnosis and undergoing a number of tests often had at least three effects on women. First, they learned about fetal abnormalities that they had never heard of before. Secondly, they learned of more tests to examine these conditions. Thirdly, however, they also came to acknowledge that care providers explicitly and repeatedly admitted that (as Elinor, the nurse mentioned earlier, put it) "*Nobody* is going to tell you after *any* test that your child is 100 percent healthy." The film shown in the explanatory classes made this point clear: "Receiving a normal result [*t'shuva tkina*] means that the fetus has no chromosomal defects, and that *most likely* there is no disability in the central neural tube. However, a normal result [*b'dika tkina*] *does not promise that the fetus is completely healthy [takin] or that no other kinds of problems may be expected.*" (emphasis added)

It is notable that the word *takin* is used generally to designate a normal result (meaning the child is not affected). *Takin* is used in Hebrew to designate machines that are working properly, usually following a repair. Interestingly, the mechanical expression used for machines is also used for fetuses, making them increasingly inhuman, even after testing shows that they are *takin*, meaning "not affected." In any case, even amniocentesis, the most accurate test available, cannot ensure that the baby is completely healthy. Explanatory classes impart a huge amount of information to their participants, but the nature of this information seems to increase anxieties rather than ease them. As Ruchama said explicitly once the class had ended, "I came with apprehensions [*hashashot*] and left with anxieties [*haradot*]." Noa, who eventually went through amniocentesis and received a normal result, concluded her account of her experience by describing a haunted state of mind: "I went through all the testing you can imagine, but I cannot say I am relaxed now. They can discover more and more things now. But I'm frightened by what they can't discover."

Interlude: Voices from the Amniocentesis Room

Aya and her husband are the first on Dr. Yuval's list this morning. They have come all the way from a modern Orthodox Jewish settlement near Jerusalem. They both keep on smiling in spite of the deeply felt tension that is apparent. Aya, twenty-seven, is pregnant for the third time, and this will be her third amniocentesis (both she and her husband are of Polish descent). In her second pregnancy a chromosomal deformation was discovered through amniocentesis, and she terminated the pregnancy. This time Aya is making sure that Dr. Yuval will conduct the test. Yuval, a woman ob-gyn in her early fifties, is well known among patients for her expertise as well as her warm smile. She is particularly skilled at making small talk during the amniocentesis procedure to distract the patient's mind from any anxieties. Yuval explained her strategy to me on one of my first observations in her clinic: "If you don't make a fuss of it [amniocentesis], it goes O.K."

When Dr. Yuval's nurse eventually arrived, Aya was already standing near the door with the forms in hand. The nurse registered her, and she got up onto the half-seat chair and raised her blouse above her belly. Then Yuval entered the room, smiling as usual. She greeted Aya and her husband, sat down in the chair beside the examination table, and said, "Good luck to us." Then she picked up the ultrasound probe and looked attentively at the screen:

YUVAL: I will tell you, there's a 90 percent [chance] that it's a girl. O.K., now we are measuring the little miss . . . here this is FEMO twenty-seven . . . here is the head [putting her hand on her head; then, to the fetus]. Oh cutie, poor thing, there's no one to pat you on the head now, but don't worry, later on you'll have someone. [To the couple] Look at her, how she is scratching her head. Nowadays they have lice in the womb [laughing]. I hope that [lice] will be the most difficult trouble in her life. Now I'm measuring the head . . . look—isn't she cool [madlik]. Look at her face: it shows she's your daughter. . . . [To the nurse] Frontal placenta. . . . [To the fetus] Come out, come out, lovey. . . . Here I see a nice pocket of amniotic fluid, I am making a mark here.

AYA (murmuring): I'm dying of fear. I've already done this twice, but I'm still afraid.

YUVAL: Of what?

AYA: Of everything.

YUVAL: Come on [yalla], you're just hysterical [stam hysterit]. You've already done this, so what are you afraid of? And you [to the husband], you are stuck there in the corner [inserts the needle].

AYA: Tell me, doctor, is electromagnetic radiation dangerous [to the fetus]? Cell phones emit them, so I thought that the equipment here . . .

HUSBAND: You're just looking for trouble again.

YUVAL: Yeah, you are looking for problems.

AYA: But does it have an effect?

YUVAL (taking the needle out): Sorry, taking out hurts the most.

AYA: Is there any chance that the needle touched the fetus?

YUVAL: There is very little chance of this happening. Now, I'll let you hear the [fetal] pulse. I haven't touched the fetus, the placenta is fine. . . . Now you must rest for a little while.

AYA: How can you be sure that you didn't touch the fetus at all?

YUVAL (folding the leg rest): That's it Aya, your time's up [zmanech avar].

Aya got off the chair, thanked Yuval with a smile and left the room. Together with her husband in the waiting room, she kept speculating about the different risks and dangers. "How nice it was," I heard her saying, "to have such a good doctor."

Conclusion: The Results of Accumulating Medical Information

Let us return to the meaning and uses that women make of medical knowledge. Regarding the first question, about the kind of "knowledge" women receive, the data above suggest that this is not really medical *knowledge* but a fragmented and fractured collection of numbers and medical terminologies that might be better termed "information." Acquiring knowledge this way is rather like learning how to pronounce certain words in a foreign language without knowing how to speak it. Hence it is fundamentally different from "knowledge," which is constituted through its holder's desire to master an inherent epistemological grammar that guides her or him to an authoritative interpretation of figures, names, and initials. So in practice, while searching for more information women find themselves engaged in a ceaseless effort to make sense of medical information by means of various explanatory models. Some women approach such information with skepticism, but the overall effect of this effort makes them more dependent on care providers to supply authoritative interpretations. Medical institutions acknowledge patients' need to contest and challenge medical information, and they create special spaces for these contestations to take place. I suggest that explanatory classes for those interested in undergoing amniocentesis, to give one example, may be understood almost as ritual loci created by institutions to contain criticism and redirect it to preserve and even strengthen their authority.

The next question was whether women act on the information they collect. However, the data suggest that the question itself is wanting, because medical information tends to represent itself as a value-free, objective, nondirective set of statistical and other data. Nonetheless, in this objectivity particularly, the metamessage of the medical information lies. This message states first, that information is a required and essential basis for decision making. Second, the decision maker must *understand* the information correctly, that is, according to the authoritative interpretation of professionals. Third, any piece of information is important and worth knowing, regardless of its recipient. Moreover, every single piece of information must be taken into account and weighed on the way to taking a decision. In this sense, women indeed act according to the metascheme that underlies information: they agree that information matters in the very act of consuming it. Nevertheless, regarding practical implications, as Lock and Kaufert suggest (1998), women are guided more by a pragmatism that goes beyond figures and medical indicators, and draws on a specific moral economy. A central factor in women's decisions is rather the metanarrative beneath the information that any fetus may carry a whole array of terrible diseases and that this is a realistic and more or less random possibility. When a younger woman decides to undergo amniocentesis she may not be acting "by the figures" but "saving her new marriage" or "saving her life"; at the same time she also supports the idea that numbers indeed "indicate" her risk of carrying an affected child, that this risk is real, and that she might very well be the one in the 1:20,000. The overall effect of the emphasis on "knowing," "understanding," "considering," and "making informed decisions" is that women may spend their pregnancies in constant mental agitation that simply increases their anxieties. That this state of mind is often understood as the price one pays for being empowered to choose one's own child is highly revealing of the restriction of reproductive choices—that it increasingly becomes less of a choice not to choose the child. This echoes the observations of Barbara Katz Rothman (Rothman 1984, 26, 32–33) and Ruth Hubbard: "As 'choices' become available, they all too rapidly become compulsions to 'choose' the socially endorsed alternative" (Hubbard, in Rothman 1984, 27).

How, in the midst of such uncertainties and turbulent processes of decision making, women set about relating to their fetuses is crucial to understanding how pregnancy is experienced.

How to Bond with an In-Utero Fetal Suspect?

Shira, an experienced birth educator, explained to her class: "Husbands should always remind their wives and keep in mind [themselves] that the birth passes [overet]. The word "fetus" [ubar] stems from the Hebrew root of passing or transience [avar]. Through birth, the fetus becomes a baby [haubar over lihyot tinok]."

Shira conceptualizes the moment of birth as a magical transition from "fetus-hood" to "babyhood," a concept that leaves the fetus suspended in "fetus-hood" up until the final stages of delivery. Shira explicitly expresses a notion that cuts throughout the narratives of many pregnant women, who showed different degrees of reluctance at being "overtly attached" to what had not yet been born. Precisely such techniques of detachment—what I call defensive emotional postures—devised to defend women from threatening catastrophe, I contend, underpin the trivialization of pregnancy, as well as the enthusiastic embrace of PND. Yet I am not saying that Israeli women never attempt to bond with their fetuses. Rather, their experiences evolve in a time-space zone that gravitates toward a particular emotional posture that surrounds their attempts with great caution. This reluctance was particularly conspicuous in women's accounts of ultrasound scans—exactly where the "fetus" becomes most visible.

Yael, a thirty-two-year-old teacher, was in her second pregnancy when I first spoke to her. She told me about her first visit to the ob-gyn after she realized that she was pregnant.

YAEL: I told the doctor, "I'm hysterical; I'm going to sit, to stick like a leech [*lehit'alek*] onto your neck. I want to have a lot of ultrasounds for my peace of mind." So he gave me an ultrasound every two weeks.

TSIPY: How did you feel seeing your baby so often?

YAEL: Well, what do you mean? The fetus? The ultrasound relaxed me, seeing the fetus, and being told that everything was O.K., but I was too busy with the ongoing things of pregnancy. I didn't let myself fantasize about the baby until very late, maybe the eighth month. I didn't let myself think about how it was going to be. I'm always so surprised at women who fantasize a lot during pregnancy. How do they dare? So many things, so many accidents, can happen.

Ultrasound might have had a "relaxing" effect on Yael, but she is still hesitant to relate to the fetus despite its enhanced visibility. Notable, too, is that far from challenging the representation of Israeli women as hysterical, Yael defines herself as such. Only later, she told me, some months after she obtained the results of the amniocentesis, did she start enjoying the sensation of the fetus kicking. "There were times when I would sit and concentrate on feeling the kicks from the inside, but this was much later, toward the end of the eighth month." For Yael, as for three more interviewees, the embodied sensations of being kicked from the inside seem to have played a more meaningful role than ultrasonic visualization in connecting herself to the fetus.

Yet for other women neither the technology of ultrasound nor embodied sensations was enough to inspire a bond if the woman was determined to stay detached. Ora, the remarried homemaker in her second pregnancy quoted previously, stated her reluctance eloquently.

ORA: I did not become attached to this pregnancy from the beginning. I felt him moving very early in the pregnancy, as early as the third month, but I ignored it. I said, "I don't want to feel anything. I want nothing. I want to know that everything is O.K. and then . . . maybe."

TSIPY: What do you mean exactly by "I did not become attached"?

ORA: The simplest thing. If I felt a movement, I ignored it, I felt nothing. It was just a muscle that moved. . . . I said, "I feel nothing," because if they told me to abort, that is, if they told me that the fetus had a terrible disease and I have to abort it, what then?

The notion of reproductive catastrophe dominates the narratives of Yael and Ora. I would say that both have assumed a defensive emotional posture through which they try to delay fetal personhood and detach themselves, for the time being, from their fetuses in order to minimize the effects of loss due to reproductive catastrophe, should it happen. Embodied sensations and ultra-sonic visions, it seems, need to be interpreted in a certain way to become a means of bonding: neither of them inherently encourages prenatal bonding in itself. Returning to Ora's narrative, soon after she speculated on what would have happened if "they told me to abort," I noticed her belly move forcefully. Ora looked down, stroked her belly, and smiled: "Morning exercises!" she exclaimed. But when I asked, "Do you speak to your fetus sometimes?" she "cor-rected" her emotional posture and answered, "I don't speak to plants, I don't speak to fetuses; I wait till they are born." Ora, it should be noted here, was one of the few Israeli women I met who arranged a special folder in which she kept all the ultrasound printouts that her doctor gave her. Nevertheless, she felt that speaking to the fetus was "going too far too soon." Although Ora makes an effort to hold herself in the defensive and detached posture, she sometimes "lets go," drifting a little to a softer posture, only to gravitate again toward defense.

This is not to say that women were not fascinated by the pictures they saw on the ultrasound screen. Deborah, twenty-seven, in the ninth month of her first pregnancy, told me at length how much she wanted to have children, and how she persuaded her husband to marry her and to stop using birth control immediately afterward. She seemed to be in a wonderful mood, and very enthu-siastic about the whole idea of having a baby soon. This is how Deborah describes the experience of her twentieth-week ultrasound: "It was astonishing, fascinating that you could really see everything, the head, the legs, the hands, all the limbs. You could really see beautifully, that it [ze] is alive and breathing, and we could hear the pulse."

Deborah's narrative is one of fascination and enthusiasm, but in describing the fetus's vitality Deborah refers to it with the Hebrew word ze. Unlike the English word "it," which is used for both animals and objects, ze only applies to objects, and even cats and dogs are referred to as he or she. The fact that Deborah depicts the fetus as breathing (although biological knowledge states that fetuses do not breathe until after they are born) suggests that she clearly understands her fetus as a living being. Nevertheless, she refers to it in terms of a nonliving object, using the word ze, even though she already knows the sex of the fetus, and therefore could say "she." The way she conceptualizes her fetus highlights its ambiguous status while it is in the womb. It can be seen, it is alive and has human characteristics, such as a human face, human hands, and so on, but it is not human yet.[7] Of course, in many years of formal and informal conversations with pregnant women, I encountered a wide range of ways to relate to the fetus; there were Israeli women and couples who invented a preterm name for the fetus, those who referred to it as he or she, and those who called it "a baby" as soon as a few weeks after they discovered the pregnancy. However, the last-named were significantly rarer cases, and they tended to "break" easily when notions of reproductive catastrophe introduced themselves. This happened once the slightest indication of anomaly appeared in the medical monitoring; or when a neighbor or family member made a point to call the woman and tell her about a friend of a friend who had an emergency cesarean section, lost her baby, or had a postdiagnostic abortion, or to ask if she had undergone prenatal diagnosis and, if not, to encourage her to make an appointment at once. A number of women told me how friends called them when they were abroad to ask if they had had amniocentesis. Though such women did not assume a defensive posture of their own volition, they were impelled to do so.

The implications of the fetus's ambiguity are highly practical. As Yael told me: "When I was in my eighth month of pregnancy, I saw a pair of wonderful bottles on sale at the supermarket. I wanted to buy them but I couldn't. So I phoned a woman friend, and she agreed to buy them for me and keep them at her house until I gave birth."

The eight month, as the reader might recall, was when Yael started "letting herself" fantasize about the baby a little more, while "meditating" on her baby's kicks. However, buying a bottle seems an excessively optimistic act, admitting, in a way, that a *real* baby is going to suck it. The fetus's ambiguity positions its mother-to-be in an equally ambiguous position. She *might* become a mother, she *might* have to use bottles, but this is not a sure thing. Therefore, while many Japanese "mothers" already prepare baby clothes for their unborn babies from the fifth month, and American expectant mothers celebrate with baby showers—events that "carry tremendous emotional importance for the nascent mother" (Davis-Floyd 1992, 36)—during the seventh month of pregnancy, Israeli pregnant women are too frightened to buy a pair of bottles even when the birth is rapidly approaching.

Carmela, who grew up in Argentina and immigrated to Israel in her twenties, was perplexed when she mentioned these aspects of Israeli pregnancy.

CARMELA: I talk to my friends in Argentina and my mother and aunts: it is so different there.

TSIPY: What, for example?

CARMELA: Like . . . real nonsense, like, the question whether people may bring things for the baby before [the birth] or not. In Argentina, the room is ready for the baby beforehand. Everything! The bed and the sheets and everything. Here, nothing. Don't open up the bed. It's wrong. [If you make an order] everything should stay at the store. With my first baby, it was strange . . . now I understand, and I live here, so I behave the way people behave here. . . . But yes, I washed the [baby's] clothes and put them in the drawers, but I won't open the bed, that's for sure; only the clothes. In the previous pregnancy I had a bed, but it was folded and I even had a mattress . . . Some people, you know, wouldn't dare even to do this . . .

TSIPY: How do you explain this?

CARMELA: I think it is superstition . . . honestly, I don't understand why. . . . I think it has to do with the fear that you will come back home without a baby, God forbid [has vehalila] . . . you know . . . as if it would hurt less . . . but honestly, I can't figure it out. It's interesting that I haven't asked about it either. I live here so I've become integrated, but I don't understand why preparing a bed for a baby is . . . Maybe it brings bad luck? . . . Maybe this way you'll be less disappointed? You see, if you're expecting the worst, then if nothing happens everything will be all right. Maybe it's wrong to expect too much, maybe you shouldn't hope. This is fear. The fewer the expectations, the fewer the disappointments.

Carmela narrates a pregnancy haunted by catastrophe. As we have seen, the arenas where pregnancy is usually negotiated supply a wide variety of vividly animated reasons for fear. It takes a *daring* individual to contest this state of mind. Even Carmela, who is intimately acquainted with a different understanding of pregnancy and does not identify with such thinking, resists quietly. Using Carmela's words, I feel that many women I interviewed did not *dare* bond with their fetuses "too much." Given such notions of risk and uncertainty, the hesitant participation of male partners and their difficulty in connecting to pregnancy becomes even more understandable.

These difficulties were especially noteworthy when men reported them in connection with ultrasound scans—precisely the kind of medical rituals that scholars working in America and Britain have marked as men-friendly. Significantly, while some of the men I interviewed in 2006 expressed their excitement at seeing their fetuses in ultrasound, many of them expressed their uneasiness. Eli, thirty-four, a lawyer, described the 3D ultrasound image as a "wax figure" or "a mummy," and Kobi, thirty, a literature student, said the sixteen-week-old fetus he saw during the scan looked to him like a bat. Clearly such experiences made it difficult for these men to "bond" with the image. Yet if it might not be simple for women, in whose bodies the fetus is growing, to bond with it, why should it surprise us that men have difficulties too? Clearly, however, for some couples, the expectant father's failing to gush with enthusiasm on seeing the fetus on the ultrasound screen could become another source of friction (Ivry and Teman 2008).

Unlike the male partners cited above, Ora's husband "fell in love" the moment he saw his son on the ultrasound screen and, as a result, tried to talk Ora out of the idea of having an amniocentesis. As Ora told me:

He cooperated [with my plan to undergo amniocentesis] . . . but he did not really; he claimed that he saw him [the fetus] on the ultrasound [screen] and he said, "Look how perfect he is, look what a perfect head. He doesn't have the head of a mongoloid, look how beautiful, and his hands . . . he's healthy, you have nothing to worry about." But I insisted: "I cannot accept your word as I don't know what you think of yourself—a healer or something? I can't take this chance." There are things that I'm not prepared to give up. So he said, "OK, if you want me to hold your hand I'll hold your hand, and if you want me to write the check I will. But I'm telling you. I saw him, and he's healthy." He really is a supportive person, but he made it very clear that he was doing it for me, he doesn't need that [amniocentesis]. . . . Then we went out to meet some friends, and you know these men, they always say that we women are so sensitive and worry too much. But then his best friend said: "Tell me, Moshe, what are you thinking of? I can't understand you. At last after three girls [from his previous marriage] you are going to have a boy, you want to have a healthy child. If he's not healthy get him out [*torid oto*] and have another one." After that he came to me and told me that we were together in this and that he realized that we couldn't take that chance.

This story of Ora's husband demonstrates how fragile enthusiasm for ultrasonic images can be in the Israeli script of reproductive catastrophe. Although Ora's husband already "fell in love," his bond with the fetus was quite easily disrupted, and the perfect-looking image rapidly returned to conditionality. Ora strongly believed that the Israeli attitude was the most logical for pregnancy.

In hospitals, even after the baby is born, they never congratulate you [say *mazal tov*]. Only after the placenta is out. I heard of a case of a mother who died during the birth because they didn't manage to get the placenta out, so the custom is that only after the placenta is out do they congratulate you. So even if the baby is out, it's only 70 percent. There's another 30 percent, so people don't like to speak, don't like to give names in advance. "We'll see, one thing at a time." I think it is very good this way. The more grief that is prevented, the better. Now it's a fetus; before it was a stinky drop [a Mishnaic expression for the sperm]; and afterward it develops and grows; and in the end it becomes your son. But in the meantime it is a fetus. You don't know how it is; you don't know how it looks; you only feel weird movement inside you . . . In my opinion it's the most logical and normal thing not to put the cart before the horse.

The attempt not to speak too much about the future baby or reveal names echoes defensive strategies against the evil eye, which I encountered almost everywhere when speaking to pregnant women, regardless of their ethnic origin or level of education.

The Israeli idea of gestating a tentative fetus lies in how conditionality potently shapes a whole range of emotional strategies to limit bonding between the pregnant woman and her fetus. Whether by devoting herself to work, ignoring physical sensations, or delaying preparations for the birth, women and their male partners carefully tried to navigate their emotions within an arena of deeply felt dangers. Conceptually and practically, the conditional status of the fetus may culminate in a division of pregnancy into two different aspects—gestation of the fetus and the pregnant woman—as two separate notions of pregnancy.

Such conceptual separation may illuminate the logic behind women's heroic stories of pain endurance. Once conceptually disconnected, the pregnant body cannot be understood as a viable mediator between the unborn baby and the outer world. Therefore, the pain or discomfort experienced by a pregnant woman is much less automatically linked to fetal distress. Thus, Israeli women and medical care providers seem relatively slower to interpret pain as "a signal from the fetus who is asking for help," as Japanese women readily interpret it.

The cultural option to understand pregnancy as a dual notion may explain how it may become trivialized. Only with physical and mental discontinuity between the fetus and the woman can the latter's physical sensations and emotional distress while pregnant be "safely" trivialized. By this means alone, trivialization cannot threaten the fetus's well-being. The consequences for some women are far-reaching. Pregnancy assumes a highly ambiguous course. It is a powerful physical experience, which changes the shape of the body considerably. However, because of the uncertainty that envelops the fetus, pregnancy can become a matter of ignoring physical sensation, and enduring emotional stress in the face of trivialization, more than of bearing children.

In Search of an Enduring Alternative

As I stated in the introductory part of this book, from the early stages of research I was actually looking for an arena of pregnancy that made possible an alternative, less frightening, more optimistic experience of pregnancy for women. When I first met Mona, thirty-seven, a mother of three children, and a sculptor, who described almost mystical pregnancy experiences, of being "overwhelmed and filled with the life that was developing inside me," I thought that I finally found what I was looking for. Her sculptures, featuring images of pregnant women, galvanized me immediately. Pregnancy was powerfully embodied in her works, but also imbued with sensuality and eroticism. Sitting together in her little house, surrounded by a nice little garden we spent four intense hours trying to uncover what it was that fascinated her about pregnancy, and what pregnancy meant for her. Mona told me how she had left a well-paid job as a pharmacist to start a new career as an artist; she would thus be able to "explore the things that interested me, to really go deep into myself and look into the important questions." The main question that Mona raised repeatedly throughout our conversation was, "How and when does life begin?" She told me: "I noticed that I was searching all the time. It's very difficult to speak about these things, because it's all a matter of sensations and feelings. I look all the time at photographs of the sperm and the egg and their moment of meeting and the creation of the fetus. So there is egg and sperm, but when and where does the soul enter all this? When does it happen? I feel as if I'm searching all the time inwardly, deeper and deeper inside the body, to find this point of becoming, this genesis, the beginning of life, and it's all happening inside my own body."

As a former pharmacist, Mona felt at home with biomedical representations of "the beginning of life" and remarked: "I can sit for hours and look at these photographs of fetuses at different stages of pregnancy, although I am aware that these are actually pictures of aborted fetuses." She stressed that she also used such biomedical representations as a source of inspiration and that the main source of her exploration was her own body. She described the "physical sensations of growing from the inside," and said that when she is pregnant, she is "overcome" by the feeling of "enclosing, encompassing, containing life inside me. I feel it here in the chest, not only in the belly—in all my physical being."

Throughout the interview, Mona kept talking about "life," not about babies. When I asked her directly about this, she commented that for her the fetus is a baby and continued to tell me the story of how she first "met" her son on the ultrasound screen: "I was alone—there was nobody with me—so when I met him on the screen, it was just me and him, and I was instantly drawn into him as if I was being vacuumed into him. It was really the feeling that his soul entered my soul and that's that, it stayed inside. I felt as if I was flying in some kind of cloud. I was so excited that I could not come down to earth long enough to take a bus or call a taxi."

Mona's narrative was about the absolute connection between herself and her unborn baby. Yet when I told her about how Japanese women talk to their unborn babies, she responded: "I could never connect with such a practice, with talking to the baby from the outside," and her narrative immediately slipped back to "life." She said that "I just enjoy this condition [being pregnant]. I don't know—it's the life growing inside my body, it simply fills me up. These are very strong sensations." In fact, throughout our conversation, the "fetus" or the unborn "baby" remained marginal to the experience of pregnancy. When she spoke about how much she longed to be pregnant again, she said it was "so I can feel and explore these sensations again"—not a matter of her longing for a baby. In a way, Mona's account of her daughter's birth suggests that her "babies" only come into being after they have been born. As she told me: "I will never forget how when we arrived at the hospital I got out of the car and knew "That's it; it's going to happen; she is going to *come into being*." I had the feeling that I was kissing death. It's not that *I'm* going to die. I'm only visiting, kissing it. It was as if I was standing on both sides of a mirror and had the opportunity to see both: *now when she is in my belly, she does not exist, and soon, she will exist*. When one dies it's exactly the opposite: what exists ceases to be. So what is it that differentiates between existence and nonexistence?" (emphasis added)

Again, Mona's narrative echoes her quest for the point where "life" begins. However, "life" and "my daughter" seem to be two distinctly different notions: "life" begins somewhere in the mists of conception, but "my daughter" only comes into being after birth. Through the birth process her daughter passed from the world of nonexistence (death) to the world of the living. Mona's account of her physical sensations after the birth suggests that before her daughter was born, she was part of Mona's body. As she recalls, "After she was born I felt a painful sensation of emptiness inside my belly, and every time people touched her [her daughter], I would feel this pain, as if somebody was pushing their hands into my insides."

Mona concluded that "giving birth to her [daughter] was like parting from one part of my body. . . . Maybe it was giving a rebirth to myself." Mona's experiences of pregnancy indeed offer an embodied and sensual alternative to the narratives that we have explored thus far. The quality of her experience stems from her ability to "reconnect" pregnancy. However, this connection is between herself and her body. I suggest that for Mona pregnancy is in fact an embodied locus of philosophical exploration, a powerful resource, an inspiration for self-discovery and artistic work. This might explain why, fascinated though Mona was with the "life" that was growing inside her, in all her three pregnancies she also made sure to take a three-hour ride from her house to undergo intensive ultrasound screening at the clinic of a leading specialist and did not skip amniocentesis either. She told me about a friend of hers whose son had died ten months after being born with a metabolic disease that had not been diagnosed prior to birth.

MONA: They [the parents] investigated the whole thing after he died. They wanted to know exactly what happened and why he died, and she realized that she could have had him diagnosed prior to birth and that she might have had an abortion if she had known. It is a loop.

TSIPY: And what do you think about it?

MONA: I think that this is indeed the proper thing to do before you really physically get to know him [the unborn baby], because the meeting [with the baby] only occurs after the birth. But from the aspect of the feeling of loss, I don't think that the feeling of loss would have been less powerful if she had aborted him before meeting him.

Mona's narratives are significant because they demonstrate that alternatives clearly exist. However, at the same time they also mark the limits of "how far" such alternatives can go. Even within a reconnected and embodied pregnancy, the idea of bonding with unborn babies remains somewhat less "digestible."

The Divided Pregnancy

The perspectives of women on their pregnancies shed a new light on the "hysterical" pregnant woman. In their personal experiences, women emerge as unrecognized heroines rather than "hysterics" who are governed by their wombs. True, anxieties dominate their narratives; yet they attempt to overcome their bodies and fears by devising degrees of detachment from bodily sensations or strategies to distract their minds. These attempts are made in a social climate that tends to trivialize pregnancy. Medical practitioners, male partners, the law, and women themselves all participate in reproducing the trivialization of the mental and physical aspects of pregnancy. In Israel, I contend, the trivialization of pregnancy feeds on local formulations of the socialist-egalitarian Zionist ethos of gender equality under which much of gender politics still takes place. Motherhood, or to be precise childbearing, may be a national mission, but the ethos of equality in its local popular formulation holds that women have other missions too. At its extreme, the equality ethos materializes into a set of denials of physical difficulties. Significantly, childbearing and motherhood do not necessarily converge within this discursive apparatus.

I suggest that the prevalent perceptions of pregnancy in Israel are deeply colored by the cultural possibility of making a conceptual and practical division between pregnancy and the fetus. That is not to say that all pregnancies are "divided" or that any specific pregnancy is "divided" at each and every moment. It means that detachment is a familiar "mental posture" that one becomes skilled in assuming, a social resource that is readily available for use. By "divided pregnancy" I do not only mean that women may experience a split subjectivity while they are pregnant, in the sense that scholars like Young (1984), Kristeva (1981), Root and Browner (2001), and others have observed. The different kinds of split that these scholars mention—between body and self, past and future (Young 1984, 46), physiology and speech (Kristeva 1981, 31), "haptic" (embodied sensations) and medical explanations (Root and Browner 2001), or between awareness of myself as body and awareness of my aims and projects (Young 1984, 51)—can be identified in whole or in part in the narratives of different women. Nevertheless, the division I point out here is a "mental posture" that is directly linked to the predominance of a *social script of catastrophe* that stretches beyond pregnancy. In fact, division is one of the defensive strategies that heroes may adopt when they are threatened. It seems to me that, as a strategy, division can be about keeping the divided person "immune" from unpleasant surprises, so that catastrophe does not befall one unexpectedly. However, research findings indicate that Israeli women who experienced pregnancy loss in various stages of gestation and birth were in no way "better" prepared for this tragedy (Gazit 2007). Yet pregnant women use techniques of detachment as preventive measures. If we imagine the social script of pregnancy as a flow chart, in the Israeli script more routes lead to division than to connectedness.

The practical meaning is that Israeli women approach the idea of bonding with their fetuses hesitantly, as if on tiptoe. A Japanese woman who "wishes" to bond with her unborn baby has plenty of scripts to use, but an Israeli woman with a similar inclination has to work hard to block ideas of catastrophe from bursting into her experience. Even when bonding is indeed established, the omnipresence of potential catastrophe makes it seem extremely fragile. In claiming that the "divided pregnancy" is a cultural possibility, I mean that division is a primary tool with which to "work through" *any* pregnancy, not explicitly "threatened" pregnancies. The majority of the Israeli women I spoke to had received no indication whatsoever of any fetal problem during their pregnancies, and they all gave birth to healthy children. Nevertheless, the notion of division cuts through most of their narratives more or less explicitly.

The conceptual division of pregnancy also explains why Israeli pregnant women too often tend to wait before they report "suspicious" bodily sensations: they are slow to associate these sensations with the fetus. From a Japanese perspective, pregnant women who are late in reporting painful or even just unusual bodily sensations would strike Japanese people as showing indifference to the unborn baby.

Interestingly, the above patterns of pain management undergo dramatic inversion in childbirth. Israeli women, who endure the burdens of pregnancy and keep working until the first contractions appear, readily use analgesics, anesthetics, and tranquilizers to relieve their pain. In fact, in many cases of uncomplicated labor the medical staff encourage women to use tranquilizers. Japanese women, who would readily seek medical advice if any suspicious sensation arose during pregnancy, are expected to endure the pain of birth without tranquilizers and are discouraged from taking them. What explains such variations in the management of pain?

I suggest that pain is managed through the same paradigms by which pregnancy as a whole is understood. In the Israeli case the division of pregnancy cuts through pain as well. When pregnancy is divided the connection between pain and the condition of the fetus is not at all obvious. Moreover, interpreted in terms of the opposition between heroines and spoiled women, pain might be easily interpreted as a whim. The same division applies to labor. Since the person in labor is the woman, and since pain is now "legitimate" (everybody knows that birth hurts), it would be logical to rid her of it completely. However, in the

Japanese context, which is one of continuity rather than division, the woman does not experience labor alone. Her unborn baby is in labor with her, and pain is readily interpreted as a vital signal that should not be silenced. The birth pains are understood as a climactic point in the process of bonding, an experience that mothers can hardly do without.

Alternatives

Clearly, even under the shadow of the key script of reproduction gone awry, alternative experiences emerge. As New Age practices and ideas spread in Israel, alternatives to medicalized pregnancy and birth present themselves. No doubt the nature, scope, and limitations of such alternatives in themselves deserve exploration (which is beyond the scope of this study). Yet from a broader perspective on reproductive practices, it is interesting that most alternatives focus their discourse and practice on the event of birth, and much less on pregnancy. In the first years of the twenty-first century a home-birth movement succeeded to draw public attention by calling for the legalization of home births. As a result, medical institutions are now increasingly trying to integrate practices of alternative medicine and incorporate them into hospital births. Can these changes alter perceptions of pregnancy? To answer this question, it will be necessary to explore local variations in the practice of alternative medicine as practiced in Israel. Although this would take us beyond the scope of the present study, I offer a few considerations here.

First, my observations suggest that alternative medicine is selectively appropriated into Israeli practice to fit Israeli paradigms of the body, pain, and birth. An example is the recent introduction of Shiatsu as a "tranquilizer" in one Israeli birthing room. The nurses who told me proudly about this new service were sure that Shiatsu was practiced during birth in Japan. They were shocked to learn that Shiatsu (and tranquilizers more generally) do not belong in birthing rooms in Japan.[8]

Secondly, I suggest that the Israeli natural-birth movement also has limited conceptual resources with which to change assumptions about pregnancy. As a birth movement, it is focused on the drama of birth and much less on the process of pregnancy. Its adherents include a high proportion of Jewish midwifes originating from America and women from highly advantaged groups in Israeli society. Although more and more Israeli-born activists are joining the movement, the majority of Israeli women seem to look with suspicion at antimedicalization messages. If pregnancy is highly risky, birth seems even more so.

With an Eye to the Evil

Israeli women who experienced their pregnancy thirty or more years ago insist that at that time pregnancy was not as haunted with anxiety as it is now for their daughters, which suggests that the divided pregnancy that we witness at the beginning of the twenty-first century is a contemporary model. Yet these women, just like their daughters, took care to remain unprepared for their new babies. Their accounts echo notions of the evil eye as much as the worst-case medical scenarios they relate. As Sered observes (2000), Jews have long used amulets for protection against the evil eye (even though many rabbis condemned this practice as idol worship). Pregnancy and birth are only particular cases of this. In her book, Sered includes a long list of amulets and incantations used specifically to safeguard pregnancy and birth from the evil eye and protect it from wicked ghosts.

The fear of worst-case scenarios seems to reside at the heart of Jewish folk religion and to cut through the pregnancy cultures of Jews of diverse ethnic origin. Medical worst-case scenarios, I suggest, are merely a recent incarnation of these anxieties. The preexisting grammar through which Jews understand themselves as living under threat serves as an especially fertile culture on which to "grow" "divided" pregnancies. Again, juxtaposition with Japanese perceptions may illustrate how deeply this understanding of reality cuts through personal perceptions, social relations, and even institutional logics. The idea of the Japanese *boshitechô*, a handbook given to the pregnant woman to fill in, which includes registration of vaccinations planned for the future child, would be inconceivable to Israelis from both the medical and folk points of view. From the medical point of view the main question is, "Who can ensure that even in the later stages of pregnancy no fetal anomaly will be diagnosed and lead to an abortion?" In the folk version it becomes, "Who would be stupid enough to tease the evil eye with the suggestion that the baby will indeed be born and the vaccination part of the handbook will be filled out?" Just as no store would try to get expectant couples to buy bottles and furniture for the baby, no bureaucrat would consider providing a record for the new baby before it is born. In this sense, the current model of pregnancy draws in its present version on a "new" medicalized script of worst-case scenarios, while at the same time resonating with Jewish history and Jewish fears.

PART THREE

Embodying Culture

Toward an Anthropology of Pregnancy

5

Juxtapositions

The Collaborative Production of Pregnancy

Now that I have explored an array of perspectives on pregnancy, I return to piece them together and use cross-cultural comparison to reexamine the metaquestions of this study. What is the range of meanings that pregnancy can take for Japanese and for Israelis at the beginning of the twenty-first century? Is it about different things? If so, what are the socio-cultural conditions that produce this difference? And what are the implications of these differences for the ways in which pregnancy can be experienced and dealt with? What are the implications of these two versions of pregnancy for anthropological studies of reproduction?

In the following discussion, my analytical strategy will operate simultaneously along the lines of integration and juxtaposition. I shall integrate the perspectives of women, their partners, birth educators, lecturers, and participants in and organizers of pregnancy days, as well as the perspectives of doctors in each locality. I shall juxtapose the two integrated entities that I call "the Japanese culture of pregnancy" and the "Israeli culture of pregnancy": this analytical operation is made possible thanks to one major finding of this study: the striking concordance between the lay perspectives of women and the medical perspectives of doctors.

Although women and doctors are often positioned differently with respect to the body of authoritative knowledge, in each locality they seem to share a distinct set of assumptions and patterns of thought. In fact, this study might serve as an example of how authoritative knowledge is locally produced through an ongoing *collaborative* social process, throughout which "common sense" ideas are juggled by different agents, and in which, as Jordan writes, "people not only accept authoritative knowledge (which is thereby validated and enforced) but also are actively and unselfconsciously engaged in its routine production and reproduction" (Jordan 1997, 57–58). Root and Browner refer to this same collaboration: the "paradoxical dependence of biomedical authority upon patient acknowledgement of its dictates" (Root and Browner 2001, 197). The Japanese practice of close weight supervision is hardly imaginable without the diligent cooperation of pregnant mothers, nor are the high detection rates of fetal abnormalities in Israel without the threatened pregnant woman. At the outset, the enterprise of prenatal care seems to require woman's collaboration as a precondition, its power drawing on its ability to "make sense," as Jordan notes (Jordan 1997, 57).

Nevertheless, by "integration" I do not mean to imply that the different agents in each arena all "think alike." I argue that they share a mutual basis for understanding, and that they operate within a common social atmosphere, within a particular state of mind. The purpose of integration is to delineate a set of ideas that *cut across* social settings and social agents, ideas with which different agents (who would not necessarily agree with each other) *negotiate*, sometimes even against their will. I see all the agents whose accounts were explored above, whether pregnant women, medical doctors, or others, as social actors who are trying to make sense of pregnancies in a most practical way, while utilizing the conceptual resources available to them, as they engage in various social interactions in different social settings. Each of these interactions is grounded in a configuration of power relations specific to it: in each social interaction professional and lay agencies, resistances, compliances, and pragmatisms are played out. Moreover, as Jordan teaches us, each of these social interactions contains a set of different kinds of knowledge about pregnancy, and a hierarchy between what counts as authoritative knowledge and other forms of knowledge can be identified. Still, from the broader perspective of cultural comparison, in each arena, the local "regime of truth" (Foucault 1980, 109–133) seems to carry the "stamp" of a cultural scheme of thinking that agents ranging from the most explicit resistor to the most conventional practitioner appear unable to escape.

To that extent, I tend to think of the perspectives of women and doctors on pregnancy as the medical and lay versions of pretty much the same ethnotheory of gestation. The social implications of the ideas and assumptions underlie both medical and lay perspectives on pregnancy that I examine in the first part of this discussion. Juxtaposed here are the two schemes of thinking, within their respective "states of mind," that inform practitioners' and patients' ideas, experiences, and actions. Each respective cultural "state of mind" is continuously reproduced by those who participate in its construction. This comparative approach to the Israeli and Japanese "realms" designates each as an interactive and interconnected process in terms of the production of knowledge and the practice of pregnancy. Each realm is made particular by local styles of reasoning that draw on socio-political histories of the body that again are both produced through this style and reproduce it at the same time. The following comparison is not a reduction of the individual voices of practitioners and women to "the

Japanese (or Israeli) case" but an integrative consideration of two whole, dynamic, and irreducible entities. Since I know of no English word that encompasses the complexity of this integrative interrelatedness, I shall alternately use expressions such as "the Japanese realm" or "the Israeli case." Nevertheless, the meaning I wish to convey is that of the Israeli, or Japanese, interactive process of producing forms of knowledge about and practices of pregnancy.

Points of Departure: Pregnancy as Limbo, Pregnancy as Parenting

Medical and lay knowledge systems, in respect of both production and practice, have different starting points: they define the protagonists of pregnancy differently and organize the relationships between them accordingly. In the Japanese arena the protagonist of pregnancy is the interconnected entity of the mother–baby, whereas in the Israeli case the protagonists are the pregnant woman and her suspect fetus. Pregnancy is conceptualized as an early stage of parenting in Japan and is all about the interdependence of mother and baby and their ongoing relationships. The Israeli model defines pregnancy as a state "in limbo" that involves two separate individuals (of whom only one is a person). Yet whether the fetus is understood as a person or not, its health is a major concern of all who are involved in the pregnancy under both formulations of gestation; but each system understands the fetus's health through a distinct conceptual set complete with its particular emphases and practical implications.

Japanese medical and folk theories are in fact a set of "etiologies" of fetal health and illness that explain how a fetus *becomes* unhealthy, thus emphasizing the pregnant body as a primary determinant of fetal health. Whether the fetus has grown too large to be born vaginally because its mother has become diabetic (to use medical vocabulary) or whether the baby cannot pass through the birth canal because of the layers of fat (to use lay imagery), both formulations agree that large babies are the result of problematic maternal behavior. In other words, Japanese lay and professional agents offer ample explanations of the various ways in which different kinds of environmental conditions matter to fetal health. This is not to say that Japanese are unfamiliar with genetic explanations but to stress that they tend to emphasize environmental factors despite this awareness. The point of departure in this thinking is the idea that the unborn baby and the mother are *interconnected* physiologically and mentally. The tendency to emphasize ecosystemic factors and interrelationships can be thought of as "somatic and mental environmentalism," here just "environmentalism" for the sake of brevity. I see "environmentalism" as a key way of thinking underlying Japanese medical and lay theories of gestation. Significantly, however, within such an ecosystemically oriented framework of thinking, the pregnant body becomes meaningful—literally as an "important body"—in respect of fetal health, not in itself.

The relative absence of etiologies and the relative meaninglessness of the pregnant body in the Israeli theory of pregnancy become visible when it is juxtaposed with the Japanese model. The Israeli theory seems to elaborate less on the reasons why a fetus should become unhealthy and tends to fear inborn abnormalities as unfortunate but realistic reproductive misfortunes that "happen," but do not necessarily result from specific actions. Abnormal fetuses *are* abnormal, they do not *become* abnormal. Genetic explanations loom large in Israeli theories of gestation, and worst-case scenarios are associated with "essential" health problems that "reside" in the initial constitution of the fetal body, that is, in the genes and chromosomes. This genetic and chromosomal determinism leaves little hope for affected individuals. Ultimately the emphasis on a predetermined genetic and chromosomal individuality stresses the instant of fertilization as the most significant moment, at which the genetic identity of the future offspring is determined. The embryo is basically either perfect or damaged on conception. It cannot be perfected in a meaningful way if a random chromosomal or genetic "accident" happened when the sperm and egg first became a zygote. The perfect baby that is aspired to can only be spoken about in terms of its not having catastrophic abnormalities. There is no vocabulary to discuss fetal health in terms other than nonillness.[1] Put differently, whereas both Japanese and Israeli models include worst-case scenarios, in the latter one can do little to bring forth a positive script. In the Israeli theories relatively few "only ifs" are present, but many "even thoughs." As one ob-gyn put it, "Even young and healthy women who are not known to be the carriers of specific genetic diseases can carry abnormal fetuses." According to this way of thinking, *any* pregnancy carries the potential to become chaotic unexpectedly. This explains why many of my Israeli women interviewees were waiting for the "verdict" of amniocentesis before organizing their emotions. The Israeli theory of gestation is inclined to fatalism: there is not much one can *do* to influence fetal health. I call this extreme case of genetic fatalism "geneticism" and see it as a key scheme of thinking that underlies both medical and lay theories of gestation in Israel. In the "geneticist" scheme of thinking gestation is relatively meaningless; the pregnant body is a receptacle for a more or less "ready-made" fetus.

Japanese and Israeli concerns with fetal health emphasize notably different kinds of "health problems." Both "kinds" of concerns are discussed in global professional literature about prenatal medical care, but in the local interactive systems of knowledge and practice only specific parts of an elaborate collection of fetal pathologies are emphasized. I suggest that each realm emphasizes the kind of health problems that "fit into" the conceptual scheme of local theories of pregnancy and that can be "solved" in "culturally correct" or socially acceptable medical procedures.

In the case of complicated deliveries of "big babies," to take one example, the intrauterine environment that gives rise to excessively large babies is understood as having been created by the pregnant woman's nutrition. Therefore, all nutritional substances entering the body must be regulated. The Japanese logic thus allocates direct *responsibility* for patrolling the entry of substances into the maternal ecosystem as dependent on the mother's cooperation. The idea that underlies such massive efforts to "filter" external "invasions" into the body is that as a rule of thumb the fetus is initially healthy.[2]

By contrast, the Israeli model aspires to achieving a healthy baby, but it has few recommendations on how to *make* one. To be exact, the distribution of hierarchies between knowledge of ideal nutritional intake and knowledge of the "prevention" of genetic and chromosomal abnormalities positions knowledge of nutrition as supplementary and marginal at best. One illustration of this hierarchy is the way the lectures by Dr. Cohen (who screened the ultrasonic horror picture show) and by Dr. Navon (who spoke about nutrition in pregnancy) were arranged in the schedule of the pregnancy day, and the way the audience related to their talks. The particular distribution of hierarchy between the different kinds of knowledge that Cohen and Navon represent reflects the privileged, even hegemonic position of "geneticist" schemes of thinking. This example echoes Jordan's insistence that authoritative knowledge does "*not* mean the knowledge of people in authority positions" (Jordan 1997, 58).

By contrast, the Japanese formal hierarchy between knowledge of environmental factors and knowledge of genetic factors in relation to fetal health is almost the opposite: it is basically a model of causality that offers prescriptions of active control as a means of achieving positive pregnancy outcomes. It does feature worst-case scenarios, but it also offers a regime of hard work through which the fetus can be *perfected*.[3] Moreover, if the woman eventually gives birth to a healthy baby (as in the majority of cases), it follows from the environmental theory that it is she who deserves praise. Nevertheless, both models harbor potential agonies for women, and in both, women are held responsible for bearing healthy children, even though they are expected to pursue markedly different strategies in achieving this goal. I shall return to this later.

"Environmentalism" and "geneticism," then, designate different emphases in the Japanese and Israeli theories of pregnancy, and the different distributions of hierarchy between two types of knowledge: knowledge dealing with environmental factors in fetal health, and knowledge of the genetic factors in fetal health.[4]

Meaningful and Meaningless Bodies

The divide between the meaningfulness and the meaninglessness of the pregnant body cuts across the Japanese and Israeli arenas, respectively, as a key principle that runs throughout medical, legislative, and lay arenas of pregnancy. What I called the "trivialization" of pregnancy in the Israeli public sphere draws on the idea that women literally merely "carry" their fetuses. It is acknowledged that working during pregnancy might be difficult for the woman, but it is seldom thought potentially harmful for the fetus. Similarly, pain felt by pregnant women could never have been dismissed so lightly (by both women and their care providers) had gestation been seen as more important for the health of the fetus. Put differently, the Israeli conceptual division between pregnancy and the fetus would not be possible if gestation did not feature so low among factors in fetal health. By contrast, the exclusion of pregnancy from the Japanese public sphere has a lot to do with the idea of women as the makers of their babies. It is widely acknowledged that pregnant bodies require a great deal of consideration because they are engaged in the hard and tiring work of making babies. In accordance with these ideas, women tend to see themselves as care providers to their unborn babies, and may become devoted and creative monitors of the quality of their own care provision.

These same basic schemes inform the outlook of Japanese medical practitioners when they provide care to pregnant women. Since "maternal ecosystems" are seen as highly important to fetal health, some doctors become committed to guiding women on the proper management of their environments but also to providing positive environments in their clinics. Dr. Sato, who was quoted above, by making sure that relaxing music is played in the waiting room of his clinic, can be understood in this light. His conduct echoes the thinking that underlies the enterprise called *taikyô*, the theory of fetal communication that predates the routinization of western medical care in Japan.

The examples of how Japanese practitioners communicate with patients about genetic and chromosomal fetal abnormalities demonstrate how, even when the fetal disorder concerned does not fit into the conceptual scheme of "environmentalism," practitioners still cling to the idea of the mother as a most vital agent whose state of mind should not be taken lightly. Although practitioners frown on patients' "misinterpretations" of statistics and probability, their reluctance to use numbers is apparently due not only to their doubts about their patients' ability to understand them properly, but also because gruesome numbers do not seem to constitute a suitable medium to discuss with mothers the health of their babies.

Regardless of whether the pregnant *body* is understood as more or less meaningful, the *pregnant patient* is a meaningful and potent factor in the design of prenatal care in both the Japanese and Israeli arenas. A common pattern that emerges in the accounts of Japanese and Israeli doctors is that both groups seem to fashion their style of practice on their understanding of patients' expectations of their care providers, their interests, and their state of mind. Yet "the patient" (though a much-quoted entity) is often reduced in practitioners' minds to an iconic image. The "hysterical woman," to take one example, does not seem an adequate depiction of the average Israeli patient in her behavior: although

Israeli women confess to their anxieties, most of them also put much effort into limiting displays of tension. How many instances of explicit "hysteria" do Israeli ob-gyns encounter in the course of their careers? Or better, what kinds of behavior do they label "hysterical"? I suggest that Israeli doctors tend to remember the rare cases of what they see as "hysterical" women.

This is illustrated by the story told by Dr. Schwartz at staff meeting that discussed whether amniocentesis should be practiced even more liberally than it is nowadays. His story about a twenty-seven-year-old patient who insisted on undergoing amniocentesis even though there were no indications of fetal problem, only for this to lead to the detection of a baby with Down's syndrome and an abortion, is in no way ordinary. Nevertheless, it was this rare case that the doctor remembered, although one can well imagine that the majority of his young patients who underwent amniocentesis had negative results, with some even miscarrying healthy fetuses following the test.

An opposite orientation of selective memory is a story I was told by a young Japanese ob-gyn. He told me how he offered amniocentesis to a forty-year-old patient, who reacted by saying that even if her child was born with Down's syndrome she intended to bring it up wonderfully. The practitioner was deeply impressed and told me, "Since then I don't suggest this test any more." Again, this seems to be quite a rare story, first, because at least some ob-gyns do not discuss prenatal diagnosis with patients of any age. Secondly, patients tend to reject prenatal diagnosis in rather passive ways that suit the hierarchical gap assumed to exist between Japanese doctors and patients. When asked directly, the same practitioner recalled a thirty-two-year-old patient who was interested in performing amniocentesis. But he recalled the story about the older woman first, and he determined his own clinical standards according to it.

Returning to the Israeli arena, the reader might recall a practitioner I called Dr. Wolli, who remembered a forty-year-old doctor who refused amniocentesis, talking in a positive way about children with Down's syndrome. However, this story remained in his memory as "weird" and did not alter his attitude to medical practice.

These examples illustrate that specific experiences with patients often become iconic when they evince the absolute necessity and appropriateness of the practitioner's medical standards. The collaborative enterprise of prenatal care is not always co-produced with "live" patients at any given moment. Often it is mediated by iconic images and stories that accord with or demonstrate the logical implications of the "truth regime" under which prenatal care is conducted. Both patients and doctors can understand and identify with these iconic images.

Throughout the ethnography the perceptions of doctors and patients seem to echo each other. Some clinical standards literally depend on the cooperation of "live" patients, not on iconic images. The strict supervision of weight and nutrition by Japanese ob-gyns largely echoes the self-perceptions of pregnant Japanese women, to whom this monitoring makes a lot of sense (although it might be stressful at times). Paradoxically, the importance of weight monitoring even justifies causing distress to the patient. Worrying the patient here is seen as instrumental, a momentary effect intended to help the patient "align" herself with optimal conduct in the best interests of the unborn baby. It seems no coincidence that the Japanese theory of pregnancy is embodied, a condition that follows from the environmental scheme. However, the fact that its strict practical implications continue to exert authority owes much to the cooperative patient. The latter's responses contribute to the doctors' understanding of the pregnant body as amenable to "taming": Israeli pregnancy, with its potential to become a reproductive catastrophe, proves hard to embody; properly "tamed" Japanese pregnancies allow embodiment. Both theories hold that pregnancy possesses a potential for chaos, but Japanese practitioners, by relying on their cooperative patients, tend to believe that this can be tamed, something Israeli practitioners are much more skeptical of.

The Israeli doctors' liberal attitude toward weight gain can be seen as one example of the kind of "freedoms" that the meaninglessness of gestation enables. The same meaninglessness is at play when a doctor straightforwardly "frightens" women with horror picture shows. Given a theory of pregnancy that disconnects fetal health from the mother's body, I suggest that Israeli ob-gyns can "afford" to frighten women because (among other reasons) their anxiety is meaningless to the development of a healthy fetus.

Clearly, freedom versus subjugation is not what the juxtaposition yields. "Environmentalism" and "geneticism" represent two distinct "truth regimes," two ways of formulating socially acceptable truth claims about gestation, complete with their practical implications and constructions of maternal responsibility.

Pragmatic Agencies and the Microphysical Grip

One of my questions throughout the fieldwork was whether specific theories of gestation shape the relationship between women and biomedicine differently. I wondered whether specific biomedical models and certain power structures are mutually constituent.

From Foucault's scholarship, one important locus for examining power relations is the body. The Japanese and Israeli prenatal realms demonstrate two considerably different "microphysical regimes" of the body. The Israeli biomedical grip tends to tighten around the fetus while "transcending" the body of the pregnant woman, as if it was an obstacle on the way to the fetus. The Japanese grip, by contrast, is preoccupied with disciplining, protecting and nourishing the maternal body for the sake of the fetus. These two different kinds of microphysical grip reflect the difference between the two distinct theories of gestation. The Japanese theory allocates to the mother's bodily and mental conduct responsibility for fetal health, so her body is an important aspect of it. By contrast, where fetal health is seen as mainly dependent on the configuration of genes and chromosomes, the woman's body can be left alone. Apparently, the more the "somatic responsibility" is allocated to the mother, the tighter the grip on her body becomes.

Yet a closer look at the Japanese "docile body" (in Foucault's idiom) reveals that the pregnant woman who inhabits it often takes *pleasure* in furthering the discipline of her body by monitoring it herself. When pregnant women enjoy keeping track of their weight gain in their private diaries or make written daily records of their eating habits and physical activities, they not only "cooperate" with the biomedical power structure, they enthusiastically initiate new ways of tightening their own grip on their own bodies. The particular kinds of pleasure taken by these women draw heavily on the prevalence of "environmental" determinism (in both its medical and folk versions) that tells them persuasively that their bodies indeed matter to fetal health. These pleasures remind one of Foucault's claim that "What makes power hold good, what makes it accepted, is simply the fact that it doesn't only weigh on us as a force that says no, but that it traverses and produces things, it induces pleasure, forms knowledge, produces discourse. It needs to be considered as a productive network which runs through the whole social body, much more than as a negative instance whose function is repression." (Foucault 1980, 119)

Obviously, not pleasure alone is at play in the Japanese power structure. When Japanese women cooperate in keeping to their doctors' dietary restrictions, they do it because they dread the consequences of not obeying, too. Doctors may even use "intimidation" as a technique to draw women back to the safe path of eating a healthy diet to produce a healthy baby. Anxieties are as prevalent in the Japanese as in the Israeli realm, although their quality and the scripts of how to alleviate them differ.

Two different kinds of agency are constructed under the "environmental" and "geneticist" truth regimes. The diligent self-monitoring of Japanese women is a form of agency that follows from the notion of interconnectedness. I call this "somatic agency" because of its focus on the importance of the management of the pregnant body. By contrast, the conceptual disconnection of fetal and maternal health in the "geneticist" model produces a situation in which the woman is not deemed "physically" responsible for fetal health: she is merely "gambling" when she gets herself into the chancy business of childbearing. Yet, as the narratives of Israeli women and doctors reveal, women are still held responsible and accountable, being expected to ensure that a healthy baby will be born. In "geneticism" meaningful agency is about sorting out healthy fetuses from potentially damaged ones. Such a form of agency emphasizes the ethos of "choice": the agent is busy "choosing" the baby who deserves to become her own. This "agency of choice" can only be played out with heavy reliance on biotechnologies, again with the imperative to choose among them and to decide.

Somatic and choice agencies are both contingent on two different kinds of "ethics of the pregnant self," to use Root and Browner's (2001) term. Somatic agency is constituted in relation to a moral economy that ultimately defines pregnant women as the responsible mothers of unborn babies. This form of pregnancy ethics builds on the vigorous promotion of the cuteness of unborn babies and cultivation of nurturing maternal emotions toward them. The practices of monitoring become mechanisms to embody maternal sentiments, and their performance is designated as the ultimate expression of responsibility that an ethical pregnant woman can display. By contrast, the moral economy in which agencies of choice are constituted has a differential commitment to fetuses, depending on their inborn quality. A responsible pregnant woman is expected to wait patiently, see whether the fetus is "worth" keeping, and be prepared to give up an unhealthy fetus. This hesitant responsibility can only be exercised if the pregnant woman avails herself of prenatal diagnosis. Through consuming the maximal number of diagnostic tests, pregnant Israeli women display their responsible and ethical pregnant selves. So while Israeli and Japanese women alike are understood as being responsible for bearing healthy children, they are expected to use different techniques: the pregnant mother in Japan is expected to make a healthy baby by disciplining her body and cultivating positive emotions toward the baby; the Israeli pregnant woman is expected to use as much biotechnology as she can to rule out the possibility of her bearing an unhealthy baby.

Not all women exercise these forms of agency in the same way, despite their appearing to follow "logically" from their respective truth regimes and subsequent moral economies; not all demonstrate equally "cultivated" "ethical selves." According to Abu-Lughod, these women's resistances should in no way be taken as "signs of human freedom" but should be used as a "diagnostic of power" (Abu-Lughod 1990, 42) to tell us about "forms of power and how people are caught up in them" (Abu-Lughod 1990, 42). Japanese and Israeli women tend to formulate their resistances by using the same vocabularies that dominate the hegemonic theories of gestation that they are resisting. Morimura the rebel, to give one example, demonstrated the most extreme form of explicit resistance that I found among Japanese women by smoking a few cigarettes a day, drinking coffee, carrying heavy loads, etc.; she justified her transgressions by recourse to an "ecosystemically" oriented rhetoric, claiming that relaxing in those ways was beneficial to her baby's well-being. By contrast, the Israeli Ora, a heavy smoker, felt no need to justify her smoking at all—she simply admitted that she was "addicted" to it. Her narratives and actions revealed that she just did not feel as threatened by the consequences of heavy smoking—bearing small babies—as she did by the idea of bearing a baby with Down's syndrome. Ora had made sure of preventing that possibility by undergoing an expensive amniocentesis. Had environmental hazards been considered more meaningful to fetal health, she might have felt a need to justify her smoking using an ecosystemic rhetoric. However, she felt secure because she was "doing her best" in "geneticist" terms. I do not see Ora's smoking as resistance; from a "geneticist" perspective resistance would be unashamedly refusing to undergo prenatal diagnosis.

A comparison of Ora's and Morimura's behavior shows that the same activity of smoking cigarettes is framed differently and carries different meanings for the two women. Clearly, each "rebel" is thinking in terms of her culture's hegemonic theory of gestation, so the ecosystemic and genetic explanations in each one's theory have to be weighed to situate her behavior along Root and Browner's spectrum of compliance versus resistance. Nor am I sure that the eating and drinking transgressions of pregnant American women that Root and Browner (2001) describe (such as having a soda every day or a beer once in a while) really deserve to be called resistances. These transgressions might be those of pregnant agents who attribute much more weight to genetic than to environmental factors (though one cannot evaluate the relative place of genetics and environment in the interviewees' thinking from the data provided by the authors).

As with Root and Browner, my own attempts to locate resistances all fall into the category of studies which, as Abu-Lughod observes, are concerned with "unconventional forms of non-collective, or at least non-organized, resistance" (Abu-Lughod 1990, 41). These accounts raise questions about the ability of the term "resistance" to capture the social and private meanings of the behaviors that it designates.

Can a pregnant Japanese woman who secretly takes a train to Kyoto and strolls slowly around the temples be considered a resistor of prenatal norms? Can a woman who feels connected to bodily sensations of the "life that is growing inside me" but nonetheless undergoes all possible prenatal diagnostic testing be considered a resistor? These cases suggest the limited ability of either Israeli or Japanese women to challenge seriously the truth regimes in which they are located, in spite of their apparent criticism, skepticism, and self-reflection.

This is where the concept of pragmatism proposed by Lock and Kaufert (1998) comes to mind. Rather than subjugation to biopower on the one hand, claim Lock and Kaufert, or inherent suspicion and resistance on the other, "women's relationships with technology are usually grounded in existing habits of pragmatism" (Lock and Kaufert 1998, 2). I suggest rather that particular pragmatic behaviors structured in accordance with the logic of local truth regimes can be identified in the various ways women choose to transgress prenatal norms. The fact that such transgressions are so seldom made explicit echoes Abu-Lughod's question: "Do certain modern techniques or forms of power work in such indirect ways, or seem to offer such positive attractions, that people do not as readily resist them? There is some evidence for this, and it is a question worth exploring comparatively" (Abu-Lughod 1990, 52). The Japanese and Israeli cases suggest that there might indeed be something hard to resist in the contemporary Japanese and Israeli power structures, although they operate through markedly different truth regimes, formulate different kinds of responsibilities, produce different forms of agency, pleasure, and resistance, cultivate different ethical selves, and place different kinds of microphysical grips on the body. The irresistibility of these forms of power seems to lie in how each of them draws on potent cultural scripts and schemes of thinking, skillfully incorporating them into the orchestration of ethical selves with microphysical grips. Irresistible to Japanese women is often the "cuteness authority" (McVeigh 2000) of the unborn baby appealing for its mother's loving attention; Israeli women find the idea of a prospective catastrophe hard to resist.

The concept of pragmatism seems to describe the behaviors of ob-gyns equally well. Many explicitly described their style of communication with the patient and their standards of practice as pragmatic solutions or reactions to social circumstances, not as deriving from medical considerations. One Israeli ultrasound expert related how "when a woman walks into my office and says, 'I'm pregnant,' I don't touch her. I don't say anything to her, I open a new card, and I write that I recommend an abortion. Then I sign her up on a paper that says that she is aware of all the testing that exists. Now we can begin to talk, to check her out."

He explained later that "I am simply being practical. All doctors know in this country that the courts are going to slaughter them, so this is my way of protecting myself." The pragmatism apparent in the attitude of this practitioner is structured in relation to the pragmatisms of Israeli patients. By contrast, a Japanese doctor who actually chose to approach his or her patient on the same issue of prenatal diagnosis would tend not to confuse her with a list of diagnostic testing. He or she would ask the pregnant woman if she was interested in a test that would tell her precisely whether or not there was any abnormality in her fetus, as against an indicative test. These doctors both act to enhance their patient's chances of achieving their goal of bearing a healthy child. However, their pragmatic ways of doing so are informed by the different forms of pragmatism they recognize in their patients.

To sum up, the diagnostics of the body and of resistance have revealed two registers of power structure. In the Japanese setting women are caught up in a "somatic agency": a collaborative enterprise of disciplining their bodies as a form of pleasure and a display of an ethical pregnant maternal self. In the Israeli setting women are intimidated by the idea of reproductive catastrophe and are caught up in an "agency of choice" and heavy reliance on the use of diagnostic technologies. The question of what can explain the inclination of each society to "ecosystemic" or "geneticist" explanations of gestation now calls for an integrated answer.

Can "Hard Numbers" Explain the Foci of Prenatal Care?

Is it not possible, I am often asked, that the inclination of Japanese and Israeli societies to "ecosystemic" and "geneticist" explanations of gestation, respectively, simply reflects their efforts to improve public-health statistics of maternal and fetal mortality and morbidity, each by combating their own local problems? My answer is that although public health statistics in each location show particular patterns, the logic that constitutes the foci of prenatal healthcare systems does not simply derive from these patterns, so it cannot be reduced to statistics. First and foremost, as my ethnographies illustrate, the dynamics that take place between pregnant women and their health-care providers, as well as the dynamics that surround pregnancy in public spheres, is crucial for understanding local patterns of prenatal care. The relationship of local traits of maternal and fetal mortality and morbidity to the foci of prenatal care are mediated through the doctor–pregnant patient interactions as they emerge vis-à-vis socio-cultural and politico-historical conceptions, which make such a relationship exceedingly complex. Local ways to interpret the "hard numbers" must be taken into account if one is to understand such complexities.

Can the large number of genetic diseases that are frequent among Jews of various ethnic origins explain the obsession of Israeli-Jewish pregnant women and ob-gyns to detect fetuses with Down's syndrome? When practitioners and pregnant women collaborate to prevent a 1:1000 chance of a young woman bearing a child with Down's syndrome by taking a 1:200 risk of the miscarriage of a healthy fetus, one cannot argue that patterns of prenatal care are simply a response to local patterns of public health. Top geneticists are indeed highly occupied with preventing (Jewish) genetic diseases; however, doctors, pregnant women and their partners are occupied with a much broader notion of anomaly that is quite vague and open-ended. Israeli doctors and pregnant women alike probably fear abnormal fetuses more than they fear the accidental death of healthy fetuses.

And what can explain why Israeli practitioners continue to "return" more embryos, compared with their European and Japanese counterparts, to the wombs of women undergoing fertility treatments, even though such practices are directly linked to the rising rates of premature birth and very low birth-weight babies in Israel, as well as to neonatal mortality and morbidity? (The more embryos implanted in the womb, the shorter the pregnancy, the lower the neonatal weight at birth, and the higher the rise in mortality and morbidity rates.)[5] The logic behind the Israeli regulations and practices is that attempting implantation with more embryos will produce the maximum rate of success in fertilization per cycle of IVF; it is the logic of a pro-natal state fighting to increase birth rates at all costs. However, by a vicious circle, the obsession with quantity again raises the dilemma about quality.[6]

Israeli ob-gyns are well acquainted with the data on morbidity and mortality rates among multifetal pregnancies and are not interested in creating pregnancies with more than two fetuses. They rely on the legitimate option of aborting "residual" fetuses if fertilization becomes "too" successful, which creates great dramas about whether to "thin out" or not, and which embryos to take out. By contrast, the Japanese regulation limiting the number of returned embryos to two seems to escape selection wherever possible.

What can possibly explain why in Japan, a country that claims the world record for the lowest neonatal mortality rates, maternal mortality rates are still behind those of other developed countries? On the issue of maternal death, doctors explained that it is caused by problems in the transport of blood. It seems easier to control women's eating habits than for medical institutions to agree on arrangements for the transport of blood.

Moreover, how can the hesitant attitudes of Japanese ob-gyns to "preventing" genetic and chromosomal abnormalities be explained in a country where maternal age is on the rise? Ob-gyns, like policy makers, apparently assume that women are already committed to their unborn babies and make themselves unreservedly available for nurturing. Raising an abnormal child often requires enormous amounts of extra effort and devotion on the part of the parents, but it takes its toll especially on mothers. Yet Japanese mothers generally are expected to put aside other activities, at least for several years, and devote themselves to providing care to their children before and after birth, whether normal or abnormal. By contrast, the assumptions behind the liberalism with which postdiagnostic abortions are practiced in Israel—a state that is desperately seeking to increase fertility rates—is that although women would not necessarily be prepared to devote themselves to any child, they would be prepared to conceive again and again.

The relationship of statistics of neonatal and maternal health with prenatal policies is complex. The general statistics of maternal and neonatal mortality and morbidity reported by the World Health Organization are insufficient to understand the logic behind local systems. First, neither death (as the Israeli logic suggests) nor chromosomal abnormality (as the Japanese logic suggests) are necessarily considered the worst-case scenario for neonates.

Secondly, managers of local health-care systems may focus on preventing particular kinds of morbidity and (willy-nilly) "paying" for it (or rather have women "pay" for it) with other kinds of mortality and morbidity. From their own socio-cultural vantage points, each prenatal health-care system is successful in terms of the direction in which effort is invested: Israelis have succeeded in decreasing the rates of genetic and chromosomal abnormalities, but not neonatal morbidity or mortality, in the nonreligious population; the Japanese have succeeded in decreasing neonatal mortality rates, but not morbidity and mortality due to inborn genetic and chromosomal abnormalities nor maternal mortality.

If statistics are insufficient tools with which to understand macro-level trends of prenatal care, they are even less adequate on the micro level. On the level of doctor–patient interactions, practitioners are aware that statistical information might be quite confusing to patients. Japanese practitioners "complain" that patients tend to look at the positive side of the statistics and conclude that their conception of probability is "underdeveloped." Israeli ob-gyns, on the other hand, observe quite the opposite, since their patients are liable to imagine themselves the unlucky ones, whose prenatal diagnosis predicts a probability of 1:20,000 of their bearing an unhealthy baby and ending up being that one. The mathematical concept of probability is a constituent of both perspectives. So although the application of probabilities in the clinic might create the illusion that "reproductive risks" can be quantified, and that "reproductive decisions" can be formed and calculated by means of statistics, my ethnographies show that both Japanese and Israeli patients could actually do without them. In the Israeli case, neither doctors who offer amniocentesis to women regardless of their age, nor young women who ask for the test, actually calculate their actions "by numbers." In the Japanese realm ob-gyns explicitly say that statistics cannot be weighed against a myriad of other considerations. Drawing on Jordan's observations on how the production of authoritative knowledge depends on specific ways of displaying it (Jordan 1997), I suggest that rather than as decision-aids for patients, probabilities serve as part of the expressive repertoires of practitioners, helping them to construct scientific gravity in the clinic.

This analysis brings us back to the ultimate challenge of incorporating the socio-cultural, political, and historical setting of gestation into the analytical effort to answer the questions at the heart of this study: Are people living in certain socio-cultural orders more inclined to use "environmental" (or "geneticist") explanations than people living in other social settings? In what kind of cultural arenas do individuals tend to find the "geneticist" (or "environmental") truth regimes more appealing and more imbued with explanatory power? The current study allows us to examine these questions in light of two contrasting cases, specifically: what renders "environmental" explanations more logical and authoritative in Japan; and what makes "geneticist" explanations more acceptable in Israel?

Japanese "Environmentalism" and the Gendered Versions of Interrelatedness

As the ethnographies here illustrate, to make sense, a theory of gestation must resonate with local schemes of thinking that are beyond gestation. In the Japanese case, biomedical and lay "environmentalism" echoes a key scheme of thinking that may be called "interrelatedness." A host of researchers into Japanese culture have described it under a variety of terms, in connection with an array of social phenomena. Studies of Japanese culture and society leave the impression that almost everything in Japanese culture, from material to mental entities, is socially constructed as relational and as dependent on context.

The Japanese social order has been described as "situationally defined" (Lebra 1976), "shifting" (Doi 1986), and "organic" (Smith 1983). "Situationalism," "relativity," and "situational shifting" have all been regarded as basic "structural principles" of Japanese society (Lebra 1976; Nakane 1970). Most important for this study, the organization of a Japanese self has been characterized as "relational" (Araki 1973; Kondo 1990; Rosenberger 1992), "indexical" (Bachnik 1992; Tobin 1992), and "dependent" (Doi 1973).[7] What all these scholars have identified is a scheme of thinking that perceives members of society not as indivisible entities but as interrelated beings in a social context. By such a scheme of thinking, one must become qualified in the arts of contextual behavior to be considered a mature "person among persons" (Ben-Ari 1997; Tobin 1992).[8] Coming of age is less about developing individuality than about learning to connect and relate to others skillfully. Interrelating is thought of as a mechanism of belonging and is explicitly taught in Japan as a key social skill, crucial to anyone who wants to belong to any unit of society (Tobin 1992). Mother–child relations became the prototypical example of interrelatedness in the second half of the twentieth century (Borovoy 2005; Yoda 2001).

That the scheme of interrelatedness feeds into notions of the physical body is quite clear, especially from Lock's (1993) accounts of the biomedical treatment of menopausal women. Her study can be read as an example of how Japanese biomedicine perceives the physical body in conjunction with its social settings. So whereas in Canada the menopausal woman is "a creature that can be made sense of solely in terms of her biology" (Lock 1996, 74), Japanese medical practitioners give expression to a local version of medicine. In their narratives, the menopausal woman is expected to be in danger of suffering from menopausal "syndromes" only under specific social circumstances (since she is positioned temporally after an intensive period of child raising and before becoming engaged in caring for an elderly parent, she might have "too much" time on her hands): "pure" biomedical indications play only a partial role in understanding the health–illness status of the body. For a full understanding of the body, it must be contextualized in relation to its social network.

Along the same lines as Lock's studies, the accounts of Japanese ob-gyns and pregnant women portray pregnancy as a socially interrelated physical and mental effort. Doctors see pregnant women, like menopausal women, as part of their social network. The patient cannot be understood solely in terms of her biology, but must be "environmentally" contextualized. In both cases a "flow chart" seems to exist that explains how physical forms of behavior and social circumstances lead to health or to illness. In both cases the woman herself is held highly responsible for her physical state, and in both cases the medical instructions tend to be environmentally oriented: pregnant women and menopausal women alike are encouraged to improve their nutrition and pursue physical activities.

Not by coincidence attitudes toward the bodies of menopausal women and pregnant women powerfully echo women's social obligations to nurture other members of their family (the elderly in the case of menopausal women and the unborn baby in the case of pregnant women). Though interrelatedness emerges as a broad cultural scheme of thinking, it reaches a new climax here, one distinctly gendered in its assumptions about the ultimate division of labor in society.

The crux of this gendered version of interrelatedness is that it figures in the understanding of the physiology of pregnancy: environmentally oriented biological theories of gestation lend themselves well to a cult of maternal domesticity. Pregnancy figures in these theories as a "corporative" project in which all the body's organs join together in the project of maintaining the health of the unborn baby. The woman governs only the outermost circle of the relationships between the body and its outer environment, yet she is held primarily responsible for the consequences. This project contains numerous ecosystems and inter-organ relationships. The concept of "environment" can be visualized here as a series of interconnected concentric circles that encompass the unborn baby. If the inner environment supplied by the womb is to be kept healthy, then the heart, lungs, liver, etc. should be kept healthy as well. This is why the *boshikenkôtechô—the mother-child health handbook, the Japanese medical record of prenatal care—*takes the trouble to register the condition of the teeth of the pregnant woman, which are as relevant as all other body organs. Understanding the body as an interrelated corporate system is dominant in "low-risk" pregnancies and throughout gestation in Japan, whereas in Israel body parts other than the fetus (even the womb) usually only become a medical concern when pregnancy becomes complicated with a threatening health problem (as in the case of pregnancy toxemia or pregnancy diabetes).

Interrelatedness is also at play in the culturally specific way in which Japanese fetuses are humanized. In the United States the rhetoric of the fetus as person is informed by religious and other pro-life rhetoric that construct it as *independent* life; Japanese ideas of the fetus draw on its *dependence* on its mother. Since life is all about the organization of relations and dependencies, dependence rather than independence is "a sign of life" (ultrasonographic depictions of fetuses are illustrations of the fetus as dependent life). Ample evidence attests that in Japan, fetuses were considered "life" and were endowed with subjectivity long before ultrasonography became popular. Fetuses were conceived more as "liquid life" (LaFleur 1992) and abortions and infanticide were widely practiced, but this did not seem to render their parents, particularly their mothers, less concerned to console their spirits. In the Buddhist liturgy cited in LaFleur's work (1992), the spirits of deceased fetuses and children are endowed with subjectivity: they are depicted as longing for their parents and siblings, and grieving for being bereft of the opportunity to live. La Fleur's historical analysis indicates that rituals to mourn deceased fetuses and children, acknowledging abortions and miscarriages as tragedies for them as well as their parents, existed prior to the 1970s commercialization of rituals to appease the angry spirits of aborted fetuses (Hardacre 1997). The difference from traditional Jewish ideas of the fetus is striking here.

According to rabbinic law, parents should not mourn fetuses that were miscarried before the fifth month of gestation (let alone aborted); nor in some cases premature babies (most rabbis rule that it is not obligatory to bury miscarried fetuses). Although rabbinic law is generally against abortions, it renders fetal life as conditional and tentative up until the actual moment of birth.[9] *Danger* to the woman's life is the circumstance under which the fetus's life can be taken.[10] The rabbis differ about what exactly constitutes "danger" to the woman's life, but all agree that the woman's life takes precedence over that of the fetus (Steinberg 2003, 5). Danger is made the parameter that indexes fetal status.[11]

Significantly, in both the Israeli and Japanese contemporary realms, fetuses are hardly endowed with "rights," unlike the American "life" rhetoric. In the Israeli context, this is because acknowledgment of fetal subjectivity is delayed, and sometimes denied. In the Japanese context, the understanding of fetal "life" as so heavily dependent on maternal agency suspends its "rights." Yet despite the absence of a "pro-life," "fetal-rights"-oriented social movement (in the American sense), women are reluctant to undergo testing that suggests selective abortion.[12] My data indicate that the essentialized emotion-saturated maternal–fetal bond is at play in this reluctance, rather than explicit religious and moralist approaches.

As scholars have pointed out (Coleman 1983; Hardacre 1997; Norgren 2001), Japanese sexual politics in the second half of the twentieth century promoted the use of abortions during the *early* stages of pregnancy as substitutes for contraception, which led to a high incidence of early abortions. This, however, should not be used as evidence of women's indifference to fetal life. Rather, the seeming contradiction between the rate of abortions and the general acknowledgment of fetuses as life points to the need for further exploration of Japanese women's *experiences* of abortion (not the politics of abortion). The ethnography presented here reveals the highly problematic nature of postdiagnostic abortions for Japanese women. In both cases (early and postdiagnostic abortions), the public discourse that surrounds abortions remains concerned with the bond created with pregnancy, and often conceives it as being difficult to sunder. Even after the unborn baby has been miscarried or aborted, the mother is expected to remain "committed" to their relationship, and several Buddhist sects have come out with renewed (and commercialized) rituals to help her appease the fetal spirit that was not given a chance to live.[13] These rituals are less about a scornful religious ethics and more a set of instrumental acts facilitating the mother's assumed psychological need to mourn her unborn child, but also to retain some kind of connection with it through perpetual visits to the graveyard. As much as the rituals of *mizuko kuyô* are cults of maternal guilt, they are also about an unbreakable bond, one that even death cannot rupture.

In fact, maternal guilt (whether about abortions, miscarriages, children born with disabilities, or even the "failures" of "normal" children) is the dark side of the Janus-faced Japanese theory of gestation. It is one of the prices that women pay for being perceived as almighty creators of life.

Israeli "Geneticism," Embodied Destinies, and the Limitations of Nurturance

It is now easier to recognize that the cultural assumptions underlying the escalation of "geneticism" in Israel revolve around notions of the person as an independent individual. Yet I do not argue that the differences between the cases stem from a contrast between "collectivist" and "individualist" societies, or between societies that are "more" or "less" oriented to collectivism, but from their embedment in two different systems of interrelated ideas about the body, its health and illness, individual fate and nurturance.

The ethnography suggests that the destiny of the fetus—the (tentative) future Israeli-Jewish person—is perceived as residing mostly in the constitution of his or her body. The body and the person are understood less in terms of a process than of a predetermined fate. I call such thinking "embodied predestination." The tendency to think about destinies as embodied emphasizes inborn talent rather than hard work. This emphasis does not exclude the notion of "molding" the body or of working hard to achieve a goal; such thinking suggests that only those who embody "proper" "initial" traits are "worth" nurturing, stressing the limited results of nurturing persons with "less favorable initial predispositions."[14]

I am not saying that Israeli parents are *less* nurturing than Japanese, or that Israeli parents feel less obliged to nurture their less-than-perfect children. But thinking within a survival-oriented frame of ideas, as set in the division of labor in Israeli-Jewish society, unlike the Japanese, they tend to perceive nurturance as a limited resource of limited effectiveness. As one pregnant Israeli woman explained to me when discussing the idea of giving birth to a Down's syndrome baby, "Why should I invest my energies, and you know how much it takes to raise a little baby into a child. . . . Why should I invest in a child that might not even smile back at me in the end? Why?" The description that the same woman gave of her relationship with her healthy son was one of absolute dedication. Her statement reflects a particular economy of nurturance whose backbone is the idea that a "destiny" written into a person's body cannot be altered to any meaningful degree—it is a verdict for life. Juxtaposing such ideas with the interconnected sense of self so heavily reliant on maternal nurturance suggests that destinies become embodied in a social context that highlights the *limitations* of maternal as well as other kinds of nurturance.

In its extreme form, the understanding of destinies as embodied disregards the powers of nurturance but also denies the importance of broader social settings in shaping the circumstances of disability. It goes unnoticed that both bodies and destinies are socially and culturally constructed. The set of values, order of priorities, and division of resources in a society construct grading systems to evaluate persons by their physical and intellectual competence, and direct their life course accordingly. But they also "stratify" the opportunities of people who inhabit different kinds of bodies. The accessibility of the public sphere to physically impaired people, to take one example, is a major factor in their ability to receive education and make a living. And to improve accessibility, a society must allocate resources to the cause.

Significantly, compared with the Japanese grassroots movements of people with disabilities, which quite successfully drew attention to disability as a social and moral issue in the mid-1990s, Israeli movements of people with disabilities at the beginning of the third millennium remain almost invisible in the public sphere. In specific connection to this study, while the Japanese movements protested the advent of prenatal testing in Japan, prevented government subsidization of PND, pushed the denunciation of the eugenic declaration in the Eugenic Protection Law, and practically brought about the outlawing of abortions of fetuses with disabilities (Norgren 2001), the Israeli movements have hardly voiced any opposition to the enthusiastic embrace of PND or to the legal status of postdiagnostic abortions in Israel. Israelis with disabilities are often quoted in the media as supporting the diagnostic endeavor to prevent the birth of other people who would suffer the kind of life that they endure (Raz 2004).

However, while Japanese disability movements have been extremely successful in changing the public image and the overall moral attitudes to people with disabilities, they have not been equally successful in persuading society to allocate more resources to support people with disabilities. A systematic review of the services provided to adults and children with disabilities in Israel and Japan, as well as the different evolutionary courses that disability legislation and institutional frameworks have taken, is beyond the scope of this study. Nevertheless, I contend that what seems to be greater readiness of Japanese mothers to bear less-than-perfect children rests less on extensive governmental support than on taking a different moral approach to disability.[15] Powerful ideas prevail about the far-reaching effects of mothers' nurturing on the ability of children and adults with disabilities to integrate in society. (These ideas are grounded at least in part on a specific gendered division of labor.) Still, the reader may ponder how these moral approaches to disability and the ecosystemically oriented prenatal care described here might be reconciled with Japan's long history of eugenic practices, and with a highly educationalist and competitive society. Keeping in mind that the daily experiences of raising children with disabilities in Japan deserve independent in-depth anthropological research, I suspect that these issues cannot be reconciled. Rather, Japanese mothers live in the tension between environmentalist ideas on how much nurturance matters to child health and development, and the realities of an educationalist achievement-oriented society. The mothers of children with disabilities are racked by this tension even more. Eugenics takes its toll on mothers, whether ecosystemically or genetically oriented.

The accounts of the Japanese and Israeli pregnant women and their families reveal that both are interested in maximizing the chances of having a perfectly healthy child, and both "environmentalism" and "geneticism" are theories of "quality control" and "human betterment." An important difference lies in the social organization of, and the power attributed to, nurturance—that is, in the set of expectations that mothers are faced with. Tolerance for children with special needs has at least as much to do with the gendered division of labor in society as with cultural notions of selfhood and disability.

It might not be a coincidence that the selective mode of responsibility that relies on prenatal diagnosis is more popular among middle-class Israeli and American working women than among Japanese homemakers. In fact, Rayna Rapp's work suggests that such correlation might exist. She describes "how close to the edge many parents feel when they imagine the juggling of work and family obligations should disability enter the already tight domestic economy. . . . The material pressures under which many families with two working parents find themselves and that serve as the matrix in which the decision to use prenatal testing is made" (Rapp 1999, 542).

So Japanese "environmentalism," assuming domesticated motherhood, produces somatic forms of agency that attribute much effect to the nurturing powers of mothers and rely on their willingness and *availability* to grant nurturing services. Israelis (whether doctors, pregnant women, or their part-ners) do not at all take for granted the availability and willingness of busy moth-ers for nurturing tasks. I presume Israeli mothers are "busy" in this context not only because they are expected to contribute to their families and society as productive laborers along with their mothering roles, but also because they are expected to bear more children. Thinking within a framework of existential dif-ficulties and myriad kinds of threat, maternal nurturance capacities are imag-ined as limited resources. With the limitations of nurturance and the busy life of working mothers in mind, the only form of control left is using technologies of choice.

Notions of choice and of being chosen in the context of religious-national continuity indeed loom large in traditional Jewish texts. In fact, selection and rejection are a most prominent motif throughout major parts of the book of Genesis, as a host of Jewish commentators on the Bible have pointed out (Breuer 1998, 506). God chooses Noah to survive his sinful generation. Later Abraham is chosen from among his siblings, the sons of Terah, and is instructed by God to choose Isaac and reject Ismael; and then, out of Jacob and Esau, the sons of Isaac, Jacob is chosen and Esau rejected. But in Jacob this series of selections and rejections comes to an end when all his twelve sons are chosen to succeed him, only to be chosen later (from among the gentiles) as God's nation. Jewish Bible commentators have been engaged in debates over whether one or another pro-genitor was chosen because of his righteous deeds (e.g., Nachmanides on Genesis 12:2) or due to an inherited attribute or birthright (e.g., Rabbi Yehuda Halevi in *Sefer Hakuzari* on God's choice of Abraham), as implied by the scrip-tures (e.g., the reason for choosing Noah: Genesis 7:1; Abraham: Genesis 26:5, Genesis 22:18). In any event, the progenitors' bodies in such contexts are rarely the reason for preferring them to others. Quite the contrary: Isaac is blind, Jacob is physically less able than his twin brother, Esau, a successful hunter, and Moses, the greatest leader and prophet in the Hebrew Bible, had a stammer and could only speak to his people with the help of Aaron, his elder brother. Indeed, the centrality of selection and choice as key concepts in the Jewish tradition is an important cue for interpreting the Israeli ethnography. However, this cen-trality (echoing the traditional Jewish preoccupation with righteousness) can-not easily explain the patterns emerging from the present ethnography, which unfolds around *physical* selections. The latter, argues Weiss (2002), echo the eugenic concerns of nineteenth-century Zionism and the physical selections characteristic of the military.

Local Versions of Eugenics, Militarism, and Pro-natalism

Japanese people and Jewish European Zionists at the turn of the nineteenth century were equally preoccupied with eugenic ideas as part of their nation-building efforts, as were many western countries at that time. However, unlike Europeans, the Japanese and the Jews developed their eugenic theories while constantly comparing their own physiques with that of western nationals, and their ideas of race betterment echo an innate feeling of physical inferiority. Japanese and Jews developed complexes about their ethnically marked bodies, although these complexes differed in several significant ways and inspired two different orientations to eugenic thinking that to this day resonate in the body politics of each nation as well as in each nation's style of pro-natalism.

In the Japanese case, as Rotem Kowner points out (2002), a wave of inferiority feelings on the collective and individual levels followed after the forced opening of Japan in 1854 in the midst of progressive colonization of the surrounding East Asian nations. These feelings of inferiority found expression in the physical body. In the books and articles from that period that Kowner reviews, Japanese express their disquiet with their skin color and their bowlegs, as well as myriad other features, but mostly with the *size* of their bodies. Japanese eugenicists aspired to a bigger and stronger Japanese race, and contemplated a range of eugenic strategies, as indicated in the introduction to chapter two. But they were equally concerned with preserving the "Japanese spirit" (*yamatodamashi*), as government slogans of that period indicate ("Japanese spirit, western technology" [*wacon yôsai*] is one example). In fact, cultivating a "Japanese spirit" was narrated (especially in the case of Japanese soldiers) as compensation for a smaller and weaker body.

A general educational effort was launched to persuade the Japanese people, who ate mainly rice, fish, and vegetables, to "improve" the nutritional quality of their food by consuming meat and milk products: in one symbolic historic instance, the Meiji emperor was photographed in 1871 eating a beef steak and drinking milk (Kowner 2002, 72). Yet this general effort turned a more gender-specific focus on improving women's health and education in particular. Gynocentric nonfeminist (Robertson 2002b) and ecosystemically oriented eugenics took the lead, while successive governments laid ever heavier emphasis on women's importance as the nation's child bearers and child raisers, *alongside* the importance of their productive labor (Nolte and Hastings 1991). The cult of maternal domesticity materialized only well after World War II (see the introductions to chapters two and three).

Almost a century later, Japanese prenatal care echoes a preoccupation with physical dimensions, accompanied by a fear of women's incompetent reproductive performance and the identification of a "solution" in the form of ultimate nutrition and the exercise of mental strength. The concentration on pregnant women's own bodies and health as a eugenic strategy is overwhelming. However, the case of pregnant Japanese women also reflects the flip side of the Japanese concern with body dimensions. In their case, growing "too" big represents a threat to the health of both mothers and babies. In the realm of national imagery, pregnancy may represent not only the problem of "taming" the chaotic potentials of nature but also the inherent incongruence between the desire to become "bigger" and more competent while still retaining one's Japanese national identity, which is still conceived in terms of a strong spirit endowed with a relatively "smaller" body. The politics of pregnancy body size might be a reflection of the actual transition in national body size, if "smaller" Japanese women are to become the bearers of "bigger" future generations. In any case, pregnant women seem to embody an inner contradiction that is inherent to the modern Japanese politics of national identity as it materializes in the body.

Turning now to Zionist ideas of the Jewish body, several writers have pointed out that in precisely the same historical period, the Zionist social movement went to extremes to distance itself from the iconic image of the Diaspora Jew (Almog 1997; Biale 1986; Weiss 2002). Like the Japanese national body image, the Jewish body stereotype was found wanting compared with its gentile counterpart. However, in the case of the iconic body of the Diaspora Jew, the problem was not only its size. In the minds of nineteenth-century Jewish nation builders, the Diaspora Jew was not just shrunk, deformed, and unattractive, but profoundly diseased and in need of healing (Weiss 2002, 1–4). In setting forth an image of the healthy, masculine, and vigorous *sabra*—a Jew born in Palestine (later to become Israel)—the Zionist system of body imagery "formally" and "openly" rejected the iconic body of the deformed Jew and reinvented the "new Jew" instead.[16] The attempt to "get rid" of the old Jewish body, with its "Jewish" diseases reverberates in the professional endeavors of Israeli geneticists in the second half of the twentieth century (Falk 2006).

So in both places, pro-natalism, that is, the desire to enlarge the size of the population, was colored with specific concerns about the body. While Japanese frustrations with their body centered largely on its dimensions, the Jews were dismayed by its inherent constitution, its "character." Strategies to remedy the national complex over the physical body were derived accordingly. The Japanese launched gynocentric, ecosystemically oriented eugenic policies aimed at bearing a bigger and stronger generation while retaining its Japanese-ness; the Zionists, who became engaged in inventing a "new Jew" while symbolically and practically *rejecting* major aspects that characterized Jews for two thousand years, emphasized geneticist eugenic strategies of selection.

At the beginning of the twenty-first century, Israeli body politics openly and formally rejects the diseased body by supporting postdiagnostic abortions. By contrast, ecosystemic gynocentric Japanese body politics manages postdiagnostic abortion with a secrecy and sense of shame that recalls the general shame and renunciation with which Japanese public discourse approaches World War II ideologies (even though, according to Otsubo and Bartholomew 1998, eugenic abortions and sterilizations were relatively few in Japan compared with other western countries in that period).

Significantly, these body politics and eugenic orientations inhabit two different regimes of state pro-natalism, giving rise to the particular tensions of each. In fact the data lead us to think of pro-natalism not simply in terms of "state encouragement of fertility" but as a set of tensions that surround the bearing of children (Ivry 2010). Japanese pro-natalism, shaded with its gynocentric ecosystemically oriented eugenics, tends to exert on women the long-term tensions of continuously creating the child—a burden women take so seriously that most refuse to bear more than one child. Israeli pro-natalism, with its emphasis on genetic selections and catastrophic scripts, produces a paradoxical situation in which a woman may spend much of her pregnancy—a state so desired from a pro-natalist perspective—in anxiety.

Whether societies deeply involved in armed conflicts incline more to physical selection is a question that arises. Explicit eugenic sterilization and abortion laws emerged throughout the Euro-American world, as well as in Japan, during the first decades of the twentieth century precisely when these states were involved in military conflicts (Rose 2001). Israel, in which the current law allows the abortion of a fetus with an anomaly without specifying the nature of the anomaly or any threshold of gestational age at the time of abortion, has been involved in continuous military conflict.

A host of scholars have pointed out the overwhelming centrality of the military in Israel and the militarization of Israeli society—a state where the majority of Jewish-Israeli men and women are conscripted to military service. Scholarly work of the last two decades in particular has shifted "from an analysis centered on Israel's unique status as a society that maintains democracy under conditions of protracted war and the centrality of the military, to more complex inquiries about this society as an instance of how democracy normalizes militarism" (Ben-Ari and Lomsky-Feder 1999; Ben-Ari, Rosenhek, and Maman 2001, 3; Ben-Eliezer 1998), and how militarism as a cognitive structure (Kimmerling 1993) figures in the everyday life-worlds of Israelis. The ideal body image that Weiss (2002) calls "the chosen body," the one whose quest she identifies among Israelis throughout the life cycle, emanates to a great degree from the military ideal of the strong and fit body of the combat soldier.

From Weiss's analysis, the connection between militarism and physical selection lies in the privileged and idealized status that soldiers and their bodies are accorded in a society where the military occupies a central place. Can one conclude that selective attitudes to fetuses correlate with idealized body images generated in militaristic societies? Considering the maternal–fetal relationships in the heyday of militarized Japan suggests that such a connection might not be that obvious. How can one explain the recommendation to the pregnant Japanese woman at the height of World War II to read hero stories to her fetus in order to develop his or her sense of patriotism in utero (Dingwall, Tanaka, and Minamikata 1991, 424)? Hero stories are a familiar form of socialization in militaristic societies, and telling them to an unborn baby signifies its inclusion as a part of the collective: through the assumed maternal–fetal *connection*, the collective attempts to mold the unborn baby into patriotism regardless of any "initial preconditions." Militarism, as well as forms of maternal–fetal relations under militaristic regimes, clearly take local forms.

Returning to Israeli society, the pregnant Israeli women in this study, most of whom had experienced military service, explained their decisions to undergo invasive testing not so much in military terms or values. Their explanations had much to do with preserving their marriages, with saving their lives from unbearable difficulties, and most of all with *fear*.

The kind of geneticist selectivity found in Israel, I argue, heavily depends on a continuous generation of fear of reproductive catastrophes (as well as doctors' fears of lawsuits), whether through technological illustrations of reproduction gone awry or folk practices to combat the evil eye. The imminence of catastrophe is a multilayered idea in contemporary Israeli society. Fear of a potential catastrophe is indeed an ideal substrate for militarism but cannot be reduced to it. In any case, the strong connection between pregnancy and anxiety does not simply "follow" from history; for "geneticism" to make sense, anxieties must be continuously generated through daily practices and technological illustrations.

Similarly, Japanese "environmentalism" relies on the continuous daily engagement in sense-making. One can hardly imagine Japanese "environmentalism" working so powerfully without the constant narration and practices of prenatal child raising as illustrated by imaging technologies, perpetuated in medical instructions about ultimate body maintenance, and reiterated in lay prohibitions and advice. I have tried to illuminate throughout this study precisely these daily processes of meaning-making, and the evocation of the atmosphere they generate and in which they are generated. Most important to bear in mind is that regardless of whether pregnancy suggests a risk-taking behavior—an ordeal of survival in the face of a threatening catastrophe (as is likely to happen in Israel) or a nurturing activity associated with child rearing (as is likely in Japan)—in neither case is pregnancy a matter of "expecting," with its implication of a state of waiting for the drama of the birth to come. In both cases, pregnancy is a mentally and physically demanding way of being, and often an energy-consuming project of meaning-making. Thus pregnancy is pregnant with meaning: it emerges as a key site for understanding wider dimensions of the embodiment of culture.

6

Pregnant with Meaning

Now that this study has been "brought to term," so to speak, I shall conclude by exploring what it might give birth to.

Rethinking Biomedical Systems with "Environmentalism" and "Geneticism"

The typology of "environmentalism" and "geneticism" suggests that the local biomedicines often described in medical anthropology can be understood within much broader models and can be used to decode health-related forms of behavior in cultures around the globe.[1] While Japanese and Israeli prenatal care systems are merely quite extreme cases of environmentalism and geneticism, respectively, other medical and lay regimes of pregnancy can be arranged on a paradigmatic scale stressing the importance of the "environment" at one end and the importance of "genetics" at the other. Different prenatal care models might be understood as different combinations of "environmental" and "geneticist" thinking. In fact, the global science of gestation is a diverse arena in which environmentally and genetically oriented ideas compete, challenge, and complement each other. In fact the distinctions between the "genetic" and "environmental" effects on health are becoming increasingly porous in various parts of biological research (Lock 2005). But this does not preclude local prenatal care systems' emphasis on genetic or environmental origins of health, as such emphases agree with local ethno-theories of procreation. In any event, I have not been trying to make a claim about the adequacy of the truth claims of "environmental" or "geneticist" scientists but to point out the social circumstances and consequences of each emphasis.

Cultures of Pregnancy, Local Politics, and Emotions

Throughout this study I have attempted to show how cultures of pregnancy form the conceptual and practical basis on which power structures draw to organize gestation in a way that "makes sense" to people. I was trying to convey the ongoing processes of sense-making by paying attention to two experiential loci: the physical body and the emotions. Here, I would like to point out the analytical potential in the latter.

Clearly the social arenas in which pregnancy is negotiated (whether private or professional) emerge from the ethnographies as highly charged with emotions. I suggest that examining the correlations between these emotions and the social and national nexuses of power within which they are shaped could benefit our analysis of reproductive relations. I suggest that we view the construction and management of emotions as an important aspect of reproductive politics. In proposing this analytical direction I am inspired by Abu-Lughod and Lutz, who counsel us to see emotions as both "discursive practices" (Abu-Lughod and Lutz 1990, 10) and socio-cultural constructs (Abu-Lughod and Lutz 1990, 7). As they explain, "The focus on discourse allows not only for insight into how emotion, like the discourse in which it participates, is informed by cultural themes and values, but also how it serves as an operator in a contentious field of social activity, how it affects a social field, and how it can serve as an idiom for communicating, not even necessarily about feelings. . . . Rather than seeing them as expressive vehicles, we must understand emotional discourses as *pragmatic acts* and communicative performances" (Abu-Lughod and Lutz 1990, 11; emphasis added).

In suggesting an analysis of the politics of emotions in reproductive relations, I attempt to draw attention to at least two levels of interconnected phenomena. At one level, the issue is how local reproductive political regimes assume and encourage specific emotional postures in pregnant women while drawing on cultural conceptions and national political discourses. On the other level, the question is how pregnant women "work" with the emotional postures that they are supposed to adopt "naturally."

The Israeli biomedical narration of reproductive catastrophe (as manifested in the "ultrasonic horror picture show") may serve as an example of the first level. Although this medical discourse presents itself as scientifically "objective" and detached, it fits Abu-Lughod and Lutz's definition of "emotional discourse," in the sense that it *arouses* fear in its audience, with the practical implication that patients will consume more prenatal tests. In the same way, Japanese biomedical narrations of the unborn baby as cute and dependent can be understood as "emotional discourses" that arouse nurturant sentiments in their audience, with the practical implication that patients will watch their diets, etc. Each emotional discourse indicates a set of practical implications that are correlated with national politics and the local politics of the body. In fact, I have shown here that while body politics in Israel depends on the production of emotional postures of fear, in Japan it depends on the production of emotional postures of nurturance. In each arena, therefore, biomedical practitioners try to stimulate specific emotional postures in pregnant women in order to induce the practical implications that they (the practitioners) regard as suitable. "Scientific" discourses may be particularly powerful in arousing emotion, precisely because they present themselves as so detached, thus making the emotions that they arouse in the audience seem "natural" and "innate." Put differently, emotions may appear to follow "logically" from scientific truth regimes.

On another level, pregnant women do "emotion work," in Hochschild's idiom (Hochschild 1983), while pragmatically using the feelings that they are supposed to feel: for example, Japanese women who use narratives of interconnectedness with their baby as emotional techniques to conquer the inconvenience of morning sickness and the pain of childbirth. In the same way, the strategies of detachment from bodily sensations that some pregnant Israeli women employ are also emotional techniques designed to conquer fear. At both levels emotional strategies are pragmatically used. Nevertheless, in identifying this "emotional pragmatism" I am not trying to imply the existence of a conspiracy through which pregnant women's emotions are manipulated to "serve" the local body politic—even though at times manipulations do indeed take place. Rather, I am trying to draw attention to an intricate dynamic in which biomedical practitioners and pregnant women draw on a common pool of emotional postures that are available and comprehensible in their culture, one in which biomedical practitioners are as "moved" by emotions as pregnant women. In both Japan and Israel professional discourses of reproduction are as saturated with emotion as lay discourses: Israeli ob-gyns are as emotional as their patients in showing their alarm at the idea that imperfect children might be born, while Japanese doctors are as emotional about the need to nurture unborn babies as their patients.

Identifying the emotional aspects of hegemonic discourses (whether biomedical discourses, national discourses, or others) means uncovering an important way in which these discourses speak to pregnant women as well as to medical practitioners, shaping their pragmatisms along socially endorsed routes of action. Therefore, I suggest that we might benefit from theorizing reproductive politics as being concerned not only with "disciplining bodies" but also with arousing emotions.

However, regardless of whether a local reproductive politics encourages emotional postures of nurturance or fear, a central theme in emotional reproductive discourses, whether implicit or explicit, is responsibility. Many Japanese women understand themselves literally as the makers of their babies and enact their agency through the "bodybuilding" of a nurturant body; for many Israeli women selection remains a highly meaningful form of agency. In both cases women themselves share with society generally the idea that *they* are assigned the responsibility for exercising reproductive agency in the best interests of society, their families, and themselves. Scholars like Rapp and Landsman have theorized this point by using concepts like "woman's accountability" (Rapp 1999) or "mother's guilt" (Landsman 1999). This study provides a comparative framework that further strengthens their observations by showing that reproductive responsibility remains mostly within female domains under both "environmentalism" and "geneticism," within social scripts of both bonding and catastrophe, and under both external and internal social grasps on the body.

Nevertheless, male partners play a crucial role in women's experiences of pregnancy.

Male Partners and Pregnancy

Classical anthropologists were concerned with fathers and their roles in pregnancy, birth, and child rearing as part of their more general attempts to probe theories of procreation and local concepts of kinship among the cultures they investigated (see, for example, Barnes 1961; Malinowski 1927). Modern anthropological studies of men and reproduction have only started to emerge very recently, and relatively little has been written about men as the partners of pregnant women. Typically, men as partners emerge in the literature usually in relation to special events and dramas, most of which take place in medical settings and are orchestrated by different kinds of health-care providers. Men are described as being involved in dramas of decision making, for example, whether to go for amniocentesis (Rapp 1999), in medical spectacles like ultrasound screenings (Draper 2002; Georges 1996; Sandelowski 1994), in birth education courses (Reed 2005; Sargent and Stark 1989), and in the birth event itself (Jordan 1978, 1997; Reed 2005). In other words, the very emergence of men in the scene of pregnancy is a sign that a drama is happening or is about to happen.

In this sense the medicalization of pregnancy contributes to its dramatization, "providing" more events and thus more opportunities for men to participate in pregnancy. Biotechnologies of imaging, in particular, seem to carry a special promise for men, since they are supposed to "connect" them as never before to their unborn children as reflected on the ultrasound screen. This makes ultrasonography an attractive field in which to investigate the pregnancy experiences of male partners.

However, I suggest that examining the participation of men only through the lens of technology means collaborating in the implicit assumptions that men are only "there" at grand events, thus overlooking the broader frames through which pregnancy is experienced by both sexes. My ethnography suggests that we approach questions of men's participation in pregnancy from the analytical perspective provided by *cultures of pregnancy*. From this perspective,

I suggest, it may be easier to pose questions about the conceptual opportunities and limitations on men's participation in pregnancy and its implications for men's and woman's experiences of gestation.[2] As we have seen, the relative exclusion of Japanese men from pregnancy has much to do with the dominance of the "environmental" theory of embodied bonding. Within the domains of "female monogenesis" men are understood as being far removed from pregnancy, since it does not occur in their bodies. So men are officially "exempt" from "maternity courses," medical checkups, and sometimes even from the birth event itself. They are only called to the clinic if the doctor has diagnosed a fetal abnormality—again, for a decision-making drama. Certainly some Israeli men accompany their partners to checkups and ultrasound screens quite frequently, and even participate in birth-education courses and in the delivery of their children. Nevertheless, their presence has to do with an Israeli ethos of gender equality that highlights the limitations of maternal powers of nurturance. Men's presence rather tends to complicate and sometimes add tensions to women's experiences of pregnancy, in part because their roles in the (often medicalized) situations in which they participate are unclear.

But what would happen if we shifted our focus from medicalized events to locating male partners in the everyday life of pregnancy? I suggest that an anthropology of pregnancy should explore pregnancy within a context of *relationship*, and move further to examine sexuality as it figures in local cultures of pregnancy. For this, the male experience of female gestation—almost terra incognita—needs exploration. Men's pregnancy experiences are crucial for understanding gestation, but also early parenthood: for the most part, we have only vague ideas about the process of becoming a father.

Cultures of Pregnancy and Biotechnology

As pointed out previously, a number of scholars have emphasized the power of biotechnology to *transform* both the experience of pregnancy and our fundamental ideas about reproduction. Whether amniocentesis makes pregnancy tentative (Rothman 1986) or transforms pregnant women into moral pioneers (Rapp 1999), whether ultrasound transforms fetuses into human patients with rights (Petchesky-Pollack 1987), whether assisted conceptive technologies change the ways we understand kinship, nature, and culture (Franklin 2003)—all such theorizings depict technologies as powerful agents of social change. By contrast, the cultural comparison offered here illuminates the role of socio-cultural schemes of thinking in facilitating the inculcation of certain technologies, thus introducing or even blocking them in any given socio-cultural-historical setting.

Specifically, in Israel ultrasound seems to succeed much less in transforming fetuses into humans; Israeli fetuses may remain suspended under heavy suspicion until well after birth. Likewise in Japan, prenatal diagnosis has not quite succeeded in making pregnancy more tentative. To become powerful, biotechnological images must resonate with cultural perceptions. The Japanese and Israeli ethnographies illustrate that the particular political uses of cultural images and social scripts "license" technology to assign meaning, and that it is individuals who connect or separate pregnancies using technologies, not technologies that separate or connect pregnancies in spite of individuals.

The Move from Reproducing Reproduction toward Anthropologies of Pregnancy

Through this study I sought to create an integral understanding of a complex and multifaceted phenomenon called pregnancy, not "reproduction." Pregnancy is much more than "reproduction." Webster's dictionary shows that the term "reproduction," with its overtones of "duplication" and "imitation," its Fordist connotations (to use Martin's terminology, 1991) of the repetitive mechanical processes of industrial "production," its detached, biological associations can hardly capture the meanings of "having a child"—the first definition that this same dictionary gives for "pregnant." "Pregnancy," according to Webster's, is "a state, condition, or quality of being pregnant," while "pregnant" also means "fertile, rich . . . full of meaning . . . of great importance or potential." In citing this definition, I do not mean to promote the romanticization of pregnancy. I suggest that the anthropology of reproduction—magnificent, inspiring and innovative though it is—tends to lose sight of pregnancy precisely because its focus is so much on "reproduction" to the exclusion of other perspectives.

As Rapp observes, over the past twenty years feminist concerns have pushed reproduction to the center of social theory (Rapp 2001). I am indeed fortunate to have conducted this research in an era when themes concerning reproduction are considered "legitimate" in anthropology, and I feel indebted to all those anthropologists in whose footsteps I follow. Nevertheless, I suggest that while "reproduction" has been pushed to the center, the ongoing experiences of pregnancy remain marginalized in the domain of "woman's talk."

As I pointed out in the introduction to this study, an increasing number of studies in the anthropology of reproduction focus on new, cutting-edge reproductive technologies, mainly assisted conception, and/or on reproductive dramas such as birth. This scholarly emphasis emerged even though most pregnancies around the world are still conceived without any technological assistance; in most places technologies of assisted conception are still mainly accessible only by socio-economically privileged individuals.

The high incidence of anthropological study of human reproduction in high-tech contexts can be attributed to the fact that many influential studies in the field have been carried out by feminist sociologists and anthropologists as forms of resistance. Through their studies, feminist scholars have protested against the exclusion, division, subversion, and silencing of women's bodies, women's power, and women's forms of experiential knowledge. These scholars made public the anguish of women caught up in the power relations that surround reproductive social arrangements. However, following the lead of Lila Abu-Lughod, who urges us to use resistance as a diagnostic of power (Abu-Lughod 1990), I ask what this form of resistance can tell us about the registers of power within which it is formulated. What is the implicit statement that anthropologists of reproduction, including myself, make when they emphasize the technological aspects of reproduction?

I suggest that anthropologists do at least three things. First, we highlight reproductive dramas rather than attend to ongoing processes. Secondly, we highlight the representation of the reproductive body through technological devices rather than the embodied experience of gestating. Thirdly, we highlight the power of technology over cultures of pregnancy. In a way, anthropologies of the "cutting edge" cut out the huge and diverse arena of human experience that lies outside technological domains. When we highlight the power of technology, do we, as anthropologists, collaborate with the hegemonic structures of power? Do we duplicate (reproduce) these same structures when we insist that technologies dominate and shape our experiences to such high degrees? Do we in fact help to promote the hegemonies of these privileged systems of knowledge in the very act of fervently criticizing them? Or do we perhaps need this focus on technology to push ourselves into the center of social theory as researchers in the "truly serious" domains of scientific knowledge?

At a point where the anthropology of reproduction has already acquired a place of honor in the social sciences, I believe we can afford to bring pregnancies back into the analysis of "reproduction," emotions into the analysis of reproductive politics, and—most importantly—continue to bring women and men into both.

NOTES

INTRODUCTION

1. The names of all informants cited in this study have been changed.

2. Biopower is a concept coined by Michel Foucault to designate a modality of power bent on fostering life, which emerged, he claims, during the seventeenth century. This new mode of power gradually substituted the ancient sovereign mode epitomized by the sovereign's right to decide matters of life and death. By biopower, Foucault means an interrelated array of techniques, technologies, procedures, and institutions, as well as entire bodies of knowledge and discourses, used by modern nation-states to discipline and subjugate individual bodies and to maximize the regulation, monitoring, and control of populations. For a detailed explanation of Foucault's notion of biopower see part five of the first volume of his *The History of Sexuality* (1978).

3. I use the concept of life-world in Schutz and Luckman's sense (1973). These scholars define life-world as "a world which is for me taken for granted and self-evidently 'real.'. . . the unexamined ground of everything given in my experience, as it were the taken-for-granted frame in which all the problems which I must overcome are placed . . . my life-world is not my private world but, rather, is intersubjective; the fundamental structure of its reality is that it is shared by us." (Schutz and Luckman 1973, 4)

CHAPTER 1   A RISKY BUSINESS

1. Israelis are familiar with the political rhetoric communicated in the Israeli media that explicitly points to fertility as a site where the demographic struggle between Israeli Jews and Palestinians is being played out. For example, the late Palestinian leader Yasser Arafat was often quoted in the Israeli media as saying that the best weapon of the Palestinian people is the womb of the Palestinian woman. Examples of this discourse are discussed in Rhoda Kanaaneh's ethnography (2002) of Palestinian women's birth strategies in the north of Israel. The cover of her book, entitled *Birthing the Nation*, illustrates this point, as it depicts a rash of people being born from a Palestinian woman's womb.

2. For a discussion of abortion debates in the Knesset, see Sered (2000).

3. The privileged status of "IDF-disabled persons" in the eyes of decision makers is reflected in the special benefits granted to them under Israeli law. The legal orientation in fact differentiates disabled people according to their relationship to the nation-state through participation in the military, and silences other categories (such

as their ability to live a meaningful life, enrich human experience, etc.) that have voices in the United States. Other disability movements do exist in Israel, but operating within the above set of binary categories (IDF-/non-IDF-disabled person), they are hard-pressed to elicit attention in the public sphere. In 2002 a group of disabled people embarked on a "strike of the disabled" and did win a fair amount of public attention through the media; however, their public concerns focused on government budgetary issues and not on changing Israeli social perceptions of disabled people and deconstructing the binary categorization code.

4. Roy Duster provides a list of the ethnic distribution of disease in appendix C of his book (Duster 2003, 195). The list of "Japanese diseases" amounts to three conditions; the list of "Jewish diseases" that follows has forty-seven items.

5. An equally important cultural perspective to deconstruct is the gap between physical conditions and their cultural definition and management as "disabilities." Such themes arise when I discuss Japanese attitudes to children with Down's syndrome, but a thorough examination of this subject is beyond the scope of this book.

6. Interestingly the connection between female reproduction and hysteria exists in the word "hysteria" itself, which is formed from the root *hyster* or "womb." The irrationality that is depicted by hysteria was associated with the idea of a "wandering womb."

7. For a discussion of the state of people with disabilities in the socio-cultural context of Israeli society, see Weiss (2002, 88–91).

8. In the same spirit, Professor Glazman, who gave a lecture on "the development of life" at another pregnancy event in May 1999, used the Hebrew military term *kaplad* (acronym for *kova plada*, steel helmet) to describe the acrosome, the top part of the sperm cell's head. He then proceeded to portray the sperm's journey in the cervix as the advance of a "sperm platoon" in "the killing fields" [*sde ketel*]. Such images echo Martin's famous essay about the representation of male and female gametes in gynecology textbooks. Martin shows how scientific texts replicates gender roles in their descriptions (Martin 1991). The gender relations in Glazman's version of the story suggest explicitly a conflict between egg and sperm: this corresponds to neither the romantic representation of an egg as a passive princess and the sperm as her beloved knight, nor the image of the egg as a femme fatale seducing the sperm. It is more reminiscent of Martin's account of "the body at war" in the context of AIDS (Martin 1994). But like Navon, Glazman managed to make his audience laugh. The images that he elicited, however, are part of army jargon that also permeates popular Israeli culture in areas not directly associated with the military.

9. This attitude contrasts with those of American genetic counselors described by Rapp (1999) who would withdraw and not try to convince patients who gave religious reasons for their refusals.

10. This echoes Rapp's discussion of the scientific illiteracy of patients from disadvantaged socio-economic backgrounds (Rapp 1999).

11. Zaken's observation is confirmed by Weiss's account of the abandonment of newborn babies in Israel (Weiss 1994).

12. Kahn's narrative echoes Rothman's observation that technological progress renders past "choices" practically irrelevant (Rothman 1984).

13. Practitioners who refused to be quoted, even under a pseudonym, told me that they had a number of cases of high-ranking ultra-orthodox patients, who refused to undergo screening tests in the earlier stages of pregnancy, and showed up in later

stages, after a severe fetal abnormality was diagnosed, and demanded late abortions. The doctors explained that these patients were in particular alarmed by the damage that the birth of an affected child would cause the family's reputation and managed to find a rabbi who was willing to give them his approval.

CHAPTER 2   THE TWOFOLD STRUCTURE
OF JAPANESE PRENATAL CARE

1. During the Tokugawa era (1600–1868), following several conflicts with Christian missionaries, the shogunate (military regime) enacted a foreign relations policy known as *sakoku* (locked country), under which foreigners would enter or Japanese would leave the country on pain of death. (An exception was Dutch merchants, who were not suspected of missionary activity; they were allowed to reside in strictly demarcated areas around the ports of Hiroshima and Nagasaki.)

2. The category of "unfit" included concepts such as *furyô* and *retsujaku naru soshitsu*—inferior disposition, or inferior quality; *ijô*—abnormal; *akushitsu naru iden*—hereditary bad quality. These concepts belong to a eugenic thinking in which biology and culture conflate. "Unfit," writes Robertson, "was an ambiguous term that included alcoholics, "lepers," the mentally ill, the criminal, the physically disabled, and the sexually alternative among other categories of people" (Robertson 2002b, 196).

3. According to the statistics of the Japanese Ministry of Health and Welfare, the rate of abortions carried out for eugenic reasons decreased from 0.17 percent of all induced abortions in 1956 to 0.02 percent in 1995 (Professor Anesaki Masahira, Nihon University, personal communication).

4. One key ob-gyn informant suggested that Japanese doctors' preoccupation with monitoring weight gain was inspired by a famous article by an American ob-gyn published in 1979 (Naeye 1979).

5. The international medical literature ponders whether short stature may be considered an independent risk factor for arrested birth due to "cephalo-pelvic disproportion"—a baby that is too big to pass through the woman's pelvic outlet. First, the literature shows a correlation between "short" maternal stature and the incidence of emergency cesareans due to a prolonged second stage of labor in a diversity of populations including New Zealand, Tanzania, and Denmark. A range of maternal heights is calculated—from 140 cm for New Zealander women (McGuinness and Trivedi 1999) through 154 cm for Nigerian women (Brabin, L., Verhoeff, and Brabin, B. J. 2002) and 156 cm for Danish women (Kappel et al. 1987) to 160 cm for Zimbabwean women (Tsu 1992)—where the risk involved in shortness increases according to diverse criteria (the risk doubles or triples as against that of women taller than the threshold). Second, in some cases the woman's "short stature" might be associated with other health factors such as calcium deficiency (Brabin, L., Verhoeff, and Brabin, B. J. 2002). Third, these studies are based on a retrospective analysis of patients who underwent cesarean sections, assuming that the birth was not "progressing" because of "cephalo-pelvic disproportion," and not on measurements of the pelvic outlet versus the baby's size in women of different statures.

6. If we consider the loathing of laziness in doctors' discourse about pregnant women from the perspective of Garon's concept of "social management" (1997), we must discuss the role of medical doctors as cooperative agents in state intrusions into social values and morality in modern Japan. Nevertheless, any discussion of social management should include women's perspectives. It should be borne in mind that, while the

state has proved successful in convincing women and their caretakers of the importance of their roles as wives and mothers (as evident in the medical discourse on pregnancy), it has been very unsuccessful in persuading women to bear more children. A full discussion of social management in the context of pregnancy is beyond the scope of this book.

7. In many countries in the postindustrial world, some of the rise in premature birth clearly has to do with growing numbers of multifetal pregnancies, which are increasing due to a rise in the use of assisted conceptive technologies such as IVF. However, in Japan, where assisted conception is not subsidized by the government, it becomes a health service that few can afford, so multifetal pregnancies due to assisted conception contribute relatively little to the rate of premature births in Japan.

8. In Japan, the positioning of the woman's *body* on the obstetrical chair is arranged so as to minimize the "shameful" aspects of the vaginal examination. Usually a curtain hangs over the chair separating the woman's upper body from the lower part, where the examination is being performed. So while the woman's upper body dwells in a kind of twilight, her lower body is illuminated in bright light. Japanese doctors claimed that this helped them get a clearer view of the "color of the cervix" (which some of them mentioned), thus increasing the diagnostic value of the vaginal examination.

9. According to an internal report by the Japanese Ministry of Health and Welfare, between 1955 and 1998 the number of abortions due to inherited genetic disorders in the pregnant woman herself or in her relatives dropped from 1,960 (0.17 percent of all abortions) in 1956, to 556 in 1963 (0.05 percent of all abortions) and then fell to 81 abortions in 1995 (0.02 percent of all abortions), just before the Maternal Body Protection Law was enacted in 1996 (personal communication from Professor Anesaki Masahira of Nihon University). The percentage of eugenic abortions might be even lower if we consider Hardacre's cautionary remark that during the early postwar years the actual rate of abortion was probably double the rate formally reported (Hardacre 1997). By comparison, according to the statistical report released in 2007 by the Israeli Ministry of Health, from 2000 to 2007 the overall number of abortions performed on the grounds of fetal anomaly ranged between 3210 and 3511 (between 15.8 percent and 17.7 percent of all abortions). An average of 200 late abortions (after the twenty-third week of gestation) was approved each year by a special committee. Of these, 79 percent that took place in 2000, and 89 percent that took place in 2007, were due to fetal disabilities. Late abortions amount to 1 percent of all abortions in Israel (Bureau of Information and Computing, Israel Ministry of Health, November 2008). The number of eugenic abortions in Japan never reached Israeli proportions even when eugenic abortions were legal. In considering the above numbers, recall that in 1997 Japan's population (125 million) was more than twenty times that of Israel (7 million). The numbers suggest that the eugenic clauses in the Japanese law during the war and in the postwar period do not necessarily reflect wider public opinion about selective abortions. An in-depth consideration of this matter is beyond the scope of this study.

10. This use of words recalls Lock's account of a Japanese internist who told a family that their son was quite brain-dead (*hobo nôshi*) (Lock 2000, 254).

11. For detailed analysis of the cultural and political forces that are at play in the emergence of the cult of *mizuko*, see Hardacre 1997 and LaFleur 1992.

12. Lock's account of a twenty-eight-year-old woman who gave birth to a baby with Down's syndrome is of special importance here (Lock 1998). Lock describes how her

informant's husband "has suggested that Kenji's problem may have resulted from something his wife did during pregnancy. Such an attitude is common in Japan. . . . Yamada-san herself has gone over her memories of nine months before the birth of her son, for she too is fearful that her behavior may have influenced the fate of her child" (Lock 1998, 212).

CHAPTER 3   THE PATH OF BONDING

1. Root and Browner similarly note that pregnancy "offers multiple opportunities for biomedical and other surveillance to be experienced" (Root and Browner 2001, 206).

2. Under Japanese law, women take maternity leave when they enter their eighth month of pregnancy. Therefore most working women spend some weeks at home before the birth.

3. In the same vein, being busy is emphasized in respect of new mothers: whereas new Israeli fathers often depict their wives as "tired," new Japanese fathers often say that their wives are "busy" (with the baby).

4. Uchino makes sure to "move her body." Unlike jerky movements, which are considered dangerous to pregnant women, physical activities such as walking and swimming are highly recommended. This makes it clear that the problem with jerking is not the movement itself but the agent that causes the movement. When the agent is a "responsible" woman who is adjusting physical activities to her pregnancy and monitoring them, movement is perceived as contributing to good health.

5. Classic Japanese literature is known for its genres of personal diaries, beginning with well-known medieval diaries. Interestingly, these early literary masterpieces, which are dedicated to detailed descriptions of the material world, were written mostly by female courtesans at the emperor's court.

6. Since four weeks are counted as a month, a forty-week gestation period is counted as ten months.

7. An onomatopoeic word describing floating on water

8. An onomatopoeic word describing knocking at a door.

9. In their analysis of Japanese pregnancy guides published during the 1980s, Dingwall, Tanaka, and Minamikata point out that they depict women as subordinate to their doctors. They observe that this line of illustrations depicts doctors as elderly men giving lectures to women on the development of the embryo, while the woman takes a submissive position: "With her head turned and eyes cast down . . . [she] does not meet his gaze" (Dingwall, Tanaka, and Minamikata 1991, 434–435). Interestingly, a wide range of guides published during the later 1990s tends to disguise power relations by conveying a growing amount of medical knowledge and medical directions as being spoken by the unborn baby.

10. The discussion about authoritative knowledge in the anthropology of reproduction initiated by Jordan (1978) relates to the opposition and inconsistencies between the experiential knowledge that women have of their bodies and scientific knowledge. But the Japanese style of assigning authority to the baby presents a new form of staging authoritative knowledge.

11. Onomatopoeic expression describing floating on water.

12. Keeping the umbilical cord seems to be rare worldwide. The wealth of ethnographic studies that focus on the treatment of the afterbirth reveals that in most places the placenta is buried together with the whole umbilical cord.

13. When I tell these stories to Israeli mothers, they always wonder why these couples could not have hired the services of a babysitter. However, babysitters are extremely rare in Japan precisely because of the dominant theories that see the mother as the only person suitable to provide care to a baby. Caring for a baby is acknowledged as a demanding physical and mental role, and care providers who are not mothers should be highly qualified people. While care providers in Israeli daycare centers are usually poorly paid high school graduates whose job is rated of low status, teachers in daycare centers in Japan are well-paid university graduates enjoying the status of *sensei* (Ben-Ari 1997, 4). Nevertheless, mothers are reluctant to send their children to these institutions because, according to bonding theories, a mother may ideally share the role of caring with no one. As Eri-san put it, "I cannot trust a stranger to open her heart to my child."

14. Studies actually show that female labor participation decreased in the 1990s and early twenty-first century, from 50.2 percent in 1994 to 48.3 in 2004. The tendency for women to work in part-time jobs also continued, and there has actually been an increase in their concentration in such low-paid jobs, with the wage gap between full-time and part-time work further widening (Usui 2005, 58). In fact, studies also show that the majority of husbands still hope that their wives will stop working when a child is born and go back to work once the child is older (personal communication, Ofra Goldstein-Gidoni).

15. As Amy Borovoy's (2005) work poignantly shows, women can extend very similar nurturant behaviours to husbands as well. Moreover, they tend to blame themselves for the failures of the latter, just as they take responsibility for the success or failure of their children.

CHAPTER 4   THE PATH OF AMBIGUITY

1. The Conscription Law 1959 provides for the exemption of women—and not men—on the grounds of religious belief, marriage, pregnancy, or motherhood. This is not to say that Jewish men may never be exempted from army service on various grounds, including religious ones and reasons of pacifism. Many have, in fact, attained exemption from military service on these and other grounds over the years and to this very day. Ultra-religious men who proclaim that Torah study is their only occupation [*torato umanuto*] are one group that have stood at the focus of public debates. The Tal Law of 2002 provides for complex arrangements regarding the military service of ultra-orthodox men.

2. According to Israeli law, a woman who works full time is entitled to forty hours of absence from her work throughout pregnancy for medical examinations and routine pregnancy tests.

3. This does not hold for classes for the ultra-orthodox, in which it is assumed that only women will participate. Also, I have not examined the special courses given to Russian-speaking and Ethiopian immigrants, some of which might also be separate for women. However, I have seen some immigrant couples participating in the Hebrew courses mentioned above.

4. Similarly, Browner and Press note that "In the United States today, prenatal care is about getting and giving information" (Browner and Press 1997, 116).

5. According to health ministry recommendations, any woman with triple-test results higher than 1:350 should be referred for amniocentesis, regardless of her age. The

reason for choosing this figure is that the statistical rate of Down's syndrome babies in women over thirty-five is 1:400. Therefore, when the risk of bearing a Down's syndrome baby according to the triple test equals that of women over thirty-five, whose tests are subsidized, the woman concerned is automatically referred for amniocentesis as well. That the risk of losing the fetus is higher than 1:400 does not enter the health ministry's considerations.

6. Elinor's narratives remind one of the descriptions of genetic counsellors explaining the meaning of statistics in Rapp's account of amniocentesis in America (Rapp 1999).

7. This echoes the ambiguous status of the fetus in Jewish Halacha, as shown in Ir-Shai 2007.

8. In the Israeli case, the use of Shiatsu demonstrates the understanding of pain as an undesirable sensation that one has to get rid of. Interestingly, while Japanese practitioners of Shiatsu use pain to heal the patient (they locate painful points and push them to unblock energy blockages), in Israel Shiatsu is often used to ease pain.

CHAPTER 5   JUXTAPOSITIONS

1. Adelson argues, in her *Being Alive Well*, that in contrast to western biomedical schemes of thinking, the Cree Indians have a concept of health, not of non-illness (Adelson 2000).

2. This echoes the observations of Ben-Ari and others about Japanese people's refusal to designate "bad intentions" or initial bad character to children: if children misbehave it must be due to a misunderstanding. For examples, see Ben-Ari 1997, 135–136; Singleton 1989, 8–15.

3. Smith calls Japanese society as a whole "the perfectible society," claiming that perfectibility through hard work is a paradigmatic Japanese pattern of thinking (Smith 1983, 106–136).

4. "Environmentalism" and "geneticism" can be understood as the extension of "nurture" and "nature," respectively, back into gestation, and they may also call to mind the debates prevalent in the 1950s on the role of (social) environment versus heredity in a person's intellectual skills and social position. Here these concepts are used in the same sense as in the narratives of Japanese and Israeli doctors and pregnant women, that is, in the context of theories about gestation. Whereas in the environment–heredity and nature–nurture debates, environment and nurturing stand for "postpartum" conditions such as the socioeconomic environment into which a person is born and the educational opportunities he or she is given, in this study "environmentalism" and "geneticism" are both seen as informing medical and lay theories of the "prenatal stage," which center on the *physical body.*

5. In a 1998 working paper of the Israeli Association of Obstetricians and Gynaecologists, the number of returned embryos for women under thirty-five is three. For women over thirty-five and for those who have undergone three unsuccessful IVF treatments the number is unspecified. The paper simply says that "it is possible to return more." The paper states that more embryos can be returned in any cycle of treatment (even in first cycles) if the couple requests this. Since the majority of IVF patients undergo more than three IVF treatments, in practice in most cases the number of returned embryos is much higher than three.

6. In a way, Israel has been locked in this cycle of quantity versus "quality" since the early days of the state. Although birth has been encouraged in general, it was always

"the wrong" populations that were fruitful and multiplied, either Mizrahi Jews or ultra-orthodox communities. The "Zionist" population was never as enthusiastic as the state might have wanted.

7. Exploring the psychological logic of Japanese interactions, Doi suggests that dependence [amae] is a key concept in Japanese culture (Doi 1973). Again, this key concept is all about relationships, not individuals. Doi claims that amae is not only a key to understanding the psychology of Japanese individuals: society as a whole is organized according to the principle of amae. He explains the logic of dependence through the central role that the mother–child relationship plays as a model for human interactions that are far removed from the home and from the family of blood relatives.

8. Hamaguchi (1985) points out the lack of an appropriate understanding of contextualization as the methodological obstacle that researchers of Japanese culture tend to be confronted with. Even a "contextual" attitude to Japanese society, argues Hamaguchi, is not contextual "enough" and cannot completely "encompass the emics inherent to Japan" (Hamaguchi 1985, 295). To do that, one should refrain from analyzing individuals within contexts. Instead one should analyze "contextuals," defined as "the 'man-in-his-nexus'" (ibid., 305) within his contextual relationships. In fact he proposes that the basic unit for analysis should be the aidagara, which he defines as containing "not only contextuals themselves but also the connections among them" (ibid., 317). Hamaguchi calls his methodology "methodological contextualism" (ibid., 318).

9. The tentative status of the fetus clearly emerges from the mishnah in Oahlot 7:6: "If a woman was in hard travail, the fetus must be cut up while it is in the womb and brought out member by member, since her life has priority over his [the fetus's] life, but once his head has appeared, it may not be touched, since the claim of one life cannot override the claim of another life." Hashiloni-Dolev (2006) uses the first part of this ruling to illuminate what she calls the nonstatus of fetuses in Jewish doctrine, and she contrasts it with the Catholic perception of "life" from the moment of conception (see also Hashiloni-Dolev 2007). In the Mishnaic text, birth clearly figures as the turning point in the status of the fetus (again, making the whole process of gestation only tentatively natal). To complement these observations I wish to draw attention to this text being an extremely vivid and gruesome sketch of a reproductive catastrophe happening, complete with practical directions as to how to handle it.

10. According to Maimonides's explanation, a fetus comes under the category of "pursuer" [rodef]; its life should not be spared, in the context of a doctrine whereby the effort to save a human life supersedes all the Torah's commandments, both "Do" and "Do not do" (the only exceptions are the "Do not do" commandments: idolatry, murder, and forbidden sexual relations).

11. For a thorough analysis of fetal status in Jewish law in the context of rabbinic rulings on abortions, see Ir-Shai 2007.

12. Although apparently abortion debates exist in Japan (one can find descriptions of such debates in Hardacre 1997, Norgren 2001, and others), LaFleur notes that "in today's Japan, in spite of problems, the abortion issue does not polarize society" (LaFleur 1992, xiii).

13. For a thorough description and analysis of the politics of Buddhist rituals to console the spirits of aborted fetuses [mizuko kuyô], see Hardacre (1997).

14. See also Weiss's (1994) analysis of the relations between Israeli parents and their physically impaired children during the mid-1980s before the PND boom. Also, the notion of limited powers of nurturance that I point out here in the context of Israeli-Jewish

pregnant women at the turn of the century should be distinguished from those described by Nancy Scheper-Hughes (1992), in which the cultural factors and economic pressures were different.

15. To give one example, while Israeli families that raise a child with Down's syndrome are eligible for a disability stipend paid by the national health insurance, in Japan such families are not entitled to such a stipend. Eligibility is granted on the basis of a categorization of disabilities according to the degree of mobility, which for people with Down's is usually not a problem.

16. In the second half of the twentieth century, the word *sabra*, Hebrew for prickly pear, became the epithet for a Jew born in Israel. The allusion is to a tenacious, thorny desert plant with a thick peel that conceals a sweet, softer interior, that is, rough and masculine on the outside but delicate and sensitive on the inside,

CHAPTER 6   PREGNANT WITH MEANING

1. It might be tempting to substitute the "geneticism-environmetalism" terminology with "nature-nurture." Yet such substitution requires taking into consideration the multiple meanings of "nature" and "nurture" in the context of discussions in different disciplines and social and historical contexts that are too numerous to elaborate here.

2. The work of classical anthropologists on the ritual of couvade, whereby men claim ownership of the baby, may potentially contribute greatly to the analysis of men's position in relation to their wives' pregnancies, as Richard Reed (2005) clearly shows in his study of men's experiences of birth.

BIBLIOGRAPHY

Abramovich, H., G. Ohel, M. Etinger, V. Insler, Y. Itskovitch, Y. Bokovsky, Y. Bait, R. Becher, Sh. Blas, G. Ben-Baruch, M. Ben-Ami, Z. Ben-Refael, Y. Barkan, A. Golan, M. Glazerman, M. Glasner, Y. Dor, Y. Diamant, Sh. Zohar, Ch. Zakut, Z. Hagai, B. Hen, Ch. Yafe, M. Katz, N. Laufer, Ch. Levavi, Y. Lesing, N. Mazor, A. Melvitzki, Sh. Mashiah, Sh. Segal, A. Samuelov, M. Fisher, A. Shalev, and M. Shtark. 2000. *Niyar Emda* 6: Nihul Ma'akav Herayon Besikun Namuch [Working Paper No. 6: Management of a Low-Risk Pregnancy]: The Israeli Association of Obstetrics and Gynecology.

Abu-Lughod, L. 1990. "The Romance of Resistance: Tracing Transformations of Power through Bedouin Women." *American Ethnologist* 17 (1): 41–55.

Abu-Lughod, L., and C. A. Lutz. 1990. "Introduction: Emotion, Discourse, and the Politics of Everyday Life." In *Language and the Politics of Emotion*, eds. C. A. Lutz and L. Abu-Lughod, 1–23. Cambridge: Cambridge University Press.

Adelson, N. 2000. *Being Alive Well: Health and the Politics of Cree Well-Being.* Toronto and Buffalo: University of Toronto Press.

Allison, A. 1991. "Japanese Mothers and Obentôs: The Lunch-Box as Ideological State Apparatus." *Anthropological Quarterly* 64 (4): 195–208.

Almog, O. 1997. *Hatsabar-Dyokan* [The Sabra: A Portrait]. Tel Aviv: Am Oved.

Amanuma, K. 1987. *Gambari No Kôzô: Nihonjin No Kôdô Genri* [The Structure of Gambaru: A Principal of Japanese Behavior]. Tokyo: Yoshikawa Kobunkan.

Amir, D. 1995. "Achrait, Mechuyevet, Unevona: Kinun Nashiyut Yisraelit Beva'adot Lehafsakat Herayon" [Responsible, Committed and Wise: The Establishment of Israeli Femininity in Committees to Terminate Pregnancy]. *Teoria VeBikoret* 7:247–254.

Araki, H. 1973. *Nihonjin No Kôdôyôshiki* [Japanese Patterns of Action]. Tokyo: Kodansha.

Arditti, R. R. Klein, and S. Minden, eds. 1984. *Test-Tube Women: What Future for Motherhood?* London and Boston: Pandora Press.

Asahi Shinbun. 1996. *"Ijônara Chûzetsu" Zôka No Yôsô* ["If There Is an Anomaly I Will Do an Abortion": Post-Diagnostic Abortions are on the Rise]. May 1, p. 21.

———. 1997a. *Onaka Ni Shôgaiji? Anata Nara* [A Handicap in Your Belly? What Would You Do?]. December 16, p. 19.

———. 1997b. *Shusseimae Shindan-Inochi Erabimasuka?* [Prenatal Diagnosis—Would You Choose a Life (a Baby?)]. December 17, p. 21.

Azmon, Y., and D. N. Izraeli. 1993. "Introduction: Women in Israel—A Sociological Overview." In *Women in Israel*, ed. Y. Azmon and D. N. Izraeli, 1–21. Studies in Israeli Society 6. New Brunswick, NJ: Transaction Publishers.

Bachnik, J. M. 1992. "Kejime: Indexing Self and Social Life in Japan." In *Japanese Sense of Self*, ed. N. R. Rosenberger, 152–172. Cambridge: Cambridge University Press.

Bachnik, J. M., and C. J. Quinn, Jr., eds. 1994. *Situated Meaning: Inside and Outside in Japanese Self, Society, and Language.* Princeton, NJ: Princeton University Press.

Barnes, B., and D. Bloor. 1982. "Relativism, Rationalism, and the Sociology of Knowledge." In *Rationality and Relativism*, ed. M. Hollis and S. Lukes. Cambridge, MA: MIT Press.

Barnes, J. A. 1961. "Physical and Social Kinship." *Philosophy of Science* 28 (3): 296–299.

Baroon. 1998. *Ninshin, Shussan Daizenka* [The Encyclopedia of Pregnancy and Birth]. Tokyo: Shufu no Tomo Seikatsu Shiriizu.

Becker, G. 2000. *The Elusive Embryo: How Women and Men Approach New Reproductive Technologies*. Berkeley, Los Angeles, London: University of California Press.

Ben-Ari, E. 1990. "A Bureaucrat in Every Japanese Kitchen?" *Administration and Society* 21 (4): 472–492.

———. 1997. *Body Projects in Japanese Childcare: Culture and Emotions in a Preschool*. London: Curzon Press.

Ben-Ari, E., and E. Lomsky-Feder. 1999. "Introductory Essay: Cultural Constructions of War and the Military in Israel." In *The Military and Militarism in Israeli Society*, ed. E. Lomsky-Feder and E. Ben-Ari, 1–34. Albany, NY: State University of New York Press.

Ben-Ari, E., Z. Rosenhek, and D. Maman. 2001. "Introduction: Military, State and Society in Israel: An Introductory Essay." In *Military, State, and Society in Israel*, ed. D. Maman, E. Ben-Ari, and Z. Rosenhek, 1–39. New Brunswick and London: Transaction Publishers.

Ben-Eliezer, U. 1998. *The Making of Israeli Militarism*. Bloomington: Indiana University Press.

Ber, A., and T. Rosin. 1998. *Hamadrich Hayisraeli Leherayon Veleida* [The Israeli Guide for Pregnancy and Birth]. Tel-Aviv: Zmora Bitan.

Berkovitch, N. 1997. "Motherhood as a National Mission: The Construction of Womanhood in the Legal Discourse in Israel." *Women's Studies International Forum* 20 (5–6): 605–619.

Bernstein, D., ed. 1992. *Pioneers and Homemakers: Jewish Women in Pre-State Israel*. Albany, NY: State University of New York Press.

Bernstein, G. L. 1991. "Introduction." In *Recreating Japanese Women, 1600–1945*, ed. G. L. Bernstein, 1–16. Berkeley: University of California Press.

Biale, D. 1986. *Power and Powerlessness in Jewish History*. New York: Shocken Books.

Bird-David, N. 1996. "Hunter-Gatherer Research and Cultural Diversity." In *Cultural Diversity among Twentieth-Century Foragers: An African Perspective*, ed. S. Kent, 297–304. Cambridge and New York: Cambridge University Press.

Birenbaum-Carmeli, D. 2004. "'Cheaper than a Newcomer': On the Political Economy of IVF in Israel." *The Sociology of Health and Illness* 26 (7): 897–924.

Birenbaum-Carmeli, D., Y. S. Carmeli, and R. F. Casper. 1995. "Discrimination against Men in Infertility Treatment." *The Journal of Reproductive Medicine* 40 (8): 590–594.

Birenbaum-Carmeli, D., Y. S. Carmeli, Y. Madjar, and R. Wessenberg. 2001. "Hegemony and Homogeneity: Donor Choices of Israeli Recipients of Donor Insemination." *Material Culture* 7 (1): 73–95.

Bonne-Tamir, B. and A. Adam. 1992. *Genetic Diversity among Jews*. New York: Oxford University Press.

Borovoy, A. 2001. "Not 'A Doll's House': Public Uses of Domesticity in Japan." *U.S.-Japan Women's Journal*, English Supplement (20–21): 83–124.

——— 2005. *The Too Good Wife: Alcohol, Codependency, and the Politics of Nurturance in Postwar Japan*. Berkeley, Los Angeles, London: University of California Press.

Brabin, L., F. Verhoeff, and B. J. Brabin. 2002. "Maternal Height, Birthweight, and Cephalo Pelvic Disproportion in Urban Nigeria and Rural Malawi." *Acta Obstetricia et Gynecologica Scandinavica* 81 (6): 502–507.

Breuer, M. 1998. *Pirqe Bereshit II Bereshit 18–50* [Chapters from Genesis II Genesis 18–50]. Alon Shevut: Tevunot Press.

Browner, C. H., and N. A. Press. 1995. "The Normalization of Prenatal Diagnostic Screening." In *Conceiving the New World Order: The Global Politics of Reproduction*, ed. F. D. Ginsburg and R. Rapp, 307–322. Berkeley: University of California Press.

Browner, C. H., and N. Press. 1997. "The Production of Authoritative Knowledge in American Prenatal Care." In *Childbirth and Authoritative Knowledge: Cross-Cultural Perspectives*, ed. R. Davis-Floyd and C. F. Sargent, 113–131. Berkeley: University of California Press.

Carmeli, Y. S., and D. Birenbaum-Carmeli. 1994. "The Predicament of Masculinity: Towards Understanding the Male's Experience of Infertility Treatments." *Sex Roles* 30 (9–10): 663–677.

Coleman, S. 1983. *Family Planning in Japanese Society*. Princeton, NJ: Princeton University Press.

Cordero-Fiedler, D. 1996. "Authoritative Knowledge and Birth Territories in Contemporary Japan." *Medical Anthropology Quarterly* 10 (2): 195–212.

Corea, G. 1985. *Man-Made Women: How New Reproductive Technologies Affect Women*. London: Hutchinson.

———. 1986. *The Mother Machine: Reproductive Technologies from Artificial Insemination to Artificial Wombs*. New York: Harper & Row.

Cromer, G. 2006. "Analogies to Terror: The Construction of Social Problems in Israel during the Intifada Al Aqsa." *Terrorism and Political Violence* 18 (3): 389–398

Cunningham, F. G., and J. W.Williams. 1997. *Williams Obstetrics*. Stamford, CT: Appleton & Lange.

Daston, L. 1995. "The Moral Economy of Science." *Osiris* 10:2–24.

Davidov, B., B. Goldman, E. Akstein, G. Bankai, C. Legum, I. Dar, Y. Romem, A. Amiel, H. Cohen, G. Bach, Z. Appelman, and M. Shohat. 1994. "Prenatal Testing for Down's Syndrome in the Jewish and Non-Jewish Population in Israel." *Israeli Journal of Medical Science* 30:629–633.

Davidovich, N., and S. Shvarts. 2004. "Health and Hegemony: Preventive Medicine, Immigrants and the Israeli Melting Pot." *Israel Studies* 9 (2): 150–179.

Davies, J. 1999. *Din Upsika Bamishpat Harefui: Betosefet Hebetim Refui'im Umishpatiim Begenicologia Vemeyaldut* [Medicolegal Case Law in Obstetrics and Gynecology]. Jerusalem: Avi Law Books.

Davis-Floyd, R. 1992. *Birth as an American Rite of Passage*. Berkeley: University of California Press.

———. 1994. "The Technocratic Body: American Childbirth as Cultural Expression." *Social Science and Medicine* 38 (8): 1125–1140.

Davis-Floyd, R., and E. Davis. 1997. "Intuition as Authoritative Knowledge in Midwifery and Homebirth." In *Childbirth and Authoritative Knowledge: Cross-Cultural Perspectives*, ed. R. Davis-Floyd and C. F. Sargent, 315–349. Berkeley: University of California Press.

Davis-Floyd, R., and J. Dumit, eds. 1998. *Cyborg Babies: From Techno-Sex to Techno-Tots*. New York: Routledge.

Diemer, G. 1997. "Expectant Fathers: Influence of Perinatal Education on Coping, Stress, and Spousal Relations." *Research in Nursing and Health* 20:281–293.

Dingwall, R., H. Tanaka, and S. Minamikata. 1991. "Images of Parenthood in the United Kingdom and Japan." *Sociology* 25 (3): 423–446.

Doi, T. 1973. *The Anatomy of Dependence*. Tokyo, New York, San Francisco: Kodansha International.

———. 1986. *The Anatomy of Self*. Tokyo: Kodansha International.

Draper, J. 2002. " 'It Was a Real Good Show': The Ultrasound Scan, Fathers and the Power of Visual Knowledge." *Sociology of Health and Illness* 24 (6): 771–795.

———. 2003. "Blurring, Moving and Broken Boundaries: Men's Encounters with the Pregnant Body." *Sociology of Health and Illness* 25 (7): 743–767.

Dundes, A. 1987. *Cracking Jokes: Studies of Sick Humor Cycles and Stereotypes.* Berkeley: Ten Speed Press.

Duster, T. 2003. *Back Door to Eugenics.* New York and London: Routledge.

Falk, R. 2006. Zionut Ve'habiyologia shel Hayehudim *[Zionism and the Biology of the Jews].* Tel Aviv: Resling Publishing.

Foucault, M. 1978. *The History of Sexuality. Vol. I:* An Introduction. New York: Vintage Books.

———.1979. *Discipline and Punish: The Birth of the Prison.* New York: Random House.

———.1980. *Power/Knowledge: Select Interviews and Other Writings,* 1972–1977, ed. C. Gordon. Brighton, UK: Harvester Press.

Fox, R. G., and A. Gingrich. 2002. "Introduction." In *Anthropology, by Comparison,* ed. A. Gingrich and R. G. Fox, 1–24. New York: Routledge.

Franklin, S. 1997. *Embodied Progress: A Cultural Account of Assisted Conception.* London and New York: Routledge.

———. 1998. "Making Miracles: Scientific Progress and the Facts of Life." In *Reproducing Reproduction: Kinship, Power, and Technological Innovation,* ed. S. Franklin and H. Ragone, 102–117. Philadelphia: University of Pennsylvania Press.

———. 2003. "Re-Thinking Nature-Culture." *Anthropological Theory* 3 (I): 65–85.

Franklin, S., and H. Ragone, eds. 1998. *Reproducing Reproduction: Kinship, Power, and Technological Innovation.* Philadelphia: University of Pennsylvania Press.

Frechter, V. 2003. "Hatinok Met. Efshar Haya Limnoa Zot" [The Baby Is Dead. It Could Be Prevented]. In *Ha"aretz.* February 24, pp. 1,16.

Frühstück, S. 2003. *Colonizing Sex: Sexology and Social Control in Modern Japan.* Berkeley: University of California Press.

Fujita, M. 1987. " 'It's All Mother's Fault': Childcare and Socialization of Working Mothers in Japan. *Journal of Japanese Studies* 15 (I): 67–91.

Gameltoft, T. 2007. "Sonography and Sociality: Obstetrical Ultrasound in Urban Vietnam." *Medical Anthropology Quarterly* 21 (2): 133–153.

Garon, S. 1997. *Molding Japanese Minds: The State in Everyday Life.* Princeton, NJ: Princeton University Press.

Gaskin, I. M. 1977. *Spiritual Midwifery.* Summertown, TN: The Book Publishing Company.

Gazit, Z. 2007. "Missing Motherhood: Reconstruction of Self-Identity Following Pregnancy Loss or the Death of a Newborn." Master's thesis, Hebrew University-Jerusalem.

Geertz, Clifford. 1968. *Islam Observed: Religious Development in Morocco and Indonesia.* New Haven, CT: Yale University Press.

Georges, E. 1996. "Fetal Ultrasound Imaging and the Production of Authoritative Knowledge in Greece." *Medical Anthropology Quarterly* 10 (2): 157–175.

Gingrich, A., and R. G. Fox, eds. 2002. *Anthropology, by Comparison.* New York: Routledge.

Ginsburg, F. 1989. *Contested Lives: The Abortion Debate in an American Community.* Berkeley, Los Angeles, London: University of California Press.

Ginsburg, F., and R. Rapp. 1991. "The Politics of Reproduction." *Annual Review of Anthropology* 20:311–343.

———, eds. 1995. *Conceiving the New World Order: The Global Politics of Reproduction.* Berkeley: University of California Press.

Goffman, E. 1959. *The Presentation of Self in Everyday Life.* Garden City, NY: Doubleday.

Goldstein-Gidoni, O. 2007. " 'Charisma Housewives' and 'Fashionable Mothers': Symbols of Ideological Change in Contemporary Japan?" Paper presented at the AJJ Conference.

Goodman, R. M. 1979. *Genetic Disorders among the Jewish People.* Baltimore: Johns Hopkins University Press.

Goodman, R. M., and A. G. Motulsky, eds. 1979. *Genetic Diseases among Ashkenazi Jews.* New York: Raven Press.

Gooldin, S. 2008. "Technologiyot Shel Osher: Nihul Piryon Bemedinat revacha Meodedet Yeluda" [Technologies of Happiness: Fertility Management in a Welfare State That Encourages Birth]. In *Pearei Ezrachut: Hagira, Piryon, Vezehut Beyisrael [Citizenship Gaps: Migration, Fertility and Identity in Israel]*, ed. Y. Yonnah and A. Kemp, 167–206. Jerusalem: Van Leer/Hakibbutz Hameuchad.

Hacking, I. 1990. The Taming of Chance. Cambridge: Cambridge University Press.

Hamaguchi, E. 1985. "A Contextual Model of the Japanese: Toward a Methodological Innovation in Japan Studies." *Journal of Japanese Studies* 11 (2): 289–321.

Hardacre, H. 1997. *Marketing the Menacing Fetus in Japan*. Berkeley: University of California Press.

Hashiloni-Dolev, Y. 2006. "Between Mothers, Fetuses and Society: Reproductive Genetics in the Israeli-Jewish Context." *Nashim: A Journal of Jewish Women's Studies and Gender Issues* 12:129–150.

———. 2007. *What is a Life (un)Worthy of Living? Reproductive Genetics in Germany and Israel*. Dordrecht: Springer-Kluwer.

Hazleton, L. 1977. *Israeli Women: The Reality Behind the Myths*. New York: Simon & Schuster.

Hendry, J. 1986. *Becoming Japanese: The World of the Preschool Child*. Manchester: Manchester University Press.

Henneborn W. J., and R. Cogan. 1975. "The Effect of Husband Participation on Reported Pain and Probability of Medication During Labor and Birth." *Journal of Psychosomatic Research* 19 (3): 215–222.

Herzog, H. 1994. "Irgunei Nashim Bachugim Haezrachiyim: Perek Nishkach Bahistoriographia Shel Hayishuv" [Women's Organizations in Civilian Circles: A Forgotten Chapter in the Historiography of the Yeshuv]. *Katedra* 70:111–133.

Hiroi, M., and E. Saitô. 1996. "Seishokuiryô Gijutsu No Shintenkai Wo Meguru Shomondai." [Questions That Surround the New Reproductive Technologies]. *Sanfujinka no Sekai* 48 (7): 23–27.

Hirsch, D. 2006. "Banu Hena Lehavi et Hama'arav: Hanchalat Repertuar 'Higieny' Bekerev Hachevra Hayehudit Bepalestina Bitkufat Hamandat" [We are Here to Bring the West: Hygiene Education Within the Jewish Community of Palestine during the British Mandate]. PhD diss., Tev-Aviv University.

Hochschild, A. R. 1983. *The Managed Heart: Commercialization of Human Feelings*. Berkeley: University of California Press.

Holstein, J., and J. Gubrium. 1997. "Active Interviewing." In *Qualitative Research: Theory, Method, and Practice*, ed. D. Silverman, 92–113. London; Thousand Oaks, CA: Sage Publications.

Holy, L., ed. 1987. *Comparative Anthropology*. Oxford and New York: Blackwell.

Howe, L. 1987. "Caste in Bali and India." In *Comparative Anthropology*, ed. L. Holy, 135–152. Oxford and New York: Blackwell.

Inhorn, M. C. 2003. *Local Babies, Global Science: Gender, Religion, and in Vitro Fertilization in Egypt*. New York and London: Routledge.

Ir-Shai, R. 2007. "Piryon, Migdar, Vehalacha: Hebetim Migdariyim Bepsikat Hahalacha Bat Yamenu Beshe'elot shel Piryon (Emtsaei Menia, Hapalot, Hazra'a Vehafraya Melachutit, Vepundeka'ut)" [Fertility, Gender and Halakha: A Feminist Perspective on Modern Response Literature (Contraception, Abortion, Artificial Insemination, In Vitro Fertilization and Surrogate Motherhood)], PhD diss., Bar Ilan University.

Israel Ministry of Health. Bureau of Information and Computing. "Hafsakot Herayon Alpi Hachok 1990–2007" [Legal Pregnancy Terminations 1990–2007]. November 2008.

Ivry, T. 2006. "At the Back Stage of Prenatal Care: Japanese Ob-Gyns Negotiating Prenatal Diagnosis." *Medical Anthropology Quarterly* 20 (4): 441–468.

——. 2007a. "The Politics of New Reproductive Technologies at the Intersection between Observant Judaism and Biomedicine." Research report submitted to the Israel Science Foundation.

——. 2007b. "Embodied Responsibilities: Pregnancy in the Eyes of Japanese Ob-Gyns." *Sociology of Health and Illness* 29 (2): 251–274.

——. 2009a. " 'We are Pregnant': Israeli Men and the Paradoxes of Sharing." In *Reconceiving the Second Sex in Reproduction: Men, Sexuality and Masculinity*, ed. M. Inhorn, T. Tjørnhøj-Thomsen, H. Goldberg, and M. La Cour Mosegaard. New York: Berghahn.

——.2009b. "The Ultrasonic Picture Show and the Politics of Threatened Life." *Medical Anthropology Quarterly* 23(3): 189–211.

——. Forthcoming 2010. "Ultrasonic Challenges to Pronatalism." In *Kin, Gene, Community: Reproductive Technology among Jewish Israelis*, ed. D. Birenbaum-Carmeli and Y. Carmeli. New York: Berghahn.

Ivry, T., and E. Teman. 2008. "Expectant Israeli Fathers and the Medicalized Pregnancy: Ambivalent Compliance and Critical Pragmatism." In *Culture Medicine and Psychiatry* 32 (3): 358–385.

Izraeli, D. 1997. "Gendering Military Service in the Israeli Defense Forces." *Israel Social Science Research* 12 (1): 129–167.

Jolivet, M. 1997. *Japan: The Childless Society?* Trans. Anne-Marie Glashin. London and New York: Routledge.

Jordan, B. 1978. *Birth in Four Cultures: A Crosscultural Investigation of Childbirth in Yucatan, Holland, Sweden, and the United States*. Montreal; St. Albans, VT: Eden Press Women's Publications.

——. 1997. "Authoritative Knowledge and Its Construction." In *Childbirth and Authoritative Knowledge: Cross-Cultural Perspectives*, ed. R. Davis-Floyd and C. F. Sargent, 55–79. Berkeley: University of California Press.

Kahn, S. M. 2000. *Reproducing Jews: A Cultural Account of Assisted Conception in Israel*. Durham, NC: Duke University Press.

Kamata, H., K. Miyasato, H. Suganema, H. Hurukawa, and Y. Sakakura, eds. 1990. *Nihonjin No Koumi Kosodate* [Japanese Childbirth and Child Rearing]. Tokyo: Keisô Shobô.

Kanaaneh, R. A. 2002. *Birthing the Nation: Strategies of Palestinian Women in Israel*. Berkeley: University of California Press.

Kaneda, I. 2007. Boshi Hoken no Omonaru Tôkei [Maternal and Child Health Statistics]. Tokyo: Boshi Hoken Jigyôdan.

Kappel, B., G. Eriksen, K. B. Hansen , L. Hvidman, B. Krag-Olsen, J. P. Nielsen, and M. Wohlert. 1987. "Short Stature in Scandinavian Women. An Obstetrical Risk Factor." *Acta Obstetricia et Gynecologica Scandinavica* 66 (2): 153–158.

Katriel, T. 1999. *Milot Mafteah: Defusei Tarbut Vetikshoret Beyisrasel*. [Key Words: Patterns of Culture and Communication in Israel]. Tel Aviv: Haifa University Press/Zmora Bitan.

Kaufman, S. R., and L. M. Morgan. 2005. "The Anthropology of the Beginnings and Ends of Life." *Annual Review of Anthropology* 34:317–341.

Kimmerling, B. 1993. "Patterns of Militarism in Israel." *European Journal of Sociology* 34:196–223.

Kleinman, A. 1988. *The Illness Narratives: Suffering, Healing, and the Human Condition*. New York: Basic Books.

Kondo, D. 1990. *Crafting Selves: Power, Gender, and Discourses of Identity in a Japanese Workplace*. Chicago: University of Chicago Press.

Kotets-Bar, H. 2002. "Herayon Betashlumim" [Pregnancy in Long-Term Payments]. In *Ma'ariv (Sofshavua)*. December 20, pp. 35–42.

Kowner, R. 2002. "Ha'acher Kemofet: Tfisat Haguf Beyapan Beikvot Hamifgash Im Hama'arav" [The Other as Paragon: The Conception of the Body in Japan Following the Encounter with the West]. *Zmanim: A Quarterly of History* 78:65–81.

Kristeva, J. 1981. "Woman's Time." *Signs: Journal of Women in Culture and Society* 7:13–35.

LaFleur, W. R. 1992. *Liquid Life: Abortion and Buddhism in Japan.* Princeton, NJ: Princeton University Press.

Landsman, G. 1999. "Does God Give Special Kids to Special Parents? Personhood and the Child with Disabilities as Gift and as Giver." In *Transformative Motherhood: On Giving and Getting in a Consumer Culture,* ed. L. L. Layne, 133–165. New York and London: New York University Press.

Laqueur, T. W. 2000. " 'From Generation to Generation': Imagining Connectedness in the Age of Reproductive Technologies." In *Biotechnology and Culture: Bodies, Anxieties, Ethics,* ed. P. Brodwin, 75–98. Bloomington: Indiana University Press.

Layne, L. L. 2003. *Motherhood Lost: A Feminist Account of Pregnancy Loss in America.* New York and London: Routledge.

Lazarus, E. 1997. "What Do Women Want? Issues of Choice, Control, and Class in American Pregnancy and Childbirth." In *Childbirth and Authoritative Knowledge: Cross-Cultural Perspectives,* ed. R. Davis-Floyd and C. F. Sargent, 132–158. Berkeley: University of California Press.

Lebra, T. 1976. *Japanese Patterns of Behavior.* Honolulu: University of Hawaii Press.

———. 1984. *Japanese Women: Constraint and Fulfillment.* Honolulu: University of Hawaii Press.

Leissner, O. M. 2000. "Jewish Women's Families' Names: A Feminist Legal Analysis." *Israel Law Review* 34 (4): 560.

Lipman, A. 1991. "Prenatal Genetic Testing and Screening: Constructing Needs and Reinforcing Inequities." *American Journal of Law and Medicine* 17 (1–2): 15–50.

Lock, M. 1993. *Encounters with Aging: Mythologies of Menopause in Japan and North America.* Berkeley: University of California Press.

———. 1996. "Centering the Household: The Remaking of Female Maturity in Japan." In *Re-Imaging Japanese Women,* ed. A. E. Imamura, 73–103. Berkeley: University of California Press.

———. 1998. "Perfecting Society: Reproductive Technologies, Genetic Testing, and the Planned Family in Japan." In *Pragmatic Women and Body Politics,* ed. M. Lock and P. A. Kaufert, 206–239. New York: Cambridge University Press.

———. 1999. "Menopause and the Politics of Aging." *American Journal of Human Biology* 11 (1): 145.

———. 2001. "The Tempering of Medical Anthropology: Troubling Natural Categories." *Medical Anthropology Quarterly* 15 (4): 478–492.

———. 2002. *Twice Dead: Organ Transplants and the Reinvention of Death.* Berkeley: University of California Press.

———. 2005. "The Eclipse of the Gene and the Return of Divination." In *Current Anthropology* 46 (suppl.): S47–S70.

Lock, M., and P. A. Kaufert, eds. 1998. *Pragmatic Women and Body Politics.* New York: Cambridge University Press.

Lock, M., A. Young, and A. Cambrosio, eds. 2000. *Living and Working with the New Medical Technologies: Intersections of Inquiry.* Cambridge: Cambridge University Press.

Magara, M., and T. Araki. 2000. *Saishin Sankagaku* [The Newest Obstetrics]. 2 vols. Tokyo: Bunkodo.

Mainichi Shinbunsha. 2004. "Japan Almanac." Tokyo: *Mainichi Newspapers.*

Malinowski, B. 1927. *The Father in Primitive Psychology.* New York: W. W. Norton.

Marcus, G. E. 1995. "Ethnography in/of the World System: The Emergence of Multi-Sited Ethnography." *Annual Review of Anthropology* 24:95–117.

Markens, S., C. H. Browner, and N. Press. 1997. "Feeding the Fetus: On Interrogating the Notion of Maternal-Fetal Conflict." *Feminist Studies* 23 (2): 351–372.

Martin, E. 1987. *The Woman in the Body: A Cultural Analysis of Reproduction.* Boston: Beacon Press.

——. 1991. "The Egg and the Sperm: How Science Has Constructed a Romance Based on Stereotypical Male-Female Roles." *Signs: Journal of Women in Culture and Society* 16 (3): 485–501.

——. 1994. *Flexible Bodies: The Role of Immunity in American Culture from the Days of Polio to the Age of Aids.* Boston: Beacon Press.

Matsubara, Y. 1997. "Yûsei Mondai Kangaeru(4)- Kokumin Yûsei Hogohô" [Rethinking the Problem of Eugenics: The Eugenic Protection Law]. *Fujin Tsûshin* 466:42–43.

——. 1998. "Senjidai Nihon No Danshu Seisaku" [The WWII Japanese Policy of Sterilization]. *Japan Journal for Science, Technology and Society* 7: 87–109.

——. 2000. "Nihon-Sengono Yûsei Hogohô to Iunano Danshuhô" [The Eugenic Protection Law and Sterilization in Postwar Japan]. In *Yûseigaku to Ningen Shakai [Eugenics and Human Society]*, ed. S. Yonemoto. Tokyo: Kodansha.

McGuinness, B. J. and A. N. Trivedi. 1999. "Maternal Height as a Risk Factor for Caesarean Section Due to Failure to Progress in Labour." *The Australian and New Zealand Journal of Obstetrics and Gynaecology* 39 (2): 152–154.

McVeigh, B. 2000. *Wearing Ideology: State, Schooling and Self-Presentation in Japan.* Oxford and New York: Berg.

Mitchell, L. M. 2001. *Baby's First Picture: Ultrasound and the Politics of Fetal Subjects.* Toronto: University of Toronto Press.

Miyake, Y. 1991. "Doubling Expectations: Motherhood and Women's Factory Work Under State Management in Japan in the 1930s and 1940s." In *Recreating Japanese Women, 1600–1945*, ed. G. L. Bernstein, 267–295. Berkeley: University of California Press.

Molony, B. 2005. "Why Should a Feminist Care about What Goes Behind Japan's Chrysanthemum Curtain? The Imperial Succession Issue as a Metaphor for Women's Rights." In *Japanese Women: Lineage and Legacies*, ed. A, McCreedy Thernstrom, 44–56. Washington: Woodrow Wilson International Center for Scholars Asia Program.

Moore, L. J. 2002. "Extracting Men from Semen: Masculinity in Scientific Representations of Sperm." *Social Text* 73:1–46.

——. 2003. "Billy, the Sad Sperm with No Tail: Representations of Sperm in Children's Books." *Sexualities* 6 (2–4): 279–305.

Morgan, L. M. 1998. "Making the Modern Fetal Body." Paper presented at the American Anthropological Association Meeting, Philadelphia, PA.

Mosk, C. 1996. *Making Health Work: Human Growth in Modern Japan.* Berkeley, Los Angeles, London: University of California Press.

Motulsky, A. G. 1979. Epilogue. In *Genetic Diseases among Ashkenazi Jews*, ed. R. M. Goodman and A. G. Motulsky, 425–427. New York: Raven Press.

Nader, L. 1994. "Comparative Consciousness." In *Assessing Cultural Anthropology*, ed. R. Borofsky, 84–94. New York: McGraw-Hill.

Naeye, R. L. 1979. "Weight Gain and the Outcomes of Pregnancy." *American Journal of Obstetrics and Gynecology* 135 (1): 3–9.

Nakajima, K. 1992. "Shusseizen Shindan No Wagakuni Ni Okeru Genjô" [The State of Prenatal Diagnosis in our Country]. In *Seishokugijutsu Kenkyû Temu Kenkyû Hôkokusho "Shusseizenshindan Wo Kangaeru"* [Research Report about Reproductive Technologies

"Considering Prenatal Diagnosis"], ed. Seimeirinri Kenkyûkai Seishokugijutsu Kenkyû Temu, 23–44. Seirinken Rebyû & Risachi: Shimei Rinri Kenkyûkai.

Nakane, Ch. 1970. *Japanese Society*. Berkeley and Los Angeles: University of California Press.

Nakatani, E. 1996a. "Seishoku Gijutsu No Tenkai to Seimei Rinri; Sôron" [The Development in Reproductive Technologies and the Ethics of Life: General Considerations]. *Sanfujinka no Sekai* 48 (7): 3–11.

———. 1996b. "Seishokuiryô Wo Meguru Hô to Rinri" [The Laws and Ethics That Surround the Reproductive Technologies]. *Pharma Medica* 14 (10): 91–100.

Negashi, K. 1991. *Iryô Minzokugakuron* [Medical Folklore Studies]. Tokyo: Kensankaku.

Nihon Kôseishô, ed. 2000. Kôshû Eisei Hôsoku IV [The Laws of Public Health]. Tokyo: Kodansha.

Nolte, S. H., and S. A. Hastings. 1991. "The Meiji State's Policy toward Women, 1890–1910." In *Recreating Japanese Women, 1600–1945*, ed. G. L. Bernstein, 151–174. Berkeley: University of California Press.

Norgren, T. 2001. *Abortion before Birth Control: The Politics of Reproduction in Postwar Japan*. Princeton, NJ: Princeton University Press.

Oe, K. 1969. *A Personal Matter*. New York: Grove Press.

Ogasawara, Y. 1998. *Office Ladies and Salaried Men: Power, Gender, and Work in Japanese Companies*. Berkeley: University of California Press.

Ohinata, M. 1995. "The Mystique of Motherhood: A Key to Understanding Social Change and Family Problems in Japan." In *Japanese Women: New Feminist Perspectives on the Past, Present, and Future*, ed. K. Fujimura-Fanselow and A. Kameda, 199–212. New York: Feminist Press.

Ohnuki-Tierney, E. 1984. *Illness and Culture in Contemporary Japan: An Anthropological View*. Cambridge and New York: Cambridge University Press.

Otsubo, S., and J. R. Bartholomew. 1998. "Eugenics in Japan: Some Ironies of Modernity, 1883–1945." *Science in Context* 11 (3–4): 545–565.

Overing, J. 1987. "Translation as a Creative Process: The Power of the Name." In *Comparative Anthropolgy, ed.* L. Holy, 70–87. Oxford and New York: Blackwell.

Parens, E., and A. Asch. 2000. "Introduction." In *Prenatal Testing and Disability Rights*, ed. E. Parens and A. Asch, ix–xvi. Washington, DC: Georgetown University Press.

Peel, J.D.Y. 1987. "History, Culture and the Comparative Method: A West African Puzzle." In *Comparative Anthropology, ed.* L. Holy, 88–118. Oxford and New York: Blackwell.

Petchesky-Pollack, R. 1987. "Fetal Images: The Power of Visual Culture in the Politics of Reproduction." *Feminist Studies* 13 (2): 263–292.

Portuguese, J. 1998. *Fertility Policy in Israel: The Politics of Religion, Gender, and Nation*. Westport, CT: Praeger.

Press, N. A., and C. H. Browner. 1994. "Collective Silences, Collective Fictions: How Prenatal Diagnostic Testing Became Part of Routine Prenatal Care." In *Women and Prenatal Testing: Facing the Challenges of Genetic Technology*, ed. K. H. Rothenberg and E. J. Thomson, 201–218. Columbus: Ohio State University Press.

Raday, F. 1995. "Al Hashivyon" [On Equality]. In *Ma'amad Haisha Bachevra Uvamishpat* [Women's Status in Israeli Law and Society], ed F. Raday, C. Shalev, and M. Liban-Kooby, 19–63. Jerusalem: Shoken.

Rapoport, T., and T. El-Or. 1997. "Cultures of Womanhood in Israel: Social Agencies and Gender Production." *Woman's International Forum* 20 (5/6): 573–580.

Rapp, R. 1999. *Testing Women, Testing the Fetus: The Social Impact of Amniocentesis in America*. New York: Routledge.

———. 2001. "Gender, Body, Biomedicine: How Some Feminist Concerns Dragged Reproduction to the Center of Social Theory." *Medical Anthropology Quarterly* 15 (4): 466–477.

Rapp, R., and F. Ginsburg. 2001. "Enabling Disability: Rewriting Kinship, Reimagining Citizenship." *Public Culture* 13 (3): 533–556

Raz, A. 2004. " 'Important to Test, Important to Support': Attitudes toward Disability Rights and Prenatal Diagnosis among Leaders of Support Groups of Genetic Disorders in Israel." *Social Science and Medicine* 59 (9): 1857–1866.

Reed, R. 2005. *Birthing Fathers: The Transformation of Men in American Rites of Birth.* New Brunswick, NJ: Rutgers University Press.

Remennick, L. 2006. "The Quest for the Perfect Baby: Why Do Israeli Women Seek Prenatal Genetic Testing?" *Sociology of Health and Illness* 28 (1): 21–53.

Roberts F.S.E. 2007. "Extra Embryos: The Ethics of Cryopreservation in Ecuador and Elsewhere." In *American Ethnologist* 34 (1): 181–199.

Robertson, J. 2002a. "Reflexivity Redux: A Pithy Polemic on 'Positionality.' " In *Anthropological Quarterly* 75 (4): 785–792.

———. 2002b. "Blood Talks: Eugenic Modernity and the Creation of New Japanese." *History and Anthropology* 13 (3): 191–216.

Root, R., and C. H. Browner. 2001. "Practices of the Pregnant Self: Compliance with and Resistance to Prenatal Norms." *Culture, Medicine and Psychiatry* 25 (2): 195–223.

Rose, N. 2001. "The Politics of Life Itself." *Theory, Culture & Society* 18 (6): 1–30.

Rosenberger, N. R., ed. 1992. *Japanese Sense of Self.* Cambridge and New York: Cambridge University Press.

———., 2001. *Gambling with Virtue: Japanese Women and the Search for Self in a Changing Nation.* Honolulu: University of Hawaii Press.

Rothman, B. K. 1984. "The Meanings of Choice in Reproductive Technology." In *Test-Tube Women: What Future for Motherhood?*, ed. R. Arditti, R. Klein, and S. Minden, 23–34. London and Boston: Pandora Press.

———. 1986. *The Tentative Pregnancy: How Amniocentesis Changes the Experience of Motherhood.* New York: Norton.

———. 1989. *Recreating Motherhood: Ideology and Technology in a Patriarchal Society.* New York: Norton.

———. 1998. *Genetic Maps and Human Imaginations: The Limits of Science in Understanding Who We Are.* New York: Norton.

Sagi, M., V. Meiner, N. Reshef, J. Dagan, and J. Zlotogora. 2001. "Prenatal Diagnosis of Sex Chromosome Aneuploidy: Possible Reasons for High Rates of Pregnancy Termination." *Prenatal Diagnosis* 21 (6): 461–465.

Saitô, Y. 1992. "Josei Shôgaisha No Shussan Wo Sasaeru" [Supporting the Birth of Women with Disabilities]. In *Seishokugijutsu Kenkyû Temu Kenkyû Hôkokusho "Shusseizenshindan Wo Kangaeru"* [Research Report about Reproductive Technologies "Considering Prenatal Diagnosis"], ed. Seimeirinri Kenkyûkai Seishokugijutsu Kenkyû Temu, 79–94. Seirinken Rebyû & Risaachi: Shimei Rinri Kenkyûkai.

Sandelowski, M. 1994. "Separate, but Less Unequal: Fetal Ultrasonography and the Transformation of Expectant Mother/Fatherhood." *Gender & Society* 8 (2): 230–245.

Sargent, C. F., and N. Stark. 1989. "Childbirth Education and Childbirth Models: Prenatal Perspectives on Control, Anesthesia, and Technological Intervention in the Birth Process." *Medical Anthropology Quarterly* 3 (1): 36–51.

Sato, K., ed. 1999. *Sanfujinka 20seiki No Ayumi* [History of 20th Century Obstetrics and Gynecology]. Tokyo: Medical View.

Schenker, J. G., and U. Elchalal, eds. 1998. *Haherayon Hayoledet Vehaleida: Sefer Yesod Bemeyaldut* [Pregnancy and Delivery: A Textbook of Obstetrics and Gynecology]. Jerusalem: Grafit Publishers.

Scheper-Hughes, N. 1985. "Culture, Scarcity, and Maternal Thinking: Maternal Detachment and Infant Survival in a Brazilian Shantytown." *Ethos* 13 (4): 291–317.

———. 1992. *Death without Weeping: The Violence of Everyday Life in Brazil.* Berkeley: University of California Press.

Scheper-Hughes, N., and M. Lock. 1987. "The Mindful Body: A Prolegomenon to Future Work in Medical Anthropology." *Medical Anthropology Quarterly* 1 (1): 6–41.

Schutz, A. and T. Luckmann. 1973. *The Structures of the Life-World.* Evanston, IL: Northwestern University Press.

Sered, S. S. 2000. *What Makes Women Sick?: Maternity, Modesty, and Militarism in Israeli Society.* Hanover, NH: Brandeis University Press (University Press of New England).

Shadmi, H. 2003. "Yugbar Hapikuach Al Tipulei Poriut Biglal Tmutat Pagim" [The Supervision on Fertility Treatments Will Tighten Because of Mortality Rates of Premature Babies]. In *Ha'aretz.* January 16, pp.1a, 9a.

Sher C., O. Romano-Zelekha, M. S. Green, and T. Shohat. 2003. "Factors Affecting Performance of Prenatal Genetic Testing by Israeli Jewish Women." *American Journal of Medical Genetics, Part A.* 120A (3): 418–422.

Shohat, M., E. Akstein, B. Davidov, G. Barkai, C. Legum, M. David, H. Dar, Y. Romem, A. Amiel, H. Cohen, G. Bach, Z. Ben-Neriah, R. N. Sheffer, Z. Appelman, J. Chemke, P. Zadka, T. Zer, and B. Goldman. 1995. "Amniocentesis Rate and the Detection of Down Syndrome and Other Chromosomal Abnormalities in Israel." *Prenatal Diagnosis* 15 (10): 967–970.

Singleton, J. 1989. "Gambaru: A Japanese Cultural Theory of Learning." In *Japanese Schooling: Patterns of Socialization, Equality, and Political Control*, ed. J. J. Shield, Jr., 8–15. University Park: Penn State University Press.

Skocpol, T., and M. Somers. 1980. "The Uses of Comparative History in Macrosocial Inquiry." *Comparative Studies in Society and History* 22 (2): 174–197.

Smith, R. J. 1983. *Japanese Society: Tradition, Self and Social Order.* Cambridge: Cambridge University Press.

Sonoda, K. 1990. *Health and Illness in Changing Japanese Society.* Tokyo: University of Tokyo Press.

Steinberg, A. 2003. Encyclopedia of Jewish Medical Ethics. Vol 1. Jerusalem and New York: Feldheim Publishers.

Steslicke, W. E. 1987. "The Japanese State of Health: A Political Economic Perspective." In *Health, Illness, and Medical Care in Japan*, ed. E. Norbeck and M. Lock, 24–65. Honolulu: University of Hawaii Press.

Strathern, M. 1992. *Reproducing the Future: Anthropology, Kinship, and the New Reproductive Technologies.* Manchester: Manchester University Press.

Swirski, B., and M. P. Safir, eds. 1991. *Calling the Equality Bluff: Women in Israel.* Elmsford, NY: Pergamon Press.

Taida, R., and S. Miyai. 1997. *Oishii Shussan* [Tasty Birth]. Tokyo: Ihatov.

Takeda, H. 2005. *The Political Economy of Reproduction in Japan: Between Nation-State and Everyday Life.* London and New York: Routledge.

Takeda, S., M. Saitoh, K. Kinoshita, and S. Sakamoto. 1992. "Himan Ninshin no Eiyô kanri ni kan suru Kisoteki, Rinriteki Kenkyû" [Studies of Diet Management and Insulin Resistance in Obese Pregnant Women]. In *Acta Obstet Gynaec Jpn* 44 (2): 229–236.

Taylor, J. S. 1992. "The Public Fetus and the Family Car: From Abortion Politics to a Volvo Advertisement." *Public Culture* 4 (2): 67–80.

———. 1998. "Images of Contradiction: Obstetrical Ultrasound in American Culture." In *Reproducing Reproduction: Kinship, Power, and Technological Innovation*, ed. S. Franklin and H. Ragone, 15–45. Philadelphia: University of Pennsylvania Press.

Teman, E. 2001. "Technological Fragmentation and Women's Empowerment: Surrogate Motherhood in Israel." *Woman's Studies Quarterly* 29 (3–4): 11–34.

———. 2003. "The Medicalization of 'Nature' in the 'Artificial Body': Surrogate Motherhood in Israel." *Medical Anthropology Quarterly* 17 (1): 78–98.

———. 2010. *Birthing a Mother: The Surrogate Body and the Pregnant Self.* Berkeley: University of California Press.

Teman, E. and T. Ivry. n.d. "God Sent Ordeals and Their Discontent: Ultra-orthodox Women and Prenatal Diagnosis."

Tobin, J. 1992. "Japanese Preschools and the Pedagogy of Selfhood." In *Japanese Sense of Self*, ed. N. R. Rosenberger, 21–39. Cambridge and New York: Cambridge University Press.

Toren, C. 2002. "Comparison and Ontogeny." In *Anthropology, by Comparison*, ed. A. Gingrich and R. G. Fox, 186–203. New York: Routledge.

Tsu, V. D. 1992. "Maternal Height and Age: Risk Factors for Cephalopelvic Disproportion in Zimbabwe." *International Journal of Epidemiology* 21 (5): 941–946.

Tsuge, A. 1992. "Shusseizen Shindan No Jushin Wo Meguru Jôkyô" [The Circumstances of Undergoing Prenatal Diagnosis]. In *Seishokugijutsu Kenkyû Temu Kenkyû Hôkokusho "Shusseizenshindan Wo Kangaeru"* [Research Report about Reproductive Technologies "Considering Prenatal Diagnosis"], ed. Seimeirinri Kenkyûkai Seishokugijutsu Kenkyû Temu, 45–78. Seirinken Rebyû & Risachi: Shimei Rinri Kenkyûkai.

Turney, J. 1998. *Frankenstein Footsteps: Science, Genetics and Popular Culture.* New Haven: Yale University Press.

Uno, K. 1991. "Women and Changes in the Household Division of Labor." In *Recreating Japanese Women 1600–1945*, ed. G. L. Bernstein, 17–41. Berkeley: University of California Press.

Usui, C. 2005. "Japan's Frozen Future: Why Are Women Withholding Investment in Work and Family?" In *Japanese Women: Lineage and Legacies*, ed. A. McCreedy Thernstrom, 57–68. Washington, DC: Woodrow Wilson International Center for Scholars.

Utsumi, Y. 1996. *Omedeta Desuyo* [I Have Concieved]. Tokyo: Seibidô.

van der Ploeg, I. 1995. "Hermaphrodite Patients: In Vitro Fertilization and the Transformation of Male Infertility." *Science, Technology and Human Values* 20 (4): 460–481.

Vogel, E. F. 1963. *Japan's New Middle Class: The Salaryman and His Family in a Tokyo Suburb.* Berkeley: University of California Press.

Vogel, S. H. 1978. "Professional Housewife: The Career of Urban Middle Class Japanese Women." *Japan Interpreter* 1 (12): 16–43.

Weiss, M. 1994. *Conditional Love: Parents' Attitudes toward Handicapped Children.* New York: Bergin & Garvey.

———. 2002. *The Chosen Body: The Politics of the Body in Israeli Society.* Stanford, CA: Stanford University Press.

White, M. 1987. *The Japanese Educational Challenge: A Commitment to Children.* New York: Free Press.

———. 1987. The Virtue of Japanese Mothers: Cultural Definitions of Women's Lives." *Daedalus* 116 (3): 149–163.

Worsley, P. 1982. "Non-Western Medical Systems." *Annual Review in Anthropology* 11:315–348.

Yoda, T. 2001. "The Rise and Fall of Maternal Society: Gender, Labor, and Capital in Contemporary Japan." *The South Atlantic Quarterly* 99 (4): 865–902.

Young, I. M. 1984. "Pregnant Embodiment: Subjectivity and Alienation." *The Journal of Medicine and Philosophy* 9:45–62.

INDEX

abdominal circumference, in Japanese prenatal care, 84, 107

abortion: decision making for, 175–176; for fetal abnormalities, 116; resistance to, 171; selective, 248

abortion, in Israel, 40, 268n. 9; for fetal abnormality, 19; late, 41, 48, 67; in rabbinical law, 248; in state law, 39

abortion, in Japan, 79, 81–82, 120, 267n. 3, 268n. 9; attitudes toward, 172–173; legalization of, 79–80; as politically incorrect, 117; in Tokugawa period, 78

abortion, postdiagnostic: in Israel, 244, 254; in Japan, 249; legal status of, 250

Abu-Lughod, Lila, 240, 241, 242, 258, 263

advertising: of pregnancy events, 29; for ultrasonography, 46

afterbirth, treatment of, 269n. 12

age, maternal, 62, 244; of Israeli mothers at first birth, 40

agency: of pregnant Israeli women, 259; somatic, of Japanese women, 239, 242–243, 251–252, 259. *See also* resistance

allergies, anxiety about, 172

Allison, Ann, 123, 183

alpha-fetoprotein (AFP) maternal blood test, 39; introduced into Israel, 38; routinization of, 206; unreliable results of, 208, 209. *See also* triple marker

alternative medicine, practices of, 227

amae (dependence), in Japanese culture, 272n. 7

Amanuma, Kaoru, 87

amniocentesis, 105, 107, 172, 177, 178, 181; decision making for, 3–4, 205–206, 209, 210; and experience of pregnancy, 261; infections caused by, 63; recommendation for, 40; refusal of, 8; and reproductive catastrophe, 53; and triple marker results, 60–61; and tyranny of PND, 66; and women's fears, 213–215

amniocentesis, in Israel: costs of, 40; as economic issue, 62, 63; explanatory classes for, 206–209, 215; health ministry's regulation of, 200, 207; indication for, 51; justification for, 64–65; liberal availability of, 237; liberal use of, 65; in "low-risk" pregnancy, 60;

miscarriage risk of, 39; patient's anxiety about, 62–63; procedure, 213–215

amniocentesis, in Japan, 215; access to, 179; and financial considerations, 177; hospitalization following, 112, 120; maternal guilt associated with, 110, 268n. 12; ob-gyn reluctance to discuss, 109

anthropology: biomedicine in, 257; comparative studies in, 18, 20; of pregnancy, 5, 261; of reproduction, 12–13, 262

anti-abortion activists, U.S., 60

anti-abortion materials, in Israel, 59

anxiety: with amniocentesis, 62–63; Israeli-Jewish, 49; Israeli-Jewish compared with Japanese, 88; in medical theory of pregnancy, 74; ob-gyn attempts to minimize, 109; for pregnant Japanese women, 171–179; prevalence of, 239; and probabilities, 112; weight gain causing, 88

anzan (safe birth), concept of, 91

Ashkenazi Jews, 41, 205

assisted conceptive technologies, 8; in anthropology of reproduction, 262; and experience of pregnancy, 261

Association for Researchers in Obstetrics and Gynecology (Japan), 100

authoritative knowledge: access to, 11; in anthropology of reproduction, 269n. 10; collaborative social process in, 231; concept of, 10; "cute," 242; interactive production of, 9; and legitimate complaints, 198; local construction of, 10–12; local versions of, 10–11. *See also* knowledge

authority, medical: and cultural image, 190; and cultural paradigm, 74; Israeli women's concern about, 205; and women's bodies, 104, 105

Aya, Iwamoto, 114

baby: contrasted with fetus, 3; Japanese notion of, 2, 146–153; in Japanese prenatal care, 93

baby, fetus as, 223; cuteness of, 150; mother's communication with, 146–147; power over mother of, 150; in pregnancy guidebooks, 148–150; *taikyô* schedule for, 151

babysitters, in Japan, 270n. 13

ABOUT THE AUTHOR

TSIPY IVRY is a lecturer in anthropology at the Department of Sociology and Anthropology at the University of Haifa, Israel. Her current research explores the politics of prenatal diagnosis and assisted conception among observant Jewish communities in Israel.

CPSIA information can be obtained at www.ICGtesting.com
Printed in the USA
269618BV00002B/39/P